T0176891

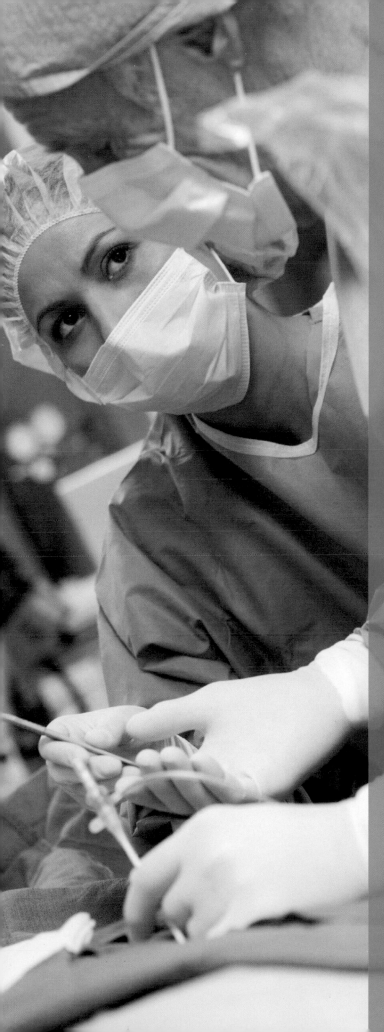

Perioperative Practice

at a Glance

Paul Wicker

MSc, PGCE, CCNS in Operating Department
Nursing, BSc, RGN, RMN
Head of Perioperative Studies,
Edge Hill University, Ormskirk
Fellow of the Higher Education Academy
Visiting Professor at the First Hospital of Nanjing,
China
Consultant Editor, the Journal for Operating
Department Practitioners

WILEY Blackwell

This edition first published 2015 © 2015 John Wiley & Sons, Ltd

Registered Office
John Wiley & Sons, Ltd, The Atrium, Southern Gate, Chichester, West Sussex, PO19 8SQ, UK

Editorial Offices
350 Main Street, Malden, MA 02148-5020, USA
9600 Garsington Road, Oxford, OX4 2DQ, UK
The Atrium, Southern Gate, Chichester, West Sussex, PO19 8SQ, UK

For details of our global editorial offices, for customer services, and for information about how to apply for permission to reuse the copyright material in this book please see our website at www.wiley.com/wiley-blackwell.

Library of Congress Cataloging-in-Publication Data
Wicker, Paul, author.
 Perioperative practice at a glance / Paul Wicker.
    p. ; cm. – (At a glance series)
 Includes bibliographical references and index.
 ISBN 978-1-118-84215-7 (pbk.)
I. Title.   II. Series: At a glance series (Oxford, England)
 [DNLM: 1. Perioperative Nursing–methods.   2. Patient Care Planning.   3. Perioperative
Care–methods.   WY 162]
 RD99.24
 617′.0231–dc23
                                        2014032711
A catalogue record for this book is available from the British Library.

Cover image: iStock © monkeybusinessimages

Set in 9.5/11.5pt Minion by SPi Publisher Services, Pondicherry, India
Printed and bound in Singapore by Markono Print Media Pte Ltd

1   2015

Perioperative Practice

at a Glance

Contents

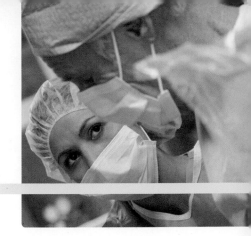

Preface vii
Acknowledgements viii
Surgical and anaesthetic abbreviations and acronyms ix
How to use your textbook xiii

Part 1 Introduction to perioperative practice 1

1 Preoperative patient preparation 2
2 Theatre scrubs and personal protective equipment (PPE) 4
3 Preventing the transmission of infection 6
4 Preparing and managing equipment 8
5 Perioperative patient care 10
6 Surgical Safety Checklist – Part 1 12
7 Surgical Safety Checklist – Part 2 14
8 Legal and professional accountability 16
9 Interprofessional teamworking 18

Part 2 Anaesthesia 21

10 Preparing anaesthetic equipment 22
11 Checking the anaesthetic machine 24
12 Anatomy and physiology of the respiratory and cardiovascular systems 26
13 Anaesthetic drugs 28
14 Perioperative fluid management 30
15 Monitoring the patient 32
16 General anaesthesia 34
17 Local anaesthesia 36
18 Regional anaesthesia 38

Part 3 Surgery 41

19 Roles of the circulating and scrub team 42
20 Basic surgical instruments 44
21 Surgical scrubbing 46
22 Surgical positioning 48
23 Maintaining the sterile field 50
24 Sterilisation and disinfection 52
25 Swab and instrument counts 54
26 Working with electrosurgery 56
27 Tourniquet management 58
28 Wounds and dressings 60

Part 4 Recovery 63

29 Introducing the recovery room 64
30 Patient handover 66
31 Postoperative patient care – Part 1 68

32 Postoperative patient care – Part 2   70
33 Monitoring in recovery   72
34 Maintaining the airway   74
35 Common postoperative problems   76
36 Managing postoperative pain   78
37 Managing postoperative nausea and vomiting   80

Part 5

Perioperative emergencies   83

38 Caring for the critically ill   84
39 Airway problems   86
40 Rapid sequence induction   88
41 Bleeding problems   90
42 Malignant hyperthermia   92
43 Cardiovascular problems   94
44 Electrosurgical burns   96
45 Venous thromboembolism   98
46 Latex allergy   100

Part 6

Advanced surgical practice   103

47 Assisting the surgeon   104
48 Shaving, marking, prepping and draping   106
49 Retraction of tissues   108
50 Suture techniques and materials   110
51 Haemostatic techniques   112
52 Laparoscopic surgery   114
53 Orthopaedic surgery   116
54 Cardiac surgery   118
55 Things to do after surgery   120

References and further reading   122
Index   144

Preface

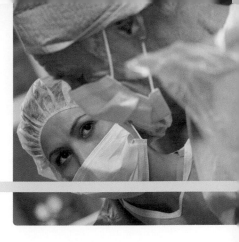

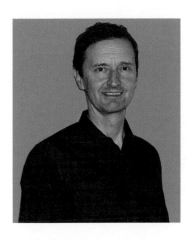

Dear reader

I hope that you really enjoy reading this book and find the content useful to underpin your practice and theory. I wrote this book to cover the 'umbrella' of perioperative practice. I have written a few books on the subject already and I am still conscious that these days technology also enables healthcare practitioners to access information quickly. Something that I have learned during my career as a theatre practitioner and a Head of Perioperative Studies is that 'time' is what theatre practitioners lack most; especially in this current healthcare climate, which is asking practitioners to do more for less, and with less support. A short, succinct and factual book like this one on perioperative practice is the solution to the problem of lack of time for all students, practitioners, teachers, mentors and medics, to ensure safe care for their patients. The chapters are short and succinct, and there are pictures, diagrams and tables full of information that will help support your reading of the chapter.

The book commences with an introduction to perioperative practice. This part covers everything from cleaning the operating room to wearing scrubs and interprofessional teamworking. These days it is crucial for interprofessional teams to work together in order to provide the best possible patient care. Surgeons and anaesthetists cannot work by themselves, and neither can practitioners!

The next parts are anaesthesia, surgery and recovery. Practitioners these days can work in all areas of the operating department, so they need to know at least the basics of each area. Working in recovery is much more different than working in surgery. These chapters cover the basics, as well as offering an advanced understanding of your roles and responsibilities when working in these areas. The following part looks at key problems in perioperative care, including hyperthermia (which is deadly), airway problems, bleeding problems, latex allergy and so on. These are also areas that are important for patient safety, which I am sure you will find useful. The final part is on advanced surgical skills. The roles of the Surgical First Assistant and the Surgical Care Practitioner are now much more common for practitioners to undertake, because of the shortage of surgeons due to the European Working Time Directive and NHS cost savings. These chapters cover items such as suturing, laparoscopies, retraction and other roles associated with the surgeon's assistant.

The reference section at the end of the book will also be of great value to you. These pages contain references for the chapter, further reading, information on websites and links to videos. So if the chapter you read does not have enough information for you, check out the relevant pages for the chapter you are reading and check up on some of the links – you will find that they contain lots more information for you.

I sincerely hope that this book is of interest to you – read, enjoy, learn and progress!

Paul Wicker

Paul Wicker

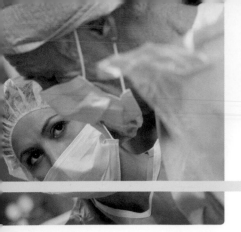

Acknowledgements

I first of all want to thank my wife Africa for all the help she has given me, and her support in reviewing the book's contents while I was writing it. And thanks to my children too, Kate, Mairi and Neil, for keeping me happy and chilled out while writing!

I also want to thank my colleagues and friends for reviewing the chapters and commenting on their contents – Ashley Wooding, Sara Dalby, Tim Lewis, Adele Nightingale and Paul Rawling.

I thank Patricia Turton and Noreen Hall from Aintree University Hospital, Liverpool, and Bob Unwin and Gill Scanlon from the Liverpool Women's Hospital, for allowing me to use photos taken within their operating department. I also thank the staff from both hospitals for allowing me to take their photos and use them in this book. Many thanks to University Hospital South Manchester for the use of the photographs taken in the cadaveric workshop entitled 'Better Training Better Care'. We very much appreciate your support for these photographs.

Finally, I also want to thank Katrina Rimmer and Madeleine Hurd from John Wiley & Sons for their help and support in getting this book published.

Surgical and anaesthetic abbreviations and acronyms

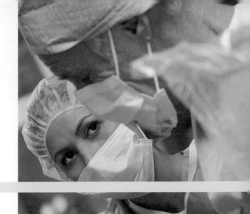

A	Ampere
AAA	Abdominal aortic aneurysm
AAGBI	Association of Anaesthetists of Great Britain and Ireland
ABC	Airways, breathing, circulation
ABG	Arterial blood gases
AC	Acromioclavicular (shoulder)
ACC	American College of Cardiology
ACC/AHA	American College of Cardiology/American Heart Association
ACD	Anterior cervical disc
ACE	Angiotensin-converting enzyme
ACL	Anterior cruciate ligament (knee)
ACS	Acute coronary syndrome
ADH	Antidiuretic hormone
AF	Atrial fibrillation
AHA	American Heart Association
AICD	Automated implantable cardiac defibrillator
ALI	Acute lung injury
APR	Abdominal perineal resection (colorectal surgery)
AR	Aortic regurgitation
ARB	Angiotensin receptor blocker
ARDS	Acute respiratory distress syndrome
AS	Aortic stenosis
ASA	American Society of Anaesthesiologists
AV	Arteriovenous or arterial-venous
AVPU	Alert, verbal, painful, unresponsive
AVR	Aortic valve replacement
Ax-fem	Axillo-femoral (axillo-bifemoral) bypass (vascular surgery)
BBSA	β-blocker in spinal anaesthesia
BiPAP	Bi-level positive air pressure
BIV	Bi-ventricular (pacemaker)
BMI	Body mass index
BNF	British National Formulary

BNP	Brain natriuretic peptide
BP	Blood pressure
BPG	Bypass graft (vascular surgery)
BSO	Bilateral salpingo-oopherectomy (gynaecological surgery)
BSSO	Bilateral saggital split osteotomy (jaw surgery)
CABG	Coronary artery bypass graft (open heart surgery)
CAD	Coronary artery disease
CARP	Coronary artery revascularisation prophylaxis
CASS	Coronary artery surgery study
CBI	Catheter-based intervention (intravascular procedure) or continuous bladder irrigation
CEA	Carotid endarterectomy (vascular surgery)
CFA	Common femoral artery
Ch	Charrière
CHF	Chronic heart failure
CI	Confidence interval
CNS	Central nervous system
CO_2	Carbon dioxide
COPD	Chronic obstructive pulmonary disease
COX-2	Cyclooxygenase-2
CPAP	Continuous positive airway pressure
CPET	Cardiopulmonary exercise testing
CPG	Committee for Practice Guidelines
CPK	Creatine phosphokinase
CRP	C-reactive protein
CS	Consensus statement or compartment syndrome
CT	Computed tomography
CVC	Central venous catheter
CVD	Cardiovascular disease
D&C	Dilation and curettage (gynaecological procedure)
DAS	Difficult Airway Society
DCU	Day case unit

DECREASE	Dutch Echocardiographic Cardiac Risk Evaluating Applying Stress Echo		**HLA**	Human leukocyte antigen
DH	Department of Health		**HNP**	Herniated nucleus pulposis (herniated disc)
DIC	Disseminated intravascular coagulation		**HR**	Hazard ratio
DIPOM	Diabetes postoperative mortality and morbidity		**I&D**	Incision and drainage (debridement)
DL	Direct laryngoscopy		**IBCT**	Incorrect blood component transfused
DSE	Dobutamine stress echocardiography		**ICD**	Implantable cardioverter defibrillators
DVIU	Direct visual internal urethrotomy (urological procedure)		**ICF**	Intracellular fluid
DVT	Deep vein thrombosis		**ICU**	Intensive care unit
ECF	Extracellular fluid		**ID**	Internal diameter
ECG	Electrocardiogram/electrocardiography		**IHD**	Ischaemic heart disease
ECT	Electroconvulsive therapy		**ILMA**	Intubating laryngeal mask airway
EEG	Electroencephalogram		**IM**	Intra-medullary (femur/humerus)
EGD	Esophagogastroduodenoscopy		**IMS**	Intra-metatarsal space (foot)
EMLA	Eutectic mixture of local anaesthetic		**INR**	International normalised ratio (of the prothrombin time)
ERCP	Endoscopic retrograde cholangiopancreatogram		**IOC**	Intraoperative cholangiogram (with gallbladder surgery)
ESC	European Society of Cardiology		**IOL**	Intra-ocular lens (eye)
ESWL	Extra-corporeal shock wave lithotripsy (for kidney stones)		**IPJ**	Intra-phalangeal joint (hand)
ET	Endotracheal		**IPPB**	Intermittent positive pressure breathing
ETT	Endotracheal tube		**IPPV**	Intermittent positive pressure ventilation
EUA	Exam under anaesthesia		**ISF**	Interstitial fluid
EVH	Endoscopic vein harvest (usually with CABG)		**ITR**	Inferior turbinate reduction (sinus surgical procedure)
EWS	Early warning score		**IV**	Intravenous
Ex Lap	Exploratory laparotomy or exploratory laparoscopy (*very* important to clarify which)		**IVC**	Inferior vena cava
Fem-fem	Femoral to femoral bypass (vascular surgery)		**J**	Joule
Fem-pop	Femoropopliteal bypass (vascular surgery)		**JVP**	Jugular venous pressure
FEV$_1$	Forced expiratory volume in 1 second		**K**	Kelvin
FFP	Fresh frozen plasma		**K**	Potassium
FiO2	Fractional concentration of oxygen in inspired gas		**kg**	Kilogram
FIO2	Fraction of inspired oxygen		**kPa**	Kilopascals
FRISC	Fast revascularisation in instability in coronary disease		**L**	Litre
FTSG	Full thickness skin graft		**Lap Appy**	Laparoscopic appendectomy
GCS	Glasgow coma score		**Lap Chole**	Laparoscopic cholecystectomy
GI	Gastrointestinal		**LAVH**	Laparoscopic assisted vaginal hysterectomy
GTN	Glyceryl trinitrate		**LBBB**	Left bundle branch block
Hb	Haemoglobin		**LMA**	Laryngeal mask airway
HbS	Sickle haemoglobin		**LMWH**	Low molecular weight heparin
HCPC	Health and Care Professions Council		**LP**	Lumbar peritoneal (shunt or drain) or lumbar puncture (diagnostic procedure)
HDU	High dependency unit		**LQTS**	Long QT syndrome
			LR	Likelihood ratio
			LV	Left ventricular
			LVH	Left ventricular hypertrophy

m	Metre
MECC	Minimal extracorporeal circulation (cardiac procedure with CABG)
MET	Metabolic equivalent
MH	Malignant hyperthermia
MI	Myocardial infarction
ML	Microlaryngoscopy (ENT procedure)
mol	Mole
mOsm	Milliosmole
MPJ	Metatarsal phalangeal joint (foot)
MR	Mitral regurgitation
MRCP	Magnetic resonance cholangiopancreatogram (scan)
MRI	Magnetic resonance imaging
MS	Mitral stenosis
MVR	Mitral valve replacement
MVV	Mitral valve valvuloplasty (valve repair)
N	Newton
NG	Nasogastric
NICE	National Institute for Health and Care Excellence
NIV	Non-invasive ventilation
NPSA	National Patient Safety Agency
NSAID	Non-steroidal anti-inflammatory drug
NSTEMI	Non-ST-segment elevation myocardial infarction
NT-proBNP	N-terminal pro-brain natriuretic peptide
O2	Oxygen
OATS	Osteochondral autograft transfer system (orthopaedic procedure)
ODP	Operating department practice/practitioner
OPUS	Orbofiban in patients with unstable coronary syndromes
Pa	Pascal
PaCO$_2$	Arterial carbon dioxide partial pressure (measured from a blood gas sample)
PAH	Pulmonary arterial hypertension
PaO$_2$	Arterial oxygen partial pressure (measured from a blood gas sample)
PAWCP	Pulmonary artery wedge capillary pressure
PCI	Percutaneous coronary intervention
PCNL	Percutaneous nephrolithotomy (usually abbreviated Perc.)
pCO$_2$	Partial pressure of carbon dioxide
PD	Peritoneal dialysis
PEG	Percutaneous endoscopic gastrotomy (inserting a feeding tube)

PETCO$_2$	End-tidal expiratory CO$_2$ pressure
PICC	Peripherally inserted central catheter
PLIF	Posterior lumber interbody fusion (spinal surgery)
pO2	Partial pressure of oxygen
PPH	Procedure for prolapsed haemorrhoids
PTA	Percutaneous transluminal angioplasty (endovascular procedure)
PVC	Polyvinyl chloride
RBC	Red blood cell
RCT	Randomised controlled trial
RFA	Radio frequency ablation
RM	Reservoir mask
ROC	Receiver operating characteristic
RPG	Retrograde pyelogram (urological procedure)
RR	Relative risk
RSI	Rapid sequence induction
SaO2	Saturation level of arterial oxyhaemoglobin
SD	Standard deviation
SF	Sapheno-femoral or superficial femoral
SHOT	Serious hazards of transfusion
SIRS	Systemic inflammatory response syndrome
SMVT	Sustained monomorphic ventricular tachycardia
SPECT	Single photon emission computed tomography
SpO2	Oxygen saturation measured by a pulse oximeter
SpO2	Saturation level of peripheral oxyhaemoglobin
SPVT	Sustained polymorphic ventricular tachycardia
STEMI	ST-segment elevation myocardial infarction survival using glucose algorithm regulation strategy
STSG	Split thickness skin graft
SVA	Supraventricular arrhythmia
SVT	Supraventricular tachycardia
SYNTAX	Synergy between percutaneous coronary intervention with taxus and cardiac surgery
TACTICS	Treat angina with aggrastat and determine cost of therapy with an invasive or conservative strategy
TEE	Transesophageal echocardiogram
TEG®	Thromboelastograph
TIA	Transient ischaemic attack
TIMI	Thrombolysis in myocardial infarction
TIVA	Total intravenous anaesthesia

TLIF	Transforamenal lumbar interbody fusion (spinal surgery)	**TVV**	Tricuspid valve valvuloplasty (valve repair)
TMJ	Temporal mandibular joint (jaw)	**UFH**	Unfractionated heparin
TMR	Trans-myocardial revascularisation (open heart procedure with a laser)	**US**	Ultrasound
		UTI	Urinary tract infection
TOE	Transoesophageal echocardiography	**VATS**	Video-assisted thoracoscopy (lung surgery)
TPN	Total parenteral nutrition	**VCO$_2$**	Carbon dioxide production
TRUS	Transrectal ultrasound	**VE**	Minute ventilation
TUI or TI	Transurethral incision	**VHD**	Valvular heart disease
TURBT	Transurethral resection of bladder tumour	**VKA**	Vitamin K antagonist
TURP	Transurethral resection of prostate	**VO$_2$**	Oxygen consumption
TVC	True vocal cord	**VP**	Vertriculo-peritoneal (shunt or drain)
TVR	Tricuspid valve replacement	**VPB**	Ventricular premature beat
		VT	Ventricular tachycardia

How to use your textbook

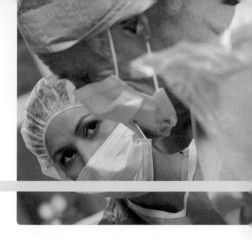

Features contained within your textbook

Each topic is presented in a double-page spread with clear, easy-to-follow diagrams supported by succinct explanatory text.

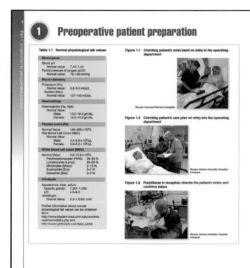

Your textbook is full of **photographs, illustrations and tables**.

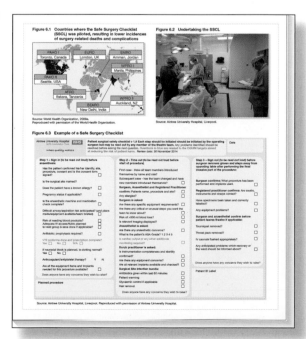

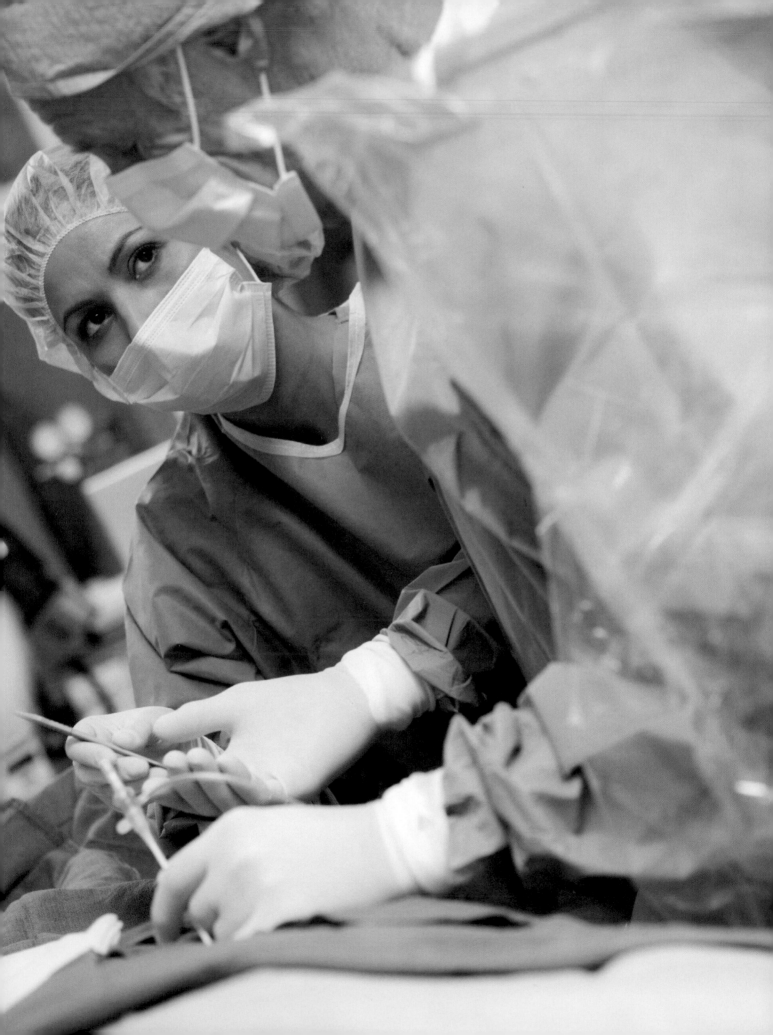

Introduction to perioperative practice

Chapters

1 Preoperative patient preparation   2
2 Theatre scrubs and personal protective equipment (PPE)   4
3 Preventing the transmission of infection   6
4 Preparing and managing equipment   8
5 Perioperative patient care   10
6 Surgical Safety Checklist – Part 1   12
7 Surgical Safety Checklist – Part 2   14
8 Legal and professional accountability   16
9 Interprofessional teamworking   18

1 Preoperative patient preparation

Table 1.1 Normal physiological lab values

Blood gases

Blood pH
Normal value: 7.34–7.44
Partial pressure of oxygen (pO2)
Normal value: 75–100 mmHg

Blood chemistry

Potassium (K+)
Normal value: 3.6–5.0 mEq/L
Sodium (Na+)
Normal value: 137–145 mEq/L

Haematology

Haemoglobin (Hg, Hgb)
Normal Value:
Male: 13.2–16.2 gm/dL
Female: 12.0–15.2 gm/dL

Platelet count (Plt)

Normal Value: 140–450 x 10^9/L
Red Blood Cell Count (RBC)
Normal Value:
Male: 4.4–5.8 x 10^6/μL
Female: 3.9–5.2 x 10^6/μL

White blood cell count (WBC)

Normal Value: 3.8–10.8 x 10^9/L
Polymorphonuclear (PMN): 35–80 %
Lymphocytes (Lymp): 20–50 %
Monocytes (Mono): 2–12 %
Eosinophils (Eos): 0–7 %
Basophils (Bas): 0–2 %

Urinalysis

Appearance: clear, yellow
Specific gravity: 1.001–1.035
pH: 4.6–8.0
Urobilogen
Normal Value: 0.2–1.0 Ehr U/dl

Further information about normal physiological lab values can be obtained from:
http://www.student.med.umn.edu/wardmanual/normallabs.php and
http://www.globalrph.com/labs_a.htm

Figure 1.1 Checking patient's wrist band on entry to the operating department

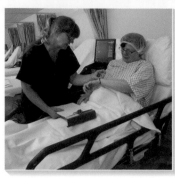

Source: Liverpool Women's Hospital.

Figure 1.2 Checking patient's care plan on entry into the operating department

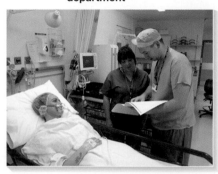

Source: Aintree University Hospital, Liverpool.

Figure 1.3 Practitioner in reception checks the patient's notes and confirms status

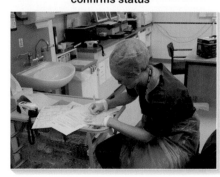

Source: Aintree University Hospital, Liverpool.

Perioperative Practice at a Glance, First Edition. Paul Wicker. © 2015 John Wiley & Sons, Ltd. Published 2015 by John Wiley & Sons, Ltd.

It is essential to prepare patients for their perioperative journey so that they experience the best care and achieve the best possible results following anaesthesia and surgery. Preoperative visiting of the patient is the first step towards providing high-quality care. Preoperative visiting by perioperative practitioners (i.e. operating department practitioners (ODP) or theatre nurses) is essential to ensure that the patient is prepared for anaesthesia and surgery, and that perioperative staff know as much about the patient as possible. Practitioners may also undertake a role in preoperative assessment clinics and it is possible to visit the patient in reception before their arrival in the anaesthetic room.

Preoperative visiting

Communication with patients includes several important areas such as confirming patient details (Figure 1.1), confirming their history of illnesses, assessing their current health, and identifying any issues the patient may have (O'Neill 2010). Educating patients is important to prepare them for surgery and provides knowledge on what is going to happen to them and why. This may also help to reduce their anxiety before anaesthesia on the day of surgery. Preoperative education includes topics such as pulmonary exercises, anaesthetic information, surgical information and leaflets about their surgery. It is also important to gain information about the patient. For example, areas such as allergies, likes and dislikes, personal issues (such as mental health problems, learning disabilities, or any abuse or addiction), religious beliefs, worries and personality traits, such as positive and negative attitudes (O'Neill 2010). Concurrent medical conditions can also have an effect on patients during surgery, for example painful joints, skin problems, tissue viability and pain. Informed consent is one of the most important areas and may include clarifying the purpose of consent, checking it is completed and valid and discussing the patient's rights (Wicker 2010). Discharge planning can further reduce anxiety, for example pick-up arrangements, postoperative care, postoperative drugs, exercises, pain relief and dressing changes. As one of the most common fears in patients is not waking up, discussing discharge planning will help the patient to develop a more positive attitude to their surgery and its results.

Preoperative assessment

The use of a perioperative care plan (Figure 1.2) is standard procedure in most operating departments (Goodman & Spry 2014). Areas that need to be explored include: **assessment of needs; diagnosis of issues; requirements for anaesthesia** (e.g. denture removal, latex allergy, pain relief, suitable time of fasting to avoid the risk of inhaling gastric fluids into the lungs); **physiological assessment** (e.g. blood pressure, heart rate and rhythm, respiration, body temperature); **fluid and electrolyte needs; psychosocial needs** (e.g. anxiety, fear, lack of understanding, maintaining dignity; Euliano & Gravenstein 2004).

Diagnostic screening determines the presence or absence of diseases or illnesses and identifies the baseline for the patient's physiological parameters, such as blood pressure, pulse, respiration and temperature (Euliano & Gravenstein 2004). Assessing these parameters during surgery helps to identify any changes, such as sudden drops in blood pressure or alteration in pulse rates

(Wicker 2010). Blood tests are normally carried out before most surgical operations to assess the patient's health. These include full blood count; cross-matching of blood; blood urea levels; blood sugar levels; and arterial oxygen saturation.

Preoperative investigations

Patients often undergo preoperative investigations to assess their health. This helps them to understand the impact of anaesthesia and surgery and to identify changes that may happen during surgery. Knowledge of these results also improves patient safety and helps to identify anaesthetic and surgical needs during the procedure (Euliano & Gravenstein 2004).

Investigations may include areas such as **radio opaque dyes** (to identify areas of the body and the flow of fluids in the body); **arteriograms and venograms** (to identify problems with the cardiovascular system); **barium swallow or enema** (to identify problems with the GI tract); **diagnostic imaging** (e.g. X ray, ultrasound, magnetic resonance imaging (MRI) or computerised tomography (CT), to provide high-quality views of body parts such as organs and any problems associated with them). There are many more investigations possible, depending on the health of the patient and the procedure being carried out.

Reducing postoperative complications

Multidisciplinary teamwork is essential to support the patient before, during and after surgery. It is also essential that practitioners consider the patient's physiological activities and understand the parameters that are within the normal range (Figure 1.3). Assessing airways and breathing is one of the most important areas, considering that patients can die within minutes of the cessation of breathing (apnoea). Such assessment needs to be undertaken and understood by all practitioners involved in the anaesthetic care of the patient, so that if a problem arises the whole team carries out the required actions (Wicker & O'Neill 2010).

Preoperative assessments by medical staff and practitioners may include, for example, **respiratory care,** including baseline observations, secretions, chest drains, pulse oximetry, cardiovascular status, jaw protrusion and head and neck distension (Goodman & Spry 2014); **joint stiffness, including** hips (regarding positioning), neck (regarding intubation), shoulder (arm boards) and back pain; u**rinary problems** such as infection, catheterisation and fluid intake; **pressure sores,** including damaged skin, excessive pressure, table fittings and Waterlow score; **deep venous thrombosis (DVT),** including risk assessment, drug therapy, DVT stockings and passive limb exercises; **nausea and vomiting, including** type of surgery, anti-emetics, predisposition to postoperative nausea and vomiting (PONV), risk assessment and reducing anxiety; **pain, including** involvement of the Pain Team, patient's expectations of pain, pain medication and patient-controlled analgesia (PCA); and **wound infection,** including preoperative skin assessment, culture swabs, dressing of lesions, cleaning of skin and removal of hair (Hatfield and Tronson 2009).

Remember: Know your patient, so you can give them the best care possible!

2 Theatre scrubs and personal protective equipment (PPE)

Figure 2.1 A practitioner prepared for cleaning the operating room and protected by personal protective equipment, including hat, gloves, mask, face shield and apron

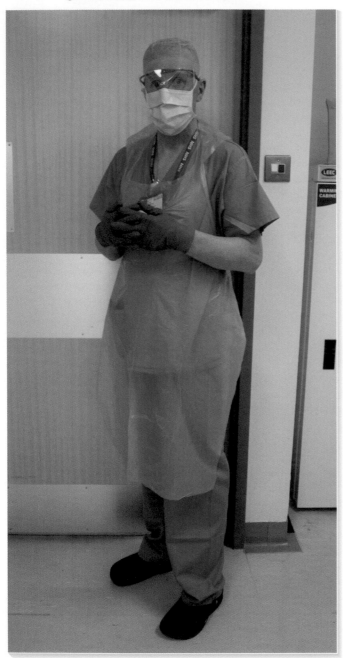

Source: Aintree University Hospital, Liverpool.

Eye protection

Glasses, visors or face shields are worn to protect from blood or body substances or fluids (e.g. bone chips or pus) splashing from the patient into the surgical team's eyes.

Eye protection includes:
- Goggles and eye glasses with side and top protection
- Anti-fog goggles to fit over prescription eyeglasses
- Combined surgical masks and visor eye shields
- Laser eye wear to protect against laser beams

Eye wear that becomes contaminated, even during a surgical procedure, should be cleaned, or discarded and replaced as soon as possible, to prevent dripping onto the face or masks.

Gloves

Non sterile gloves are normally made of latex or vinyl. Policies regarding the wearing of gloves vary between hospitals (Petty *et al*, 2005), however, essential elements should include:
- Wash hands before and after wearing gloves
- Wear gloves when handling contaminated items
- Only wear gloves when required, not during periods of non-contact with contaminated items
- Gloves shouldn't be washed, they should be removed if contaminated
- Clean items should not be handled with soiled gloves

Personnel entering an operating department need to wear suitable theatre scrubs (otherwise known as attire or theatre dress) to reduce the potential for patient infections (NICE 2008). Operating departments normally have policies and procedures identifying the need for correct theatre scrubs, with the aim of providing a barrier for microorganisms between patient and staff. Practitioners wear personal protective equipment (PPE; Figure 2.1) in specific cases where infection is a greater risk, for example due to blood spatter, infected patients or potential for inhaling microorganisms. Such theatre scrubs prevent harm to both patients and staff; it is also a responsibility of the employer to follow policies effectively (Phillips 2007).

Theatre scrubs

Perioperative practitioners need to be fully aware of the policies and procedures for correct wearing of theatre scrubs. Theatre scrubs are designed to reduce the transfer of microbes from skin and hair to the patient. Theatre scrubs also protect the perioperative staff from infection from the patient (DH 2010). By staff changing into clean scrubs when suitable, and not wearing them when going home, the hospital can ensure that the scrubs are clean and infection free. Changing rooms should have an entrance from outside the operating department and an exit into the operating department. No staff should be allowed into the operating department if they are not wearing appropriate theatre scrubs. Changing rooms require showers and sinks to support staff hygiene. Storage spaces for theatre scrubs should provide a clean and dry environment.

Theatre scrubs can include single-piece overalls or shirts and trousers. Staff should put the shirt on first and tuck it inside the trousers to prevent shedding of bacteria or skin flakes, and they should wear a plastic apron when cleaning operating rooms. Trousers are better for female staff than dresses, to prevent perineal fallout. Theatre scrubs should also be professional in appearance, made of close-knit, antistatic material, resistant to fluid strike-through, flame resistant, lint free and comfortable (AFPP 2011). Theatre staff may also wear 'warm-up jackets' to prevent shedding from arms and armpits and to keep the staff warm if the operating room is a cold environment (Goodman & Spry 2014). Practitioners should change theatre scrubs if they become soiled and if they move between operating rooms or specialities. For example, a practitioner who attended bowel surgery in the morning and then undertakes orthopaedic surgery in the afternoon should change theatre scrubs because of the risk of transfer of the microorganisms from the previous patient's bowel to the orthopaedic patient's bones.

Headwear

The purpose of headwear is to cover all hair to prevent contamination of wounds from hair and dandruff falling from heads and beards or moustaches (Goodman & Spry 2014). Surgical caps, hats and hoods are normally lint free, disposable, non-porous and non-woven. Practitioners can wear reusable woven hats, but they need to clean them daily. People with long hair need to wear bouffant-style hats. People with beards need to wear hoods. People with short hair can wear caps (Goodman & Spry 2014). Headwear can be either caps or hoods, and is dependent on hospital policies and speciali-

ties. Hoods are most often worn in orthopaedic theatres because of the high risk of bone infection from falling hair or skin flakes.

Footwear

Theatre shoes come in various formats, including clogs, leather slip-on shoes, plastic shoes and canvas shoes. The essential criteria include regular cleaning, removal if contaminated, protection against heavy equipment and insulated soles. Theatre footwear should be well fitting, supportive, protective and enclose the whole foot. The purpose of the footwear is to protect the staff member from falling equipment, spillages and infection (BSI 2004). Normally staff wear leather-topped theatre clogs, but sometimes they wear shoes instead. In each case, staff must follow hospital policy. Practitioners rarely use theatre overshoes because of the risk of infection when removing them, and because they increase bacterial infection on the floor.

Surgical masks

Contemporary surgical masks are soft and made of fine synthetic materials. They are 95% efficient in filtering microbes in exhalations and inhalations (Phillips 2007) and in preventing splashes of blood and body fluids on faces, eyes and mouths. Masks also help protect practitioners against inhaling surgical smoke or foreign particles from the air. As a minimum, masks should cover the mouth and nose; however, fluid shields can also be attached to masks to protect against splashing of fluids into the eyes (AORN 2012). There are various types of surgical masks available and practitioners need to choose the correct mask depending on the environmental conditions during the surgery. However, because the evidence base for the use of masks differs, operating department policies about the use of masks vary between hospitals. It is always important that staff know the policies and procedures for the wearing of masks that are in place for each type of operation (BSI 2006).

Patient dress

Patients normally wear theatre nightdresses, pyjamas or gowns and caps when entering the operating room. This reduces the risk of infection from their own clothing, and prevents their own clothing from being damaged during surgery. In some situations, such as minor surgery, patients may be allowed to wear their own clothes. Patients' relatives may be allowed to wear their own clothes, normally covered with a theatre gown, if observing only in the anaesthetic room. However, they would need to wear appropriate theatre attire if entering the operating room itself.

Theatre scrubs outside theatre

There is little evidence to show that wearing theatre scrubs outside theatre causes an increase in infection rates (Woodhead et al. 2002). However, common sense suggests that it is better to change theatre scrubs when going outside the theatre, or to wear a clean gown or laboratory coat over theatre scrubs when going between operating departments or out to wards. Under most circumstances it is best practice to change into clean theatre scrubs when returning to theatre. It is also unprofessional and possibly dangerous to patients to wear theatre scrubs in public places.

3 Preventing the transmission of infection

Figure 3.1 Key elements of standard precautions to help prevent infection in patients

Health-care facility recommendations for standard precautions

KEY ELEMENTS AT A GLANCE

1. Hand hygiene [1]

Summary technique:
- Hand washing (40–60 sec): wet hands and apply soap; rub all surfaces; rinse hands and dry thoroughly with a single use towel; use towel to turn off faucet.
- Hand rubbing (20–30 sec): apply enough product to cover all areas of the hands; rub hands until dry.

Summary indications:
- Before and after any direct patient contact and between patients, whether or not gloves are worn.
- Immediately after gloves are removed.
- Before handling an invasive device.
- After touching blood, body fluids, secretions, excretions, non-intact skin, and contaminated items, even if gloves are worn.
- During patient care, when moving from a contaminated to a clean body site of the patient.
- After contact with inanimate objects in the immediate vicinity of the patient.

2. Gloves
- Wear when touching blood, body fluids, secretions, excretions, mucous membranes, nonintact skin.
- Change between tasks and procedures on the same patient after contact with potentially infectious material.
- Remove after use, before touching non-contaminated items and surfaces, and before going to another patient. Perform hand hygiene immediately after removal.

3. Facial protection (eyes, nose, and mouth)
- Wear a surgical or procedure mask and eye protection (face shield, goggles) to protect mucous membranes of the eyes, nose, and mouth during activities that are likely to generate splashes or sprays of blood, body fluids, secretions, and excretions.

4. Gown
- Wear to protect skin and prevent soiling of clothing during activities that are likely to generate splashes or sprays of blood, body fluids, secretions, or excretions.
- Remove soiled gown as soon as possible, and perform hand hygiene.

5. Prevention of needle stick injuries [2]

Use care when:
- handling needles, scalpels, and other sharp instruments or devices
- cleaning used instruments
- disposing of used needles.

6. Respiratory hygiene and cough etiquette

Persons with respiratory symptoms should apply source control measures:
- cover their nose and mouth when coughing/sneezing with tissue or mask, dispose of used tissues and masks, and perform hand hygiene after contact with respiratory secretions.

Health care facilities should:
- place acute febrile respiratory symptomatic patients at least 1 metre (3 feet) away from others in common waiting areas, if possible.
- post visual alerts at the entrance to health-care facilities instructing persons with respiratory symptoms to practise respiratory hygiene/cough etiquette.
- consider making hand hygiene resources, tissues and masks available in common areas and areas used for the evaluation of patients with respiratory illnesses.

7. Environmental cleaning
- Use adequate procedures for the routine cleaning and disinfection of environmental and other frequently touched surfaces.

8. Linens

Handle, transport, and process used linen in a manner which:
- prevents skin and mucous membrane exposures and contamination of clothing.
- avoids transfer of pathogens to other patients and or the environment.

9. Waste disposal
- Ensure safe waste management.
- Treat waste contaminated with blood, body fluids, secretions and excretions as clinical waste, in accordance with local regulations.
- Human tissues and laboratory waste that is directly associated with specimen processing should also be treated as clinical waste.
- Discard single use items properly.

10. Patient care equipment
- Handle equipment soiled with blood, body fluids, secretions, and excretions in a manner that prevents skin and mucous membrane exposures, contamination of clothing, and transfer of pathogens to other patients or the environment.
- Clean, disinfect, and reprocess reusable equipment appropriately before use with another patient.

[1] For more details, see: WHO Guidelines on Hand Hygiene in Health Care (Advanced draft), at: http://www.who.int/patientsafety/information_centre/ghhad_download/en/index.html.
[2] The SIGN Alliance at: http://www.who.int/injection_safety/sign/en/

World Health Organization • CH-1211 Geneva-27 • Switzerland • www.who.int/csr

Source: World Health Organization, 2006. Reproduced with permission of the World Health Organization.

Perioperative Practice at a Glance, First Edition. Paul Wicker. © 2015 John Wiley & Sons, Ltd. Published 2015 by John Wiley & Sons, Ltd.

Infection prevention and control (IPC) has become a major area of importance in the perioperative environment. This is due to infections such as Hepatitis B, tuberculosis, meticillin-resistant *Staphylococcus aureus* (MRSA) and human immunodeficiency virus (HIV). Infection control policies therefore aim to reduce the risk of cross-infection in the operating department. Practitioners can use Standard Precautions (Figure 3.1) to assess the safety of the activities they are undertaking, regardless of whether the patient is infected or not (CDC 1998; Goodman & Spry 2014). The operating department is a high-risk environment due to the potential exposure of staff and patients to blood and body fluids and organisms. Therefore every practitioner should be aware of Standard Precautions, national guidelines (e.g. NICE 2012) and local policies on infection control.

Operating room cleaning

Wound infections often occur during surgery, rather than postoperatively. The reason is that the wound is open during surgery, but closed and covered with sterile dressing postoperatively. Wound infections can therefore arise from the patient's own flora, externally from theatre personnel or from the operating room environment. NHS Estates (2002) classifies the operating room as being high risk, therefore it is essential that the perioperative environment is clean and dust free. This is helped by positive air pressure within the operating room. A local policy for operating room cleaning should be available in every operating room. This will highlight the level of cleanliness needed and the personal protective equipment that practitioners require while cleaning (for example gloves, aprons and eye protection).

Personal protection while cleaning

Practitioners may also develop infections during cleaning, if they are not protected while doing so. Any skin cuts or grazes should have a waterproof dressing applied. If that is not possible, then occupational health needs to review the practitioner's ability to safely provide direct patient care, or to take part in cleaning activities. Hand washing is one of the main areas for concern, especially when cleaning contaminated items or coming into direct contact with the patient's blood or body fluids (Pratt *et al.* 2007). The use of the Ayliffe technique (see Chapter 21) is recommended for washing hands, as it effectively removes most soiled or contaminated particles. Even if a practitioner is wearing gloves while cleaning contaminated items, it is essential to wash hands following removal of the gloves.

Assessing the risk of splashes to the eyes, nose or mouth is also essential before undertaking a task. For example, washing contaminated items in a sink often leads to splashing and therefore eye protection should always be worn. Remove gloves as soon as possible after they have been contaminated, and if necessary double gloving may help to prevent contamination of the skin by glove perforation (Tanner & Parkinson 2002).

Cleaning equipment

Cleaning equipment normally consists of floor-scrubbing machines, mops and disposable cloths. Staff usually wear disposable plastic aprons and non-sterile gloves when cleaning to prevent contamination of theatre scrubs. While simple detergents are often used, disinfectants, such as Actichlor®, can clean blood spillages and contaminated areas.

Cleaning between cases

Normally, only surfaces that have some form of patient contact are cleaned between cases. So, for example, a wall that has blood splashes needs to be washed, but otherwise would be left until the end of the case, or the end of the week, depending on local policies. Removing all waste, laundry and used instrument trays following completion of the case is also essential to prevent contamination of the next patient. All equipment that is in use needs to be cleaned and decontaminated, to prevent the transmission of organisms between cases (AFPP 2011). The operating table should be cleaned, and if necessary dismantled, to ensure that no blood or body fluids will contaminate the next patient. Any broken equipment should be removed from the operating room and replaced with working copies, for example a ripped or torn mattress should not be used again, even if it was repaired by tape.

Cleaning at the end of cases

Under normal circumstances, staff will thoroughly clean and remove all portable equipment from the operating room (NICE 2012). Other items in the operating room that need to be cleaned include windowsills, benches, cupboards, trolleys, lights, furniture etc. Following cleaning and disinfecting by the theatre team, domestic staff may also clean the operating room later to ensure that every area is clean and dust free.

Risks to practitioners
Blood-borne viruses

Adhering to Standard Precautions reduces the risk of acquiring blood-borne infections, such as HIV, hepatitis B (HepB) and hepatitis C (HepC). All personnel should receive health checks, including, where appropriate, antibody checks and vaccines, to prevent them from acquiring such infections.

Sharps and splash injuries

Any practitioner receiving a sharps injury should report the incident to the theatre manager and complete an accident form. The manager will then liaise with the relevant departments (for example Health and Safety or Infection Control) to determine a solution to the issue. Practitioners who receive a sharps injury should also immediately encourage bleeding of the wound by applying pressure surrounding the wound site (AFPP 2011), wash well with running water and apply a waterproof dressing. Splashes to the mouth or eyes should also be washed or irrigated as needed and reported to the theatre manager. In most situations it is also advisable to go to the Accident and Emergency department (A&E) for further examination.

MRSA patients

MRSA is one of the most significant causes of hospital-acquired infection. It is often found in warm and moist areas of the body, such as the nose, armpits and groin (NICE 2012). MRSA normally causes the host no harm, but can be transmitted to others, leading to skin damage or more serious infections such as pneumonia or septicaemia. The primary mode of transmission is usually from hands to light switches, door handles and trolleys etc. Standard Precautions will help to reduce the risk of acquiring MRSA. Therefore staff should following cleaning policies and hand cleaning policies, wear appropriate personal protective equipment and follow national and local infection control policies closely (Goodman & Spry, 2014).

4 Preparing and managing equipment

Figure 4.1 Equipment checklist

This is an example of a potential checklist for equipment. The checklist in each operating theatre depends on the surgical speciality and the equipment that is present.

The purpose of this checklist is to ensure that all equipment has been checked to make sure that it is clean and working properly. Sign and date this checklist to indicate completion of the checklist.

Name(s):

Date:

General Surgery	Sign	Sign	Sign
Valleylab Electrical Surgical Units			
Birtcher 6400 Argon Beam Coagulator			
Ethicon Harmonic Scalpel			
Room Lights – Castle			
Head Lights			
Operating Room Tables – Maquet			
Operating Room Tables – Eschmann			
Amsco Gravity Flash Sterilizers			
Kendall Sequential Compression Devices			
Bear Hugger Patient Warming System			
Level I Infuser			
Stryker Video Cabinets – camera, light source, printer, insufflator			
Circon Niagra Pump			
Haemonetics Cell Saver			
Bowel Stapling Equipment			
Laser • Candella • Nd Yag • Holmium • CO2 • Novus 2000			
Gynaecological Surgery	Sign	Sign	Sign
Berkley Uterine Aspirator			
Wells Johnson Aspirator			
Storz Hysteroscopy Equipment – scope, light source			
Storz Hysteroscopy Pump			
Stirrups			
Smoke Evacuator			
Culposcope			
Video Cart – insufflator, camera, light source, printer			

Source: Adapted from School of Surgical Technology Equipment Checklist, Association of Surgical Technologists.

Equipment in the operating room is expensive and complex, with many different types of equipment available depending on the surgery taking place. It is therefore essential that practitioners have knowledge and understanding of all perioperative equipment that they use, and follow local policies on cleaning, checking and preparing the equipment before use. This ensures that it is fully working and reduces the risk of harm to patients or staff (AFPP 2011).

The theatre manager is responsible for ensuring that practitioners follow the Health and Safety at Work Regulations (HSE 1999) and that policies are in place stating the correct use and maintenance of equipment. Managers are also responsible for ensuring that there are planned maintenance programmes in operation to ensure that all equipment is safe and ready to use. Practitioners' responsibilities include checking recording equipment and following local policies as well as national guidelines. A major consideration for all practitioners is that if they are not familiar with a particular piece of equipment, they should not use it or set it up (HSE 1999). For this reason, all staff need to be adequately trained and educated in order to reduce the risk of harm to themselves and their patients.

Initial equipment checks

A checklist (Figure 4.1) is the best way to ensure that all equipment is set up and checked prior to the start of an operating list. The checklist should include areas such as selection of correct equipment, identification of any faults, calibration of equipment, testing of equipment, cleaning and so on. Electrical equipment in particular needs to be checked by authorised personnel who have been trained in its use (TNA 1999). Equipment that is sterile and packaged also has to be in date and intact.

Anaesthetic equipment

Checking anaesthetic equipment before starting anaesthesia helps to avoid critical incidents. Normally the anaesthetic machine is checked by the anaesthetic assistant, following local policies and protocols based on the Association of Anaesthetists of Great Britain and Northern Ireland (AAGBI 2012). However, the anaesthetist has responsibility for ensuring that the anaesthetic machine is fully operational. The main components of an anaesthetic machine include:

- Ventilator
- Vaporiser
- Scavenger system
- Flow control valve and meter
- Gas supply – via pipeline or cylinder
- Pressure regulator

Total intravenous anaesthesia may be used in place of general anaesthetics. Drug agents such as propofol, alfentanyl and remifentanyl are used as they have rapid anaesthetic and pain-killing effects on the patient. Target controlled infusion (TCI) devices are used to maintain and monitor the correct levels of propofol in the patient's plasma (AAGBI 2012). Drugs are injected into the patient at a particular rate or as a bolus by using a syringe pump. The syringe must fit securely in the clamp on the syringe pump and the battery needs to be checked to ensure that it is fully charged.

Secretions or vomit are extracted from the patient's airway using suction catheters. They should be checked to ensure that they are working, they are at the right setting and the tube and suction catheter are connected.

Monitoring equipment provides continual assessment of the patient during anaesthesia. Monitors include pulse oximetry, non-invasive blood pressure monitors, temperature gauges, capnography and electrocardiography. Monitors need to be tested for alarm settings, frequency of recordings and cycling times (DH 2013). Further information about anaesthetic equipment is available in Part 2 of this book.

Surgical equipment

Many items of equipment are in use during surgery, all of which need to be checked before the start of surgery to ensure that they are clean, in working condition and ready to use.

Electrosurgical generators exist in most operating rooms, as they are the best way to reduce bleeding and to cut tissues. However, this is also one of the most dangerous pieces of equipment, as it is designed to burn patient tissues. Before the start of surgery it is important to examine, test and set up all electrosurgical equipment (Cunnington 2006). Further information on electrosurgical devices is provided in Part 5.

A piece of equipment called a pulse lavage can irrigate wounds using 0.9% saline or water. Normally it is high power and can therefore cause splashing around the wound. Staff should therefore wear visors and preferably masks if they are within the vicinity of this machine when it is in use. The devices can either be electrical or air powered. In all cases, equipment needs to be checked to ensure that it is intact and operational (Goodman & Spry 2014).

Surgeons use visual display units to monitor laparoscopic procedures. These systems need to work perfectly and at a high resolution to allow the surgeon to view the necessary anatomical details during surgery. Before surgery, the laparoscope needs to be checked at both ends to ensure that the lenses are clean and scratch free. Viewing down the laparoscope helps to check for foggy, dirty, scratched or damaged parts of the laparoscope (DH 2013). Checking light cables is also important to ensure that they are fully working – broken fibres will reduce the quality of light during the laparoscopic surgery. Establishing the white balance is also necessary to ensure that the camera displays all colours correctly, which can be done using the built-in testing system and a white swab. A correct white balance supports diagnosis when looking through the camera as the tissues will show in the correct colours (Wicker & O'Neill 2010).

Several checks are needed for all laparoscopic equipment to ensure that it is fully working. Apart from those issues, checks also include:

- Checking and preparing all laparoscopic equipment
- Preparing irrigation fluids
- Checking gas supplies for insufflation
- Testing the video display unit
- Testing suction units

Efficient cleaning and checking of the laparoscopic equipment are vital before the start of surgery. Therefore it is essential that practitioners have been trained thoroughly to ensure that all the equipment is both ready for use and safe to use (DH 2013).

5 # Perioperative patient care

Figure 5.1 Sample of patient care plan

Preoperative Patient Checklist   Yes No N/A

Patient details
- Name, address, hospital number:
- Patient documents present:
- Consent form:
- Allergies:
- Operation site marked:
- Blood results:
- ECG results:
- Fasted as per policy:

Medication
- Premed:
- Medications taken:
- Anticoagulants:

Personal
- Contact lenses removed:
- Glasses removed:
- Dentures removed:
- Status of teeth:
  (caps, crowns, bridges, etc.)
- Make-up and nail varnish removed:
- Hearing aid:
- Prosthesis:
- Pacemaker:
- Patient is safe on trolley:
- Ward nurse name and signature:

Anaesthetic Care

- Anaesthetic: General, spinal, epidural, regional, local
- Airway equipment:
- Monitoring sites: ECG, pulse oximeter, arterial line, CVP, other
- Peripheral IV access:
- Airway maintenance:
- Skin integrity
- Nasogastric tube:
- Drugs used:

Intraoperative Care Plan – Circle, tick or complete using text as appropriate

Position
- Supine
- Lithotomy
- Left lateral
- Right lateral
- Prone
- Knee/elbow
- Other:

Arm position
- At side
- On arm board
- Palm down
- Palm up
- Palm at side
Concerns:

Aids used
- Arm boards
- Tissue support mattress
- Warming blanket
- Bair Hugger
- Other warming device:
- Arm retainer
- Heel support
- Lloyd Davies stirrups
- Lithotomy stirrups
- Head support
- Sacral wedge
- Lateral support
- Pillows
- Flowtron boots
- Other:

Concerns

Electrosurgery
- Monopolar Bipolar
- Patient plate site:
- Shaved:
- Concerns:

Skin preparation
- Chlorhexidine
- Betadine
- Other:

Skin closure
- Absorbable steristrips
- Clips Non-absorbable
- Other:

Dressings
  Adhesive   Melonin
  Velband   Backslab
  Crepe   Tegaderm
  Plaster of Paris
  Jelonet
- Other:

Specimens
- Specify:

  Histology   Microbiology
  Cytology   Frozen section
- Specimen sent:

Tourniquet
- Position: Left Right
- Arm
- Leg
- Finger
- Toe
- Time on:
- Time off:
- Pressure:
- Concerns:

Urinary catheter
- 2-way catheter
- 3-way catheter
- Suprapubic
- Bladder irrigation
- Balloon (ml)
- Catheter type and size:

Dressing packs
- Pack *in situ*:
- Site:

Wound drains
- Suction
- Site:
- Non-suction
- Site:
- Chest drain
- Site:
- Other:
  Specimens:
- Specify:

Postoperative inspection
- Airway status
- Skin integrity
- Diathermy site
- Tourniquet site
- Peripheral perfusion of limbs

Surgical procedure
- Final count correct: Register completed:
- Computer record completed:
- Final count incorrect (specify reasons):
- Surgeon informed: X ray taken: Incident form completed:

Comments, concerns and handover information

Perioperative Practice at a Glance, First Edition. Paul Wicker. © 2015 John Wiley & Sons, Ltd. Published 2015 by John Wiley & Sons, Ltd.

Providing perioperative care to patients throughout their perioperative journey is often managed through care planning (Figure 5.1). Care plans must be individualised to meet each particular patient's needs and individual situation, keeping in mind disease or injury prevention, health promotion, health restoration, health maintenance and palliative care. Considering cultural, religious and ethnic diversity is also important while providing perioperative care.

The practitioner must also respect the patient's expected outcomes and preferences when developing and carrying out a care plan. A primary responsibility of the practitioner is to provide patient education, enabling patients to gain enough information to make informed decisions regarding their care and treatment.

The standard approach to care planning involves assessing, planning, implementing and evaluating (Davey 2005). Under most circumstances, practitioners record a patient's care using perioperative documentation. Normally this is composed of the following sections: preoperative checklist, surgical safety checklist, anaesthetic room care, intraoperative care and postoperative care.

The preoperative checklist is often carried out on the ward and then checked on admission to the operating department. Checks include many areas such as consent form, allergies, preoperative investigations, medication, jewellery, hearing aids, dentures and so on.

The WHO Surgical Safety Checklist (WHO 2009) verifies that all discussions and checks regarding the patient's condition and treatment have been carried out. The checklist normally comprises sign in, time out and sign out procedures. Often there is also a group meeting during 'sign in' in order to clarify everybody's duties and roles and the patient's treatment. Its aim is to reduce errors during surgical and anaesthetic procedures (see Chapter 6 for more information). The following are checklists of minimum requirements.

Anaesthetic room care normally includes recording the monitoring of the patient's vital signs and identifying the type of anaesthetic required as well as any particular anaesthetic needs (Davey 2005). **Intraoperative care** involves recording such items as positioning, electrosurgery, tourniquets, skin preparation, specimens, surgical procedure, swab counts and so on. This helps to ensure that the correct actions are taken and that any problems can be identified later if there are any complications (WHO 2009). **Postoperative care** involves immediate assessment of the patient's condition on entry to the recovery area, and then regular monitoring of vital signs until the patient has recovered enough to return to the ward. Breathing, circulation, fluid and electrolyte balance and pain relief are among the most important areas to be monitored and recorded. Observations recorded include blood pressure, respiration, wound condition, drains, central venous pressure and temperature. The patient should be assessed through discharge criteria before returning to the ward in areas such as airway and breathing, cardiovascular status, comfort, surgical factors and fluid and electrolyte balance (WHO 2009).

Patient outcomes

The expected patient outcomes vary between hospitals and depend on the model of care plan used. Basic patient outcomes incorporated into care plans may include the following, adapted from University of Connecticut Health Centre (2013):

Patient Outcome 1: The patient is free from signs and symptoms of injury.

Patient Outcome 2: The patient receives appropriate prescribed medications safely.

Patient Outcome 3: The patient is free from signs and symptoms of infection.

Patient Outcome 4: The patient is normothermic following surgery.

Patient Outcome 5: The patient's physiological parameters (for example fluids, electrolytes, cardiac function, acid-base balance etc.) are within normal limits following surgery.

Patient Outcome 6: The patient is aware of the physiological and psychological impact of the surgical and anaesthetic procedures.

Patient Outcome 7: The patient is aware of nutritional and fluid requirements before and after anaesthesia and surgery.

Patient Outcome 8: The patient is aware of medication requirements, before and after anaesthesia and surgery.

Patient Outcome 9: The patient understands the need for and methods of delivery of pain relief following surgery.

Patient Outcome 10: The patient understands the need for support on discharge from the hospital.

Patient Outcome 11: The patient is informed about wound management following the surgical procedure.

Patient Outcome 12: The patient's right to privacy and dignity is maintained.

Patient Outcome 13: The patient's psychosocial values are respected and acknowledged before, during and after surgery.

While the above outcomes highlight the end result of care planning, the actual care plan documentation needs to be much more detailed. (See Figure 5.1 for an example.)

Care pathways

Care pathways were developed several years ago with the intention of providing a multidisciplinary approach to addressing a patient's needs and expectations during their perioperative journey (Lemmens 2008). Many areas use care pathways, especially day surgery and wards, where the pathway is less complex and easier to manage. A care pathway is a method for managing patient care in a well-defined group of patients during a well-defined period of time. A care pathway will explicitly state the goals and key elements of care based on evidence-based medicine guidelines, best practice and patient expectations by facilitating the communication, coordinating the roles and sequencing the activities of the multidisciplinary care team, patients and their relatives. The care pathway will document, monitor and evaluate variances and provide the appropriate resources and outcomes. The reason for using a clinical pathway is to improve the quality of care, reduce risks, increase patient satisfaction and increase efficiency in the use of resources (De Bleser et al. 2006).

Macario et al. (1998) undertook a research study into perioperative care pathways for patients undergoing knee replacement. The study concluded by stating that patient care was improved, multidisciplinary teams worked well together and hospitalisation costs were reduced significantly.

6 Surgical Safety Checklist – Part 1

Figure 6.1 Countries where the Safe Surgery Checklist (SSCL) was piloted, resulting in lower incidences of surgery-related deaths and complications

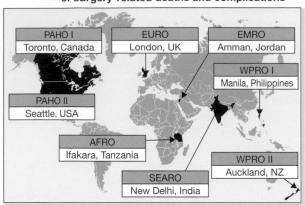

| PAHO I | EURO | EMRO |
| Toronto, Canada | London, UK | Amman, Jordan |

WPRO I
Manila, Philippines

PAHO II
Seattle, USA

AFRO
Ifakara, Tanzania

WPRO II
Auckland, NZ

SEARO
New Delhi, India

Source: World Health Organization, 2009a.
Reproduced with permission of the World Health Organization.

Figure 6.2 Undertaking the SSCL

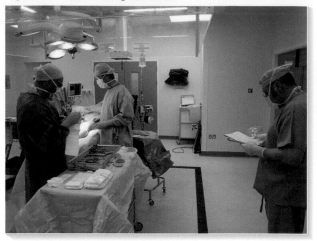

Source: Aintree University Hospital, Liverpool.

Figure 6.3 Example of a Safe Surgery Checklist

Aintree University Hospital
NHS Foundation Trust **NHS**
Where quality matters

Patient surgical safety checklist v 1.9 Each step should be initiated should be initiated by the operating surgeon but may be read out by any member of the theatre team. Any problems identified should be resolved before asking the next question. Questions in blue are related to the CQUIN targets aimed at reducing the risk of patient harm. Review date: 30 November 2014

Date

Step 1 – Sign in (to be read out loud) before anaesthesia

Has the patient confirmed his/her identity, site, procedure, consent and is the consent form signed? ☐

Is the surgical site marked?

Does the patient have a known allergy? ☐

Pregnancy status if applicable? ☐

Is the anaesthetic machine and medication check complete? ☐

Difficult airway/aspiration risk anticipated? (and plans made/equipment available/team briefed) ☐

Risk of needing blood products? ☐
Adequate IV access/fluids planned ☐
Is valid group & save done if applicable? ☐

Antibiotic: prophylaxis required? ☐

VTE proforma done and prescription complete?
Yes ☐ No ☐ N/A ☐

If neuraxial block is planned, is clotting normal?
Yes ☐ No ☐

Anticoagulant/antiplatelet therapy?   Y   N

Are all the equipment items and implants needed for this procedure available? ☐

Does anyone have any concerns they wish to raise?

Planned procedure

Step 2 – Time out (to be read out loud before start of procedure)

First case - Have all team members introduced themselves by name and role?

Subsequent case - has the team changed and have new members introduced themselves? ☐

Surgeon, Anaesthetist and Registered Practitioner confirm: Patients name, procedure and site? ☐
Any allergies? ☐

Surgeon is asked:
Are there any specific equipment requirements? ☐
Are there any critical or unusual steps you want the team to know about? ☐
Risk of >500 ml blood loss? ☐
Is relevant imaging displayed? ☐

Anaesthetist is asked:
Are there any anaesthetic concerns? ☐
What is the patient's ASA Grade? 1 2 3 4 5
Is cardiac output or any other additional monitoring required? ☐

Scrub practitioner is asked:
Is instrumentation completeness and sterility confirmed? ☐
Are there any equipment concerns? ☐
Are all relevant implants available and checked? ☐

Surgical Site infection bundle:
Antibiotics given within last 60 minutes ☐
Patient warming ☐
Glycaemic control if applicable ☐
Hair removal ☐

Does anyone have any concerns they wish to raise?

Step 3 – Sign out (to be read out load) before surgeon removes gloves and steps away from operating table after performing the final invasive part of the procedure:

Surgeon confirms: What procedure has been performed and implants used. ☐

Registered practitioner confirms: Are swabs, instruments and sharps correct? ☐

Have specimens been taken and correctly labelled? ☐

Any equipment problems? ☐

Surgeon and anaesthetist confirm before patient leaves theatre if applicable:

Tourniquet removed? ☐

Throat pack removed? ☐

IV cannula flushed appropriately? ☐

Any anticipated problems which recovery or the ward should be informed about? ☐

Does anyone have any concerns they wish to raise?

Patient ID Label

Source: Aintree University Hospital, Liverpool. Reproduced with permission of Aintree University Hospital.

The National Patient Safety Agency (NPSA) stated that in England and Wales, 129,419 surgical incidents were reported to the NPSA's Reporting and Learning System (RLS) in 2007 (NPSA 2009). In the same year there were 16 wrong-site surgery incidents reported (NPSA 2009). This shows that failure to use existing safety 'know-how' may occur within the operating department. For example, high rates of preventable surgical-site infection result from inconsistent timing of antibiotic prophylaxis. Accidental burns also occur despite improved electrosurgical technology. Anaesthetic complications are also 100–1000 times higher in countries that do not adhere to patient monitoring standards, and wrong-patient, wrong-site operations persist despite the high publicity over such events (NPSA 2009). In 2007 the World Health Organization (WHO) launched an initiative, called 'Safe Surgery Saves Lives', to ensure that surgical staff apply minimum standards of safe surgical care universally by using a checklist (Hunter & Finney 2011). In January 2009, the results of an international evaluation of this checklist were published (Haynes *et al.* 2009). Hospitals in eight cities around the globe (Figure 6.1) successfully proved that using a simple surgical checklist can lower the incidence of surgery-related deaths and complications by one third. Analysis showed a major fall in complications from 11% to 7%, a fall in unintentional death rates by 47% and a significant improvement in patient care reported at each site (WHO 2009a). Completing the WHO Safe Surgery Checklist (SSCL) has also led to a decline in injuries and deaths among patients caused by human error. This resulted in an alert issued by the NPSA to all UK hospitals requiring them to conduct the SSCL for all patients undergoing surgery (NPSA 2009).

To prevent such errors occurring, training of all staff, including surgeons, anaesthetists and practitioners, is essential to ensure the correct use of the SSCL, because practitioners are accountable to their patients, to employers, to the public and to their profession (Middleton 2007). The use of the checklist helps to identify the necessary steps to take and why they need to be taken (Figure 6.2). Carter (2009) states that all team members should join in completion of the SSCL to uphold best practice. Such best practice will give the patient a better experience and journey from anaesthetics to recovery, improve their outcomes and provide a high standard of care to the patients (Curley *et al.* 2007).

The Surgical Safety Checklist (Figure 6.3)

The SSCL has three sections: Sign In, Time Out and Sign Out. The WHO implementation manual (WHO 2013) provides suggestions for carrying out the checklist, with the understanding that different practice areas will adapt it to their own situations. By following a few critical steps in a logical and planned way, healthcare professionals can improve teamworking and minimise the most common and avoidable risks that endanger the lives of surgical patients, which in turn improves the patients' well-being. Before the start of a surgical list, it is often common practice for staff to get together in the operating room to discuss the whole list together – surgeon, anaesthetist, team leader and other staff. This is called the 'Team Brief' (NPSA 2009). Everybody introduces themselves and the surgeon and anaesthetist describe the surgical and anaesthetic procedures and any concerns. The team leader will then discuss any concerns related to patient care, equipment, instruments and so on. Team members may also raise concerns, which can then be discussed and actioned. The 'Sign In' section takes place in the anaesthetic room. This identifies patient details, anaesthetic techniques and any risks associated with the patient (NPSA 2009). The 'Time Out' section occurs in the operating room before the start of surgery. This identifies the patient and staff, anticipated critical events, correct preparation of equipment and so on. The 'Sign Out' section is normally undertaken before closing of the wound, or before any member of the team leaves the operating room.

Introducing the checklist into the operating department

Because of the checklist's complexity, it will take time for teams to learn to use it effectively and some members of the team may consider it an imposition or a waste of time (Hunter & Finney 2011). However, the checklist intends to give teams a simple, efficient set of priority checks for improving effective teamwork and communication and to encourage active consideration of the safety of patients during every operation performed. It also enables all members of the team to have their voices and concerns heard so that a mutual understanding and conclusion can be reached (WHO 2013). The checklist has two main purposes: ensuring consistency in patient safety; and introducing (or maintaining) a culture that values achieving it. To succeed, the anaesthetic and surgical consultants, theatre managers and team leaders must embrace the checklist and make it happen. Without leadership, use of the checklist can result in discontent and antagonism. With proper planning and commitment, accomplishing the checklist can make a profound difference to the safety of perioperative patients, as demonstrated by the Haynes study (Haynes *et al.* 2009).

Adjusting the checklist

The checklist should be modified to suit the particular clinical area – for example, by adapting processes or recognising the way in which the team works. However, important safety checks should not be removed, because these checks should inspire effective change that will help an operating team to comply with each and every element of the checklist. Clinical placement areas may also need to add safety checks for specific procedures.

In conclusion, the WHO SSCL has to be used proactively and has been proven to reduce errors and patient harm. Failure to implement it will result in 'never events', patient injury and possible harm to staff. As this checklist is proven to reduce errors, not conducting it could lead to a chain of events that can be seen as an 'intentional mistake' because the risks of doing so were known (Cvetic 2011: 263).

Surgical Safety Checklist – Part 2

Figure 7.1 Surgical Safety Checklist

This document can be updated and amended to conform to hospital rules and regulations within the NHS

Surgical Safety Checklist   **World Health Organization** | **Patient Safety** _A World Alliance for Safer Health Care_

Before induction of anaesthesia	Before skin incision	Before patient leaves operating room
(with at least nurse and anaesthetist)	(with nurse, anaesthetist and surgeon)	(with nurse, anaesthetist and surgeon)

Before induction of anaesthesia (with at least nurse and anaesthetist)

Has the patient confirmed his/her identity, site, procedure and consent?
- ☐ Yes

Is the site marked?
- ☐ Yes
- ☐ Not applicable

Is the anaesthesia machine and medication check complete
- ☐ Yes

Is the pulse oximeter on the patient and functioning?
- ☐ Yes

Does the patient have a:

Known allergy?
- ☐ No
- ☐ Yes

Difficult airway or aspiration risk?
- ☐ No
- ☐ Yes, and equipment/assistance available?

Risk of >500 ml blood loss (7 ml/kg in children)?
- ☐ No
- ☐ Yes, and two IVs/central access and fluids planned

Before skin incision (with nurse, anaesthetist and surgeon)

- ☐ Confirm all team members have introduced themselves by name and role.
- ☐ Confirm the patient's name, procedure, and where the incision will be made.

Has antibiotic prophylaxis been given within the last 60 minutes?
- ☐ Yes
- ☐ Not applicable

Anticipated Critical Events

To Surgeon:
- ☐ What are the critical or non-routine steps?
- ☐ How long will the case take?
- ☐ What is the anticipated blood loss?

To Anaesthetist:
- ☐ Are there any patient specific concerns?

To Nursing Team:
- ☐ Has sterility (including indicator results) been confirmed?
- ☐ Any there equipment issues or any concerns?

Is essential imaging displayed?
- ☐ Yes
- ☐ Not applicable

Before patient leaves operating room (with nurse, anaesthetist and surgeon)

Nurse Verbally Confirms:
- ☐ The name of the procedure
- ☐ Completion of instrument, sponge and needle counts
- ☐ Specimen labelling (read specimen labels aloud, including patient name)
- ☐ Whether there are any equipment problems to be addressed

To Surgeon, Anaesthetist and Nurse:
- ☐ What are the key concerns for recovery and management of the patient?

This checklist is not intended to be comprehensive. Additions and modifications to fit local practice are encouraged. Revised 1/2009   © WHO, 2009

Source: World Health Organization (2009).
Reproduced with permission of World Health Organization.

This chapter highlights important issues related to the WHO Surgical Safety Checklist (SSCL; Figure 7.1). Other risks and dangers may be present depending on the surgery and the state of health of the patient (NPSA 2009).

SIGN IN

(In the anaesthetic room, before induction of anaesthesia)

- **Has the patient confirmed their identity, site, procedure and consent?** The patient should give verbal confirmation of their identity by using the wristband, site of surgery and consent forms as evidence.
- **Is the surgical site marked?** The surgeon should mark the operative site and confirm this with the team before the start of surgery to ensure correct surgery and patient positioning.
- **Is the anaesthesia machine and medication check complete?** The completed anaesthesia safety checklist confirms inspection of the anaesthetic equipment, medications and risks to the patient before each case.
- **Does the patient have a known allergy?** Identify patient allergies and communicate issues to the team before the start of the procedure.
- **Does the patient have a difficult airway/aspiration risk?** Airway evaluation indicating high risk helps the team to prepare against any airway complications and prevents aspiration.
- **Does the patient have a risk of >500 ml blood loss (7 ml/kg in children)?** There is a risk of hypovolaemic shock intensifying when blood loss exceeds 500 ml (7 ml/kg in children). Consider venous access and availability of fluids and blood products.

TIME OUT

(Prior to start of surgical intervention, e.g. skin incision)

- **Have all team members introduced themselves by name and role?** All team members should understand who each member is, their roles and skills. This process should include all personnel, including students and visitors/observers (Curley *et al.* 2007).
- **Surgeon, anaesthetist and registered practitioner verbally confirm patient, site and procedure.** Confirmation of the name of the patient, the surgery, imaging, the site of surgery and correct positioning of the patient avoids operating on the wrong patient or the wrong site.
- **Anticipated critical events.** Communicating critical patient issues during the 'Time Out', by sharing risk assessments and plans, helps to mitigate anticipated critical risks (Middleton 2007).
- **Surgeon reviews: What are the critical, expected or unexpected issues, expected blood loss, specific needs and any special investigations?** A discussion of 'critical or unexpected steps' informs the team of the risk of rapid blood loss or of injury, and confirms specific equipment, implants, preparations and investigations that are required (NPSA 2009).
- **Anaesthesia team reviews: Are there any patient-specific concerns?** ASA Grade (identifies patient health status), risk of major blood loss, haemodynamic instability, complications, monitoring equipment and so on should be considered to highlight potential problems and their management.
- **Practitioner reviews: Has the sterility of the instrumentation been confirmed and are there any other equipment issues or concerns?** This includes verbal confirmation of the sterility of instru-

mentation, and highlighting specific concerns of the scrub team that have not been addressed by the surgical or anaesthesia team.
- **Has the Surgical Site Infection (SSI) bundle been undertaken? Antibiotic prophylaxis within the last 60 minutes?** Confirmation is required that prophylactic antibiotics have been given during the previous 60 minutes. Exceptions to this include vancomycin, which requires two hours to reach therapeutic levels; also patients whose procedure involves inflating a tourniquet; and women who need a caesarean section, when antibiotic administration is withheld until after the umbilical cord has been clamped (Hunter & Finney 2011).
- **Maintenance of normothermia.** Maintaining normothermia during surgery can reduce the rate of infection. Several studies have shown the benefits of both preoperative warming and perioperative maintenance of normothermia (NICE 2008).
- **Use of recommended hair-removal methods.** Evidence in the literature suggests (Tanner *et al.* 2011) that electric clippers should be the apparatus of choice to reduce the incidence of postoperative wound infection.
- **Maintenance of glycaemic control.** Hyperglycaemia in the perioperative period can lead to postoperative surgical site infection in patients undergoing major surgery.
- **Has venous thromboembolism (VTE) prophylaxis been undertaken?** VTE is associated with inactivity during surgical procedures.
- **Is essential imaging displayed?** Imaging is critical to ensure proper planning and conduct of many operations.

SIGN OUT

(Before any team member leaves the operating theatre)

- **Registered practitioner verbally confirms with the team the name of the procedure recorded.** Since the procedure may have changed or expanded during the operation, the procedure that has been carried out must be confirmed.
- **Verify that the instruments, swab and sharps counts are correct.** Confirmation of final swab and sharps counts must be carried out following local policy. Incidents reported to the National Reporting and Learning System (NRLS) from April 2007 to March 2008 identified 779 reports of missing or retained swabs and instruments (NPSA 2009).
- **Have the specimens been labelled correctly?** False labelling of pathological specimens is potentially disastrous for a patient and can result in a frequent source of laboratory error. 18 incidents reported to the NRLS from September 2007 to August 2008 identified 105 reports of incorrect or mislabelled specimens (NPSA 2009).
- **Have any equipment problems been identified?** Accurately identifying the sources of failure, and instruments or equipment that have malfunctioned, is important in preventing devices from being moved back into the theatre before the problem has been addressed.
- **Surgeon, anaesthetist and registered practitioner review the key concerns for recovery and management of this patient.** The team must carry out a review of the postoperative recovery and management plan, focusing in particular on intraoperative or anaesthetic issues that might affect the patient. The aim of this step is the efficient and appropriate transfer of critical information to the entire team.

8 Legal and professional accountability

Figure 8.1 Legal and professional accountability

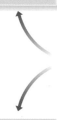 

Modes of Accountability

Professional accountability
Issues to consider:
• Code of professional conduct
• Standards of care
• Duty of care
• Vicarious liability
• Indemnity insurance

Self and others accountability
Issues to consider:
• Self
• Clients
• Healthcare team

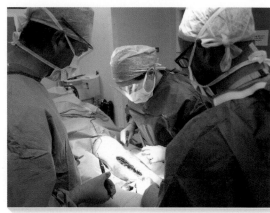

Source: Aintree University Hospital, Liverpool.

Legal accountability
Issues to consider:
• Civil actions
• Criminal actions
• Intentional torts
• Unintentional torts

Contractual accountability
Issues to consider:
• Employing institution
• Contract of employment
• Quality of work
• Discrimination
• Equality

Figure 8.2 The anaesthetic practitioner checks the patients details and discusses the actions to be taken during anaesthesia

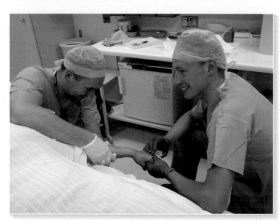

Source: Aintree University Hospital, Liverpool.

Modes of accountability

Accountability comes in four different modes: professional, self and others, legal, and contractual. 'Professional accountability' refers to a practitioner's accountability to the Health Care Professions Council (HCPC) or Nursing and Midwifery Council (NMC) as a registered practitioner. Registering bodies provide regulations and competencies that registered practitioners have to uphold. 'Self and others accountability' refers to accountability to ourselves and others as human beings. For example, people are accountable to one another for their social behaviour. This mode of accountability cannot be enforced in law and therefore the other modes of accountability are necessary to regulate public behaviour. 'Legal accountability' protects the public in general through the criminal courts and protects individuals through the civil courts. 'Contractual accountability' refers to employment law, for example contracts between an employer and an employee (both of these terms are legally defined; Highfield 2013).

Legal issues

The operating department is a well-known high-risk area and therefore there is an ever-present potential for litigation (Figure 8.1). There have been many examples of events over the years that have led to litigation. Risk assessment, the sister of quality assurance, can be used to prioritise risks in order to address them more efficiently. Civil law protects individuals and covers areas such as negligence, assault, defamation, negligent advice and false imprisonment (Dimond 2008). Negligence involves acting in a manner in which no reasonable person would act, guided by the regulations that normally guide that behaviour. It involves careless actions or omissions and may be beyond the abilities of the person undertaking the task. In asserting negligence a plaintiff must prove four points (Linda 2012):

- **A duty of care exists** – there must be some relationship between the plaintiff and defendant that leads to a duty of one to take care while interacting with the other (for example practitioner/patient, policeman/criminal, train driver/passengers).
- **The duty was breached** – something occurred that should not have occurred, or was omitted when it should have been done.
- **Harm was suffered** – negligence cannot have occurred (in the legal sense) if no damage was sustained.
- **Harm was caused by the act** – the action or omission must have been the cause of the damage (not a later action or omission, for example).

Defences against negligence

In court, asking defendants to justify their actions is called a defence. Some situations can make an act non-negligent, for example during an emergency certain actions might be acceptable that would not be acceptable during a non-emergency. The main defence that a person can make is to prove that they acted reasonably like a competent, ordinary skilled practitioner who normally undertakes that job (Dimond 2008). However, while many reasons for negligence may be understandable, they may not be an appropriate defence. For example, an overworked scrub practitioner may not have time to undertake a swab check correctly. Nevertheless,

the lack of time is not the patient's fault, and every patient deserves the same care as the previous one. Therefore, the patient would have every right to sue the hospital for negligence, despite the fact that the practitioner was working hard at the time and doing their best to cope. Other 'reasons' that are not acceptable include inexperience of staff, heavy workloads, faulty equipment, shortage of staff and emergency situations (Dimond 2008).

Assault and consent

Assault, in the civil sense, occurs whenever an individual's body is interfered with, or is in danger of being interfered with. 'Interfered with' means any contact or threat of contact at all. Assault is deemed not to have taken place if the individual gives informed consent for such actions. There are several legal requirements that must be satisfied to make consent valid (Linda 2012). Consent must be voluntary, and must be offered freely with no coercion or persuasion. However, it could be argued that a sedated patient cannot give voluntary consent if they cannot make a rational decision. Consent must be informed and the patient must be aware and understand the implications of what they are consenting to. It must cover the act, meaning that a 'blanket consent' is unlikely to stand up to scrutiny in court even if the patient agreed to it (Dimond 2008). Consent must also come from a legally competent source, which includes consent for minors, mentally ill patients and so on.

Several defences against the charge of assault are possible, for example consent is not needed in emergency situations, such as cardiac arrest, which are life threatening or likely to cause harm to the person. Other areas of defence against the charge of assault include protecting the public from an individual's reckless behaviour; the Mental Health Act where a carer needs to restrain a patient; and self-defence where the individual is being attacked or is under threat of attack (Linda 2012).

Hospital requirements

Hospital requirements are different to legal requirements, which shows the difference between legal accountability and contractual accountability. If the practitioner admitting the patient did not check for a consent form, then they would be in breach of contract and could be counter-sued by the hospital to recover any payment of damages made to the patient.

Accountability and professional practice

The regulatory bodies set the tone for the exercise of professional accountability. Formal education then sets boundaries of practice. Pre-registration education prepares the individual for the role of registered practitioner; each practitioner has a scope of practice appropriate to the individual's education, skills and competence. The practitioner, the registration body, the practitioner's employers and the law define this scope of practice.

An integrated understanding of legal and professional issues in perioperative practice will underpin professional roles and ensure that individual practitioners exercise their duties within the sphere of their responsibilities and abilities. Understanding and application of professional and legal accountability will ensure that quality patient care is enhanced and protected.

Interprofessional teamworking

Figure 9.1   Better Training Better Care

This poster refers to a pilot project entitled 'Better Training Better Care', which is being supported by Health Education England. The pilot projects involve using cadaveric workshops to train surgeons and perioperative practitioners, and also to increase collaboration between all the professions in perioperative care

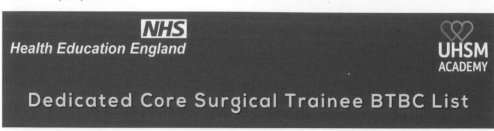

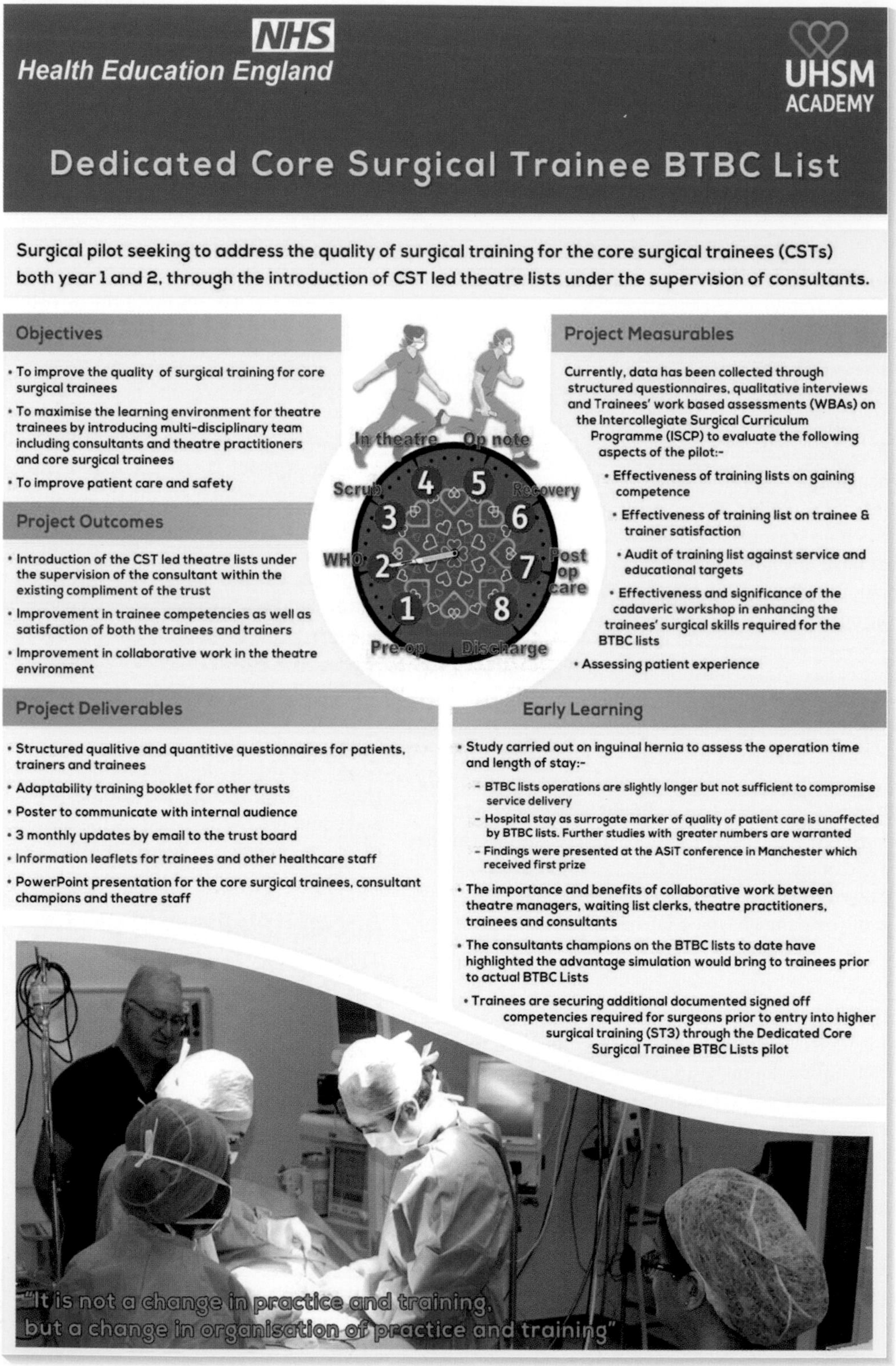

NHS
Health Education England

UHSM ACADEMY

Dedicated Core Surgical Trainee BTBC List

Surgical pilot seeking to address the quality of surgical training for the core surgical trainees (CSTs) both year 1 and 2, through the introduction of CST led theatre lists under the supervision of consultants.

Objectives

• To improve the quality of surgical training for core surgical trainees

• To maximise the learning environment for theatre trainees by introducing multi-disciplinary team including consultants and theatre practitioners and core surgical trainees

• To improve patient care and safety

Project Outcomes

• Introduction of the CST led theatre lists under the supervision of the consultant within the existing compliment of the trust

• Improvement in trainee competencies as well as satisfaction of both the trainees and trainers

• Improvement in collaborative work in the theatre environment

Project Deliverables

• Structured qualitive and quantitive questionnaires for patients, trainers and trainees

• Adaptability training booklet for other trusts

• Poster to communicate with internal audience

• 3 monthly updates by email to the trust board

• Information leaflets for trainees and other healthcare staff

• PowerPoint presentation for the core surgical trainees, consultant champions and theatre staff

Project Measurables

Currently, data has been collected through structured questionnaires, qualitative interviews and Trainees' work based assessments (WBAs) on the Intercollegiate Surgical Curriculum Programme (ISCP) to evaluate the following aspects of the pilot:-

• Effectiveness of training lists on gaining competence

• Effectiveness of training list on trainee & trainer satisfaction

• Audit of training list against service and educational targets

• Effectiveness and significance of the cadaveric workshop in enhancing the trainees' surgical skills required for the BTBC lists

• Assessing patient experience

Early Learning

• Study carried out on inguinal hernia to assess the operation time and length of stay:-

  – BTBC lists operations are slightly longer but not sufficient to compromise service delivery

  – Hospital stay as surrogate marker of quality of patient care is unaffected by BTBC lists. Further studies with greater numbers are warranted

  – Findings were presented at the ASiT conference in Manchester which received first prize

• The importance and benefits of collaborative work between theatre managers, waiting list clerks, theatre practitioners, trainees and consultants

• The consultants champions on the BTBC lists to date have highlighted the advantage simulation would bring to trainees prior to actual BTBC Lists

• Trainees are securing additional documented signed off competencies required for surgeons prior to entry into higher surgical training (ST3) through the Dedicated Core Surgical Trainee BTBC Lists pilot

Clock labels: In theatre · Op note · Scrub · Recovery · WHO · Post op care · Pre-op · Discharge · 1 2 3 4 5 6 7 8

"It is not a change in practice and training, but a change in organisation of practice and training"

Source: Health Education England. Reproduced under the Open Government Licence.

There are many ways to describe interprofessional teamworking. One definition is 'working together with one or more members of the health care team who each make a unique contribution to achieving a common goal. Each individual contributes from within the limits of her/his scope of practice' (College of Nurses of Ontario 2008: 3).

Interprofessional courses can help members of professions learn more about each other and about the extent to which knowledge is shared and where it diverges (Howkins & Bray 2008). This is now a fundamental part of most health-orientated preregistration programmes.

Clinical governance is seen as a systematic approach to preserving and improving the quality of patient care within a high-quality health environment. Interprofessional teamworking can assist in clinical governance by providing an environment in which all staff know one another and are aware of each other's responsibilities (MacDonald *et al.* 2010). Registering bodies, in particular the Health Care Professions Council and the Nursing and Midwifery Council, support autonomy and accountability for individual practitioners, while highlighting the need for interprofessional collaboration.

Several different professions carry out perioperative care, for example surgeons, anaesthetists, nurses, ODPs, healthcare workers, radiographers and so on. To provide high-quality patient care it is important that all professions work together collaboratively, with a working knowledge of the role of each member of the team (Reel & Hutchings 2007). For example, while a surgeon can undertake surgery, they may not be aware of the need to prepare particular items of equipment before the start of the case. Similarly, the anaesthetist may be able to intubate, but the practitioner assisting them must ensure that the correct equipment is available and working.

Human errors occur often during surgery, and when they do happen it is important that the whole team knows about them and why they happen. Sharing such information between team members may help to identify the cause of the error and reduce mistakes occurring in the future through better organisation and better understanding of each other's roles (Osbiston 2013). Undertaking the Surgical Safety Checklist (Chapter 6) has helped to create closer teamworking, as its use involves all members of the perioperative team.

Although interprofessional teamworking occurs wherever two or more different professionals work together, Reel and Hutchings (2007) have argued that it can take away autonomy and independence from practitioners. For example, an anaesthetist might argue that an anaesthetic machine had not been checked properly, when in fact it had. However, Hawley (2007) also suggests that interprofessional working helps professionals learn more about each other's roles and is essential for patient-centred care. Collaboration between professionals can improve patient-centred care through better understanding and respect within the team (Osbiston 2013). It is important to understand, nevertheless, that all the professionals within the team have their own range of duties and limits to their practice (MacDonald *et al.* 2010).

An example of perioperative teamworking could involve positioning a patient's arm on an arm board in the correct way. The anaesthetist will need access to the arm for invasive blood pressure monitoring, pulse oximeter monitoring and IV fluid access. The surgeon may need access to the patient's body without hyperextending the arm and causing damage to the brachial plexus. Discussion between the surgeon, anaesthetist and practitioner would support patient safety and ensure placing of the arm in the best and safest position.

Knowledge of the role of other members of the team facilitates the challenging of poor or unsafe practice that may lead to patient harm, and supports the best ways of carrying out practice to improve patient care. For example, if surgeons are aware of the knowledge and skills of the theatre practitioners, then they are much more likely to ask for help or advice in a collegial way, rather than blaming the practitioner for not informing them of a problem.

Interprofessional conflicts

Interprofessional conflicts (between surgeons, anaesthetists, ODPs and nurses) have occurred for many years (Kalisch & Kalisch 1977). Conflicts have arisen mainly because of the hierarchy, with surgeons traditionally at the top of the tree, anaesthetists underneath them, followed by nurses and finally ODPs at the root. Often the underlying professions could not solve problems because of a lack of communication and assertiveness towards the professions above them (Stein 1967). This in turn has also led to issues within teams when senior members of the team are oppressed, leading them to oppress their juniors. Tame (2012) refers to this as horizontal violence, and it is known to occur in nursing and ODP teams.

However, in many areas this situation has now eased, because of the increasingly complex workload of practitioners, high medical turnover and a high proportion of doctors arriving from other countries (Coombs 2004). The changes in the professions have resulted in boundaries becoming blurred. For example, ODP and nurses can now develop their roles as non-medical anaesthetists or surgical care practitioners, indicating that they are capable of interacting more with medical professions. A scrub practitioner who has been working in orthopaedics for 15 years will have a much better understanding of the equipment needed than a junior surgeon who has only just started. Mutual dependency therefore requires teams to work together with mutual understanding, to carry out the procedure in the best possible way (Coombs 2004).

Interprofessional education has increased over the past few years, leading to greater interaction between students from different health professions (Howkins & Bray 2008). A recent pilot, supported by Health Education England, is looking at training junior surgeons and at increased collaboration with theatre practitioners within the perioperative environment (Figure 9.1; Health Education England 2013).

Interprofessional teamworking should therefore be seen as an advantage to patients, as it assists with decision making in the patient's best interests, ensuring safer patient care.

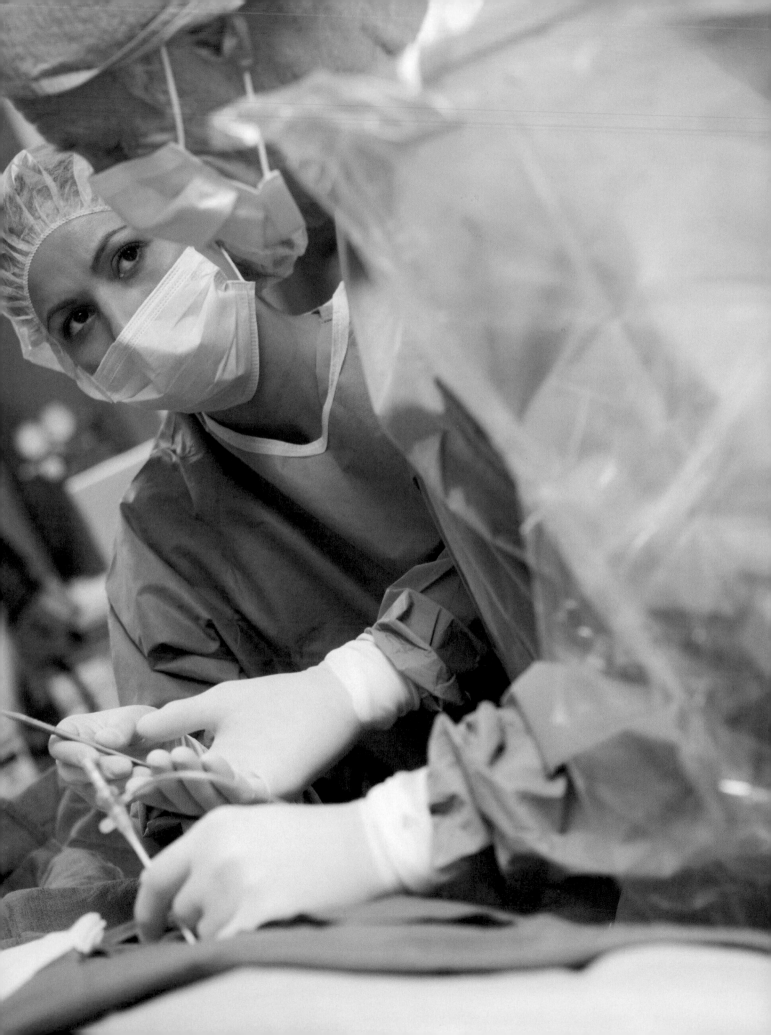

Anaesthesia

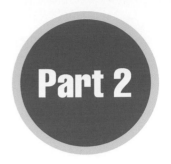

Part 2

Chapters

10 Preparing anaesthetic equipment   22
11 Checking the anaesthetic machine   24
12 Anatomy and physiology of the respiratory
    and cardiovascular systems   26
13 Anaesthetic drugs   28
14 Perioperative fluid management   30
15 Monitoring the patient   32
16 General anaesthesia   34
17 Local anaesthesia   36
18 Regional anaesthesia   38

10 Preparing anaesthetic equipment

Figure 10.1 Basic anaesthetic machine, for use in the anaesthetic room

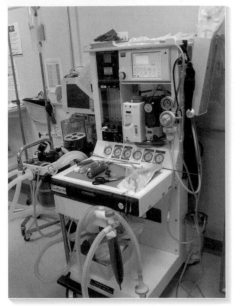

Source: Aintree University Hospital, Liverpool.

Figure 10.2 Anaesthetic machine, ECG monitor, capnograph, ventilator etc., used during surgery

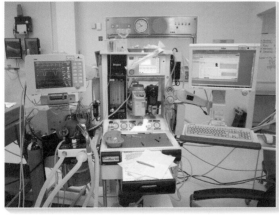

Source: Aintree University Hospital, Liverpool.

Figure 10.3 Guedal (oral) airways
These devices may be used in association with a face mask or postoperatively until the patient wakes up

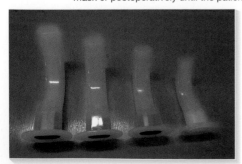

Source: Aintree University Hospital, Liverpool.

Figure 10.4 ET tubes, laryngoscope, oral airways, laryngeal mask airways (LMA)

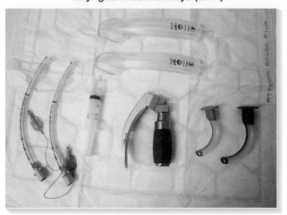

Source: Aintree University Hospital, Liverpool.

Figure 10.5 Cuffed tracheostomy tube

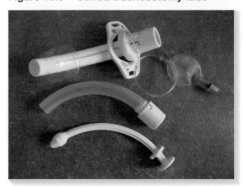

Source: Wikipedia © Klaus D. Peter, Wiehl, Germany. Reproduced under the Creative Commons Attribution 2.0 Germany License.

Airway tubes

Tracheal tubes (Figure 10.5) provide a way of securing the patient's airway. Tracheal tubes are made of polyvinyl chloride (PVC) and have a radio-opaque line that enables their position to be determined using X ray. The bevel at the tip of the tube is left facing and oval. Tracheal tubes are either cuffed or uncuffed. Cuffed tubes prevent the passage of vomit into the lungs.

Types of tracheal tubes include the Oxford tube, which is an L-shaped tube used for head and neck surgery; the armoured tube, which contains a spiral of metal wire or tough nylon, helping to prevent kinking and occlusion of the tube; the RAE tube, a preformed tube that fits the mouth or nose without kinking; and the laser-resistant stainless steel tube, used when laser surgery is being performed on the larynx or trachea. Tracheostomy tubes are short, curved plastic tubes for insertion through cartilage rings. They include cuffed and uncuffed tubes, fenestrated tubes and metal tubes. Fenestrated tubes allow patients to speak. Double lumen endobronchial tubes allow selective deflation of one lung during thoracic surgery, while maintaining standard ventilation in the other lung. An oropharyngeal (Guedel) airway is inserted through the mouth into the oropharynx to maintain patency of the upper airway.

Perioperative Practice at a Glance, First Edition. Paul Wicker. © 2015 John Wiley & Sons, Ltd. Published 2015 by John Wiley & Sons, Ltd.

Apart from the anaesthetic machine (Figure 10.1), it is also important to check other items of equipment and ensure that they are working correctly in order to provide patient safety. The Association of Anaesthetists of Great Britain and Ireland (AAGBI 2012) offers guidelines relating to the use of all anaesthetic equipment.

Consumable items

The anaesthetic room needs to contain a large number of consumable items that nowadays are in use only once per patient. Airway consumables include face masks, oxygen masks, oral and nasal airways (Figure 10.3), laryngeal mask airways (LMA), endotracheal (ET) tubes, laryngoscopes and bougies (Figure 10.4). Other small consumables include lubricants for LMA or ET tubes, tapes, ties, gauze roll for a throat pack, eye pads, gum guards and paraffin jelly to moisturise the lips. Intravenous equipment includes syringes, needles, intravenous (IV) cannulae and giving sets. These items are essential for anaesthesia and must be available and in working condition (Al-Shaikh & Stacy 2002).

Monitoring devices

Monitoring devices are becoming increasingly complex and diverse (Figure 10.2). Therefore it is important that the anaesthetic practitioner and anaesthetist are fully aware of the particular device: what it is, how it is used safely and how to check it (AAGBI 2009). Monitoring devices provide information about the physiological well-being of the patient and operate in collaboration with patient observation. Anaesthetic monitors used during general anaesthesia include, but are not restricted to, pulse oximeter, non-invasive blood pressure monitor, electrocardiography, airway monitor, airway pressure monitor, nerve stimulator, invasive arterial pressure and temperature probe. During local anaesthesia fewer monitors are required; they normally include pulse oximeter, non-invasive blood pressure monitor and electrocardiography. The anaesthetist has overall responsibility for ensuring that the monitors are working properly and that alarm limits have been set (AAGBI 2009).

Calibrating the monitors prior to use involves reading the manual prior to the patient arriving, or establishing with the anaesthetist the level of calibration required. Monitors should be attached before anaesthesia starts, in order to establish physiological parameters prior to anaesthesia. Recording data in the patient's notes provides a record of their state of health during the surgery. In situations in which a practitioner is recording vital signs, the anaesthetist has to ensure that the practitioner is capable of reading the data and interpreting it correctly, so that the practitioner knows when to inform the anaesthetist of any problems (Hughes & Mardell 2012).

A central venous pressure (CVP) line helps to monitor fluid balance, measures the filling pressure of the right atrium and gives an indication of circulating volume. The anaesthetist inserts the CVP line by first inserting a needle into the patient, next inserting the guide wire inside the needle, then removing the needle and inserting the catheter over the guide wire. X ray is used to confirm that the catheter is placed correctly. The risks to the patient include pneumothorax, air embolus, haematomas and infection. An electronic transducer that is connected to a monitor then measures the patient's CVP.

Monitoring arterial blood gases is carried out using a heparinised syringe of patient blood, which is sent off to a laboratory for analysis. The arterial blood gas results can show the level of carbon dioxide and oxygen in the blood, indicating the patient's level of respiration and also the acid base balance. The normal ranges for arterial blood results are (Hughes & Mardell 2012):

PaO_2:	12–15 KPa (90–110 mmHg)
$PaCO_2$:	4.5–6 KPa (34–46 mmHg)
HCO_3:	21–27.5 mmol/L
H + ions:	36–44 nmol/L (pH 7.35–7.45)

Medical gas cylinders

Medical gas cylinders contain a variety of different gases used for particular purposes, including for example oxygen, nitrous oxide and medical air. Therefore, it is important that practitioners know what they are used for and how to use them (AAGBI 2012). Medical gas cylinders have labels and are colour coded to help identify what they contain. Cylinders also have markings on their shoulder (top curve of the cylinder) or valve block identifying the name and chemical contents, the cylinder size and capacity, the empty cylinder weight and the maximum working pressure. Most cylinders also have plastic collars attached that identify various other areas for consideration, including directions for use, storage and handling instructions, shelf life, batch number and product license number (Hughes & Mardell 2012).

The pin index safety system prevents a cylinder from being connected to the wrong location. Attaching a cylinder to a piece of equipment requires the valve to be opened for a few seconds to blow any foreign materials out of the valve. The cylinder is then attached to the machine yoke and, once secured, the valve is slowly opened in an anticlockwise direction. Any leakage will be detected by a 'hiss' from around the area of the valve and yoke (AAGBI 2012). If this cannot be rectified, then the cylinder should be shut down and removed, and the equipment checked to ensure that it is not broken or damaged (Al-Shaikh & Stacy 2002).

Fluid warmers

Fluid warmers are used to infuse warm fluid, including blood, into patients. Dry heat warmers are made of two heated plates into which a plastic cassette is fitted, which allows the fluid to pass through the plates and be warmed. There are various models of dry heat warmers, but all are effective in warming blood and fluids. The coaxial fluid heating system consists of water heated to approximately 40 °C, which then heats the fluids being infused. Again, various methods are used, but in all cases the infusion never comes into direct contact with the warming fluid (Diba 2005; AAGBI 2009).

There are many more items of equipment used to support anaesthesia. Anaesthetic practitioners need to be fully aware of how they work and ensure that they are clean and ready to use prior to anaesthesia.

11 Checking the anaesthetic machine

Box 11.1 Checking anaesthetic equipment

- Anaesthetic machine (connections to gas and electric supplies)
- Monitoring equipment
- Medical gas supplies
- Vaporisers
- Breathing circuits
- Ventilator
- Scavenging systems
- Ancillary equipment
- Single-use equipment
- Airway equipment
- Difficult intubation trolley
- Machine failure
- Recording and audit

Source: Checklist for anaesthetic equipment 2012. Reproduced with permission of John Wiley & Sons Ltd.

Figure 11.1 Checklist for anaesthetic equipment

(a)

Checklist for Anaesthetic Equipment 2012
AAGBI Safety Guideline

Checks at the start of every operating session
Do not use this equipment unless you have been trained

Check self-inflating bag available

Perform manufacturer's (automatic) machine check

Power supply	• Plugged in • Switched on • Back-up battery charged
Gas supplies and suction	• Gas and vacuum pipelines - 'tug test' • Cylinders filled and turned off • Flowmeters working (if applicable) • Hypoxic guard working • Oxygen flush working • Suction clean and working
Breathing system	• Whole system patent and leak free using 'two bag' test • Vaporisers - fitted correctly, filled, leak free, plugged in (if necessary) • Soda lime - colour checked • Alternative systems (Bain, T-piece) - checked • Correct gas outlet selected
Ventilator	• Working and configured correctly
Scavenging	• Working and configured correctly
Monitors	• Working and configured correctly • Alarms limits and volumes set
Airway equipment	• Full range required, working, with spares

RECORD THIS CHECK IN THE PATIENT RECORD

Don't forget	• Self-inflating bag • Common gas outlet • Difficult airway equipment • Resuscitation equipment • TIVA and/or other infusion equipment

This guideline is not a standard of medical care. The ultimate judgment with regard to a particular clinical procedure of treatment plan must be made by the clinician in the light of the clinical data presented and the diagnostic and treatment options available.
© The Association of Anaesthetists of Great Britain & Ireland 2012

(b)

CHECKS BEFORE EACH CASE

Breathing system	• Whole system patent and leak free using 'two-bag' test • Vaporisers – fitted correctly, filled, leak free, plugged in (if necessary) • Alternative systems (Bain, T-piece) – checked • Correct gas outlet selected
Ventilator	• Working and configured correctly
Airway equipment	• Full range required, working, with spares
Suction	• Clean and working

THE TWO-BAG SYSTEM

A two-bag test should be performed after the breathing system, vaporisers and ventilator have been checked individually

i. Attach the patient end of the breathing system (including angle piece and filter) to a test lung or bag.

ii. Set the gas flow to 5l min^{-1} and ventilate manually. Check the whole breathing system is patent and the unidirectional valves are moving. Check the function of the APL by squeezing both bags.

iii. Turn on the ventilator to ventilate the test lung. Turn off the fresh gas flow, or reduce to a minimum. Open and close each vaporiser in turn. There should be no loss of volume in the system.

This checklist is an abbreviated version of the publication by the Associated of Anaesthetists of Great Britain and Ireland 'Checking Anaesthesia Equipment 2012'. It was originally published in Anaesthesia.
(Endorsed by the Chief Medical Officers)

If you wish to refer to this guideline, please use the following reference: Checklist for anaesthetic equipment 2012. Anaesthesia 2012; **66**; pages 662-63.http://onlinelibrary.wiley.com/doi/10.1111/).1365-2044.2012.07163.x/abstract

Making sure that the anaesthetic machine is working correctly is an essential part of the anaesthetic practitioner's role, in collaboration with the anaesthetist (Al-Shaik & Stacey 2002). During induction of anaesthesia, the patient is at one of the most vulnerable points in their perioperative care, so equipment error can put the patient at high risk of harm, for example through airway obstruction, circulatory problems, reduced blood oxygenation or even death due to errors such as flow reversal though the back bar on the anaesthetic machine (Cheng & Bailey 2002).

Practitioners and anaesthetists should check the anaesthetic machine using the checklist from the Association of Anaesthetists of Great Britain and Northern Ireland (AAGBI 2012) and the manufacturer's manual as guides to ensure that the machine is safe to use. Often the anaesthetic assistant will assemble and check the equipment in preparation for the anaesthetist (Box 11.1), who then ensures that they have the correct equipment for the anaesthetic procedure. The assistant's role is therefore to support the anaesthetist, check the equipment and ensure the patient's safety (Wicker & Smith 2008).

Errors during anaesthesia have often been associated with a lack of proper equipment checks. Kumar (1998) states that checking an anaesthetic machine using a checklist can lead to a reduction in incidents. For example, wrong assembly of the anaesthetic machine can lead to errors such as high dosages of volatile agents. A checklist also needs to be completed when equipment is returned from servicing – it cannot be guaranteed that a serviced, or brand new, anaesthetic machine is working perfectly.

Risk assessment reduces anaesthetic risks, improves patient safety and offers a cost-effective, high-quality service. The anaesthetic checklist is therefore a method of risk assessment that can help the anaesthetic practitioner identify risks to the patient from faulty equipment, and ensure the best patient care during anaesthesia (Wicker & Smith 2008).

The Association of Anaesthetists of Great Britain and Ireland published a document in 2004, updated in 2012 (AAGBI 2012), discussing the extensive checks required for ensuring the safe use of anaesthetic equipment. This document has now become the standard for establishing the best ways of pre-anaesthetic checking of anaesthetic equipment. It offers a baseline for the safe and effective checking of parts of the anaesthetic machine such as gas supply pipelines, breathing circuits, ventilators and monitors (AAGBI 2012).

This checking procedure is applicable to all anaesthetic machines and should take only a few minutes to perform. Practitioners should use this check alongside any automatic pre-anaesthetic checking procedures provided on the anaesthetic machine. They should also keep a record of the routine checking of anaesthetic machines following the checklist. Anaesthetic technicians should carry out regular full services on all anaesthetic machines, following the manufacturer's recommendations, and the equipment must have an up-to-date service record (Wicker & Smith 2008). Practitioners should also not assume that a preoperative check can completely protect the user against intraoperative failure of equipment. The following checklist (Figure 11.1) describes the procedure for checking anaesthetic machines.

Basic steps for checking an anaesthetic machine

Step 1 – Perform the manufacturer's automatic machine check.

Step 2 – Make sure the power supply is connected to an uninterrupted power supply and the back-up battery is charged.

Step 3 – Check that gas supplies and suction are working: check flowmeters, hypoxic guard, cylinders and gas pipelines.

Step 4 – Check the breathing system: identify leaks using the 'two-bag' test, check that vaporisers are leak free, soda lime is colour checked (changing from pink to white means it needs to be changed), and alternative breathing systems (e.g. Bains Circuit) are present and working.

Step 5 – Check that ventilator and scavenging systems are working properly and configured appropriately.

Step 6 – Check that monitors are connected and working. Set alarm parameters and volume limits.

Step 7 – Check that all airway equipment is ready for use and working correctly (AAGBI 2012).

The 'two-bag' test involves attaching an airway bag to the end of the circuit and turning on the fresh gas flow (AAGBI 2012). The system can then be checked to ensure that the circuit is intact and the valves are working. Turning on the ventilator will ensure that it is working correctly by observing the bags as they inflate and deflate.

This checklist shows the basic steps required for checking an anaesthetic machine at the start of each day. However, the machine should also be checked prior to the start of every case (AAGBI 2012). This check is of course less complex, but is still essential to ensure that the anaesthetic machine and airway equipment are working correctly and are available. The basic checks between patients should include:

Step 1 – Check breathing system.

Step 2 – Check ventilator.

Step 3 – Check for the full range of airway equipment.

Step 4 – Ensure that suction is clean and working.

There are, of course, many other checks that need to take place. For example, drugs must be available and in date. Similarly, equipment for giving drugs should be available, including syringes, needles, giving sets, alcoholic wipes, Band-Aids® and so on. Difficult intubation equipment should be easily accessible, and of primary concern is that the anaesthetic practitioner is qualified and experienced in the relevant speciality (AAGBI 2012).

The anaesthetic checklist is a method of systematically ensuring that the practitioner carries out a thorough check of the anaesthetic equipment. Anaesthetic assistants should therefore check and sign the anaesthetic checklist, appropriately amended to suit the equipment, as a standard practice for checking the anaesthetic machine to provide the best and safest patient care.

Anatomy and physiology of the respiratory and cardiovascular systems

Figure 12.1 Respiratory anatomy

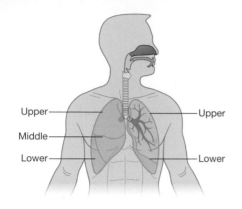

Upper — Upper
Middle
Lower — Lower

Figure 12.2 Gas exchange in the alveoli

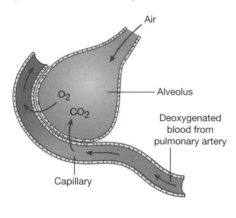

Air
Alveolus
O_2
CO_2
Deoxygenated blood from pulmonary artery
Capillary

Figure 12.3 Cardiovascular anatomy (external)

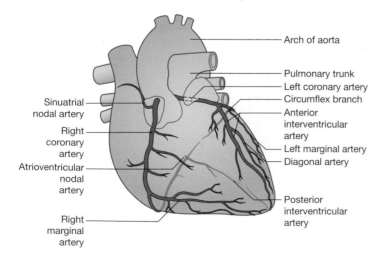

Arch of aorta
Pulmonary trunk
Left coronary artery
Circumflex branch
Anterior interventricular artery
Left marginal artery
Diagonal artery
Posterior interventricular artery
Sinuatrial nodal artery
Right coronary artery
Atrioventricular nodal artery
Right marginal artery

Figure 12.4 Cardiovascular anatomy (internal)

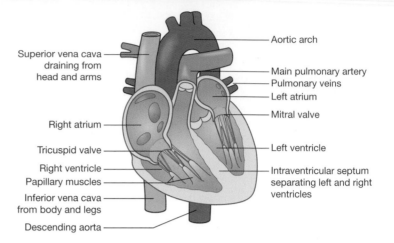

Aortic arch
Main pulmonary artery
Pulmonary veins
Left atrium
Mitral valve
Left ventricle
Intraventricular septum separating left and right ventricles
Superior vena cava draining from head and arms
Right atrium
Tricuspid valve
Right ventricle
Papillary muscles
Inferior vena cava from body and legs
Descending aorta

Figure 12.5 Cardiovascular blood flow

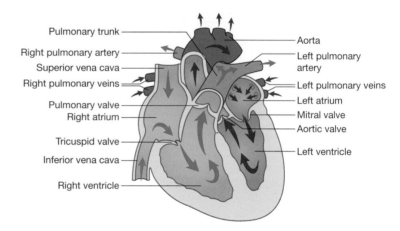

Pulmonary trunk
Right pulmonary artery
Superior vena cava
Right pulmonary veins
Pulmonary valve
Right atrium
Tricuspid valve
Inferior vena cava
Right ventricle
Aorta
Left pulmonary artery
Left pulmonary veins
Left atrium
Mitral valve
Aortic valve
Left ventricle

Figure 12.6 ECG

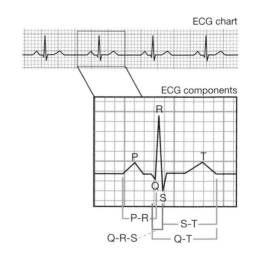

ECG chart
ECG components
R
P
Q
S
T
P-R
Q-R-S
S-T
Q-T

Respiratory system

The chest contains one lung on each side, which is made of soft tissues and is protected by the ribcage. Each lung is made up of sections called lobes. The left lung is composed of an upper and lower lobe and the lingual, which is a small part of the lung resting near to the heart. The right lung is slightly different and is composed of upper, middle and lower lobes (Figure 12.1).

The purpose of the lungs is to bring pxygen (O_2) into the body and to remove carbon dioxide (CO_2). The respiratory system therefore organises the exchange of gases between the body's circulatory system and the outside air. During inhalation, air travels through the nasal cavity, pharynx and larynx, which are the upper airways, into the trachea, primary bronchi and bronchial tree, which are the lower airways, and finally into the lungs, which contain small bronchioles and alveoli. During exhalation, the airflow is reversed (Figure 12.2).

Mechanics of breathing

The chest and diaphragm are used for breathing (Francis 2006). The diaphragm separates the lungs from the organs in the abdominal cavity, such as the intestines, stomach and liver. During inhalation external intercostal muscles contract, moving the ribcage up and out, and the diaphragm moves downwards, the lungs expand and air is drawn in due to negative pressure within the lungs. The lungs expand outwards because they are attached to the thoracic wall by the pleural membranes. During exhalation, the diaphragm relaxes; air leaves the lungs and the lungs and diaphragm move back to their original size and position.

Physiology of gas exchange

As air passes through the airways, it eventually reaches very narrow terminal bronchioles, at the end of which are the alveoli, which are very small and bunched together. Millions of alveoli are present in each lung, providing a huge surface area, and it is here that gaseous exchange occurs (Wicker 2010). A rapid exchange of gases is possible here by passive diffusion as the capillary and alveolar walls are very thin. This occurs because of concentration gradients – for example high levels of O_2 within the alveolus diffuse into the capillary, which has low levels of O_2, and high levels of CO_2 from the capillaries diffuse into the alveolus, which has low levels of CO_2.

Cardiovascular system

The heart is a pump that circulates blood around the body (Figure 12.3). The heart has four chambers – left and right atria, and left and right ventricles (Figure 12.4). The right side of the heart receives low-pressure deoxygenated blood via the veins, and pumps it to the lungs via the pulmonary circulation. The left side of the heart receives oxygenated blood from the lungs and pumps it at high pressure through the body via the systemic circulation (Figure 12.5). Cardiac muscle is a specialised form of muscle called myocardium, which consists of cells connecting with each other through electrical connections. A rise in intracellular calcium concentration leads to spontaneous depolarisation, resulting in contraction of the cell, which produces a wave of depolarisation and contraction across the entire myocardium (Wicker 2010). The sino-atrial node controls the depolarisation and contraction of the heart. This node is located in the right atrium; this group of cells are often called pacemaker cells. Depolarisation of these cells causes an electrical wave to spread across the atria towards the atrioventricular node, which is located in the wall of tissue between the left and right ventricles. The atria then contract simultaneously, pumping blood into each of the ventricles (Figure 12.3). The electrical wave passes through the atria to the atrio-ventricular node and then the bundle of His. The electrical wave travels down the bundle of His and then into the Purkinje fibres, which in turn split into the right and left ventricles and the wave travels across the lower part of the myocardium. This results in a contraction of the ventricles from the bottom to the top, pumping blood up and out into the pulmonary artery (deoxygenated blood from the right side) and aorta (oxygenated blood from the left side). The atria then refill as the myocardium relaxes and the process starts again.

The ECG

Reading the electrocardiogram (ECG) helps anaesthetists and practitioners to assess the condition of the heart and its conducting system. ECG monitors also show changes in rhythm and height of the impulses when there is damage to the myocardium. The PQRS waves demonstrates depolarisation (contraction) of the heart muscles, whereas the T wave demonstrates repolarisation (relaxation) of the heart muscles (Wicker 2010). Figure 12.6 shows a normal lead II ECG. The P wave illustrates atrial depolarisation. The reason the P wave is small is because the atria are smaller and contain less muscle than the ventricles. The Q wave identifies depolarisation around the bundle of His. The R wave represents depolarisation in the base of the ventricles, as it spreads through the base of the heart. This is the largest deflection in the ECG reading because it involves the largest number of muscles in the heart. The S wave represents depolarisation of the ventricles as the electrical current moves from the base of the ventricles upwards towards the atria. Finally, the T wave illustrates repolarisation of the myocardium after systole (the period of contraction of the heart) is complete.

The coronary circulation

As the heart contains muscles, the coronary circulation provides the necessary blood supply to feed the muscles and keep the heart beating. The left and right coronary arteries, which lie in grooves called sulci and run over the surface of the myocardium, provide most of the blood circulation for the heart. These arteries also divide further into several branches, which become arterioles and then capillaries.

13 Anaesthetic drugs

Figure 13.1 Action of inhalational agents

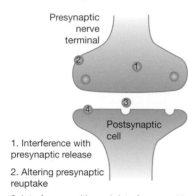

Presynaptic nerve terminal

Postsynaptic cell

1. Interference with presynaptic release

2. Altering presynaptic reuptake

3. Interference with postsynaptic binding

4. Interference with postsynaptic ionic conductance

Inhaled anaesthetics disrupt normal synaptic transmission: they may interfere with the release of neurotransmitters from the presynaptic nerve terminal, alter the reuptake of neurotransmitters, change the binding of neurotransmitters to the post-synaptic receptor sites, or influence the ionic conductance change that follows activation of the postsynaptic receptor by neurotransmitters.

Figure 13.2 Neuromuscular junction

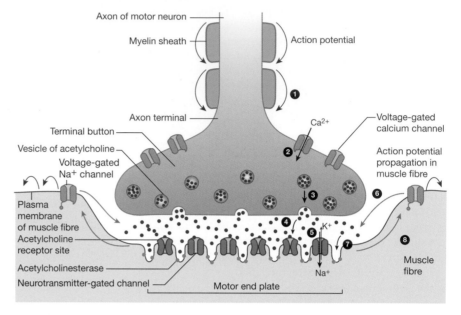

Axon of motor neuron
Myelin sheath
Action potential
Axon terminal
Ca^{2+}
Voltage-gated calcium channel
Action potential propagation in muscle fibre
Terminal button
Vesicle of acetylcholine
Voltage-gated Na^+ channel
Plasma membrane of muscle fibre
Acetylcholine receptor site
Acetylcholinesterase
Neurotransmitter-gated channel
K^+
Na^+
Muscle fibre
Motor end plate

Figure 13.3 Action of muscle relaxants

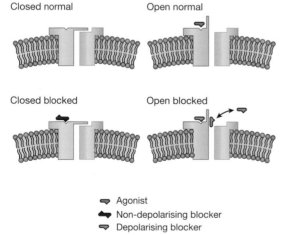

Closed normal

Open normal

Closed blocked

Open blocked

Agonist
Non-depolarising blocker
Depolarising blocker

Figure 13.4 Action of opioids

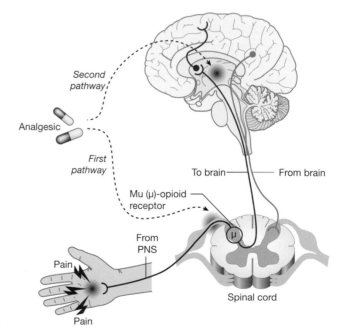

Second pathway
Analgesic
First pathway
To brain
From brain
Mu (μ)-opioid receptor
From PNS
Pain
Pain
Spinal cord

The purpose of using drugs in anaesthesia is to produce loss of consciousness, muscle relaxation and lack of response to pain. Drugs used in anaesthesia can therefore come under the following headings: induction agents, inhalation agents, muscle relaxants and analgesics. There are many more drugs used during anaesthesia, so this chapter will focus on the main drugs that implement and support anaesthesia.

Induction agents

Induction agents are intravenous drugs that are normally used to induce anaesthesia prior to the administration of inhalation agents. They can also be employed as the sole anaesthetic drug by using total intravenous anaesthesia (TIVA; Lupton & Pratt, 2012). **Thiopentone sodium** is a short-acting barbiturate that is still widely used and results in a smooth and rapid induction of anaesthesia. Side effects include cardiovascular and respiratory depression (BNF 2012). **Propofol** is supplied in 1% or 2% aqueous emulsion, containing soya oil, egg phosphatide and glycerol. It is short acting, with its onset usually between 30 and 40 seconds. Recovery from the anaesthetic is usually rapid and patients have less of a hangover effect than with other drugs. Side effects include bradycardia and hypotension due mainly to systemic vasodilation. Propofol is not recommended for neonates (BNF 2012). **Etomodate** causes less hypotension than other drugs and also provides a rapid recovery without hangover effect (BNF 2012).

Inhalation agents

Inhalation agents (Figure 13.1) are either gases or volatile liquids. Volatile liquid agents are administered via calibrated vaporisers attached to anaesthetic machines, using medical air and oxygen, or nitrous-oxide/oxygen mixtures as carrier gases for the agent. To prevent hypoxia, the inspired gas mix should always include at least 25% oxygen (BNF 2012). Gases include oxygen and nitrous oxide. Volatile liquid anaesthetic agents are used for the induction and maintenance of anaesthesia. Minimum alveolar concentration (MAC) measures the potency and strength of anaesthetic vapours. While inhalation agents are effective in producing unconsciousness, they must be used with care as they have potential side effects, including inducing malignant hyperthermia, cerebrospinal pressure increases, hepatotoxicity, cardio-respiratory depression, hypotension and arrhythmias (BNF 2012; Cox & Bhudia 2009). **Sevoflurane** is a rapidly acting volatile liquid anaesthetic. Emergence from the anaesthetic is swift and it is not irritant to the airways, so is useful in inhalational induction of anaesthesia (BNF 2012). **Isoflurane** is also a volatile liquid anaesthetic. The heart rhythm is usually stable during isoflurane anaesthesia; however, it may induce tachycardia, especially in young patients. Systemic arterial pressure may also fall and cardiac output can decrease, due to a decrease in systemic vascular resistance. Side effects include irritation of the mucus membranes, causing coughing, breath holding and laryngospasm (BNF 2012). **Desflurane** is a rapidly acting volatile agent that has around one fifth the potency of isoflurane (BNF 2010). Emergence and recovery from the anaesthetic are particularly rapid due to its low solubility. Unlike other volatile agents, the vaporiser for desflurane requires an electrically heated pressurised vaporiser. The vapour pressure of desflurane is three to four times that of others and it boils at 22.8 °C, which is close to room temperature (Andrews & Johnston 1993). Nitrous oxide is used for maintenance of anaesthesia and in subanaesthetic quantities for analgesia. During anaesthesia, nitrous oxide is used 50–66% with oxygen as part of a balanced technique, in association with other inhalation or intravenous agents. Hypoxia can occur immediately following the use of nitrous oxide and additional oxygen should be administered for several minutes after stopping the flow of nitrous oxide (BNF 2012).

Muscle relaxants

Muscle relaxants (Figures 13.2 and 13.3) are neuromuscular blocking agents that produce relaxation of the muscles of the body. This facilitates the passage of an endotracheal tube to allow adequate control of respiration and securing of the patient's airway, as well as relaxing muscles during surgery. There are two types of neuromuscular blocking drugs: depolarising muscle relaxants and non-depolarising muscle relaxants (BNF 2012; Simpson & Popat 2002). Depolarising muscle relaxants include **suxamethonium**, which has a rapid onset and brief duration of action, making it ideal for rapid-sequence tracheal intubation. Suxamethonium is normally administered after the anaesthetic induction, as paralysis is preceded by painful muscle fasciculation (BNF 2012). Non-depolarising muscle relaxants include **atracurium**, **mivacurium**, **rocuronium** and **vecuronium**. These work differently and compete with acetylcholine at the receptor sites in the neuromuscular junctions. When they are locked in place, they prevent the contraction of muscles by inhibiting depolarisation of the neuromuscular junction. This action may be reversed with anticholinesterase drugs (BNF 2012). **Atracurium** is a neuromuscular blocking agent with an intermediate duration of action of 30–40 minutes and an onset time of around 2.5 minutes. Potential side effects are bradycardia and histamine release (BNF 2012). **Mivacurium** has a short duration of action of around 15–30 minutes and onset of action is around 2.5 mins. It is metabolised by plasma cholinesterase, so muscle paralysis can be prolonged in patients deficient in this enzyme. It tends not to release histamine, although this does occur sometimes (BNF 2012). **Rocuronium** is a rapid-onset muscle relaxant that works within 2 minutes. It is also reported to have minimal cardiovascular effects (BNF 2012). Sugammadex is used to reverse its actions. **Vecuronium** has an onset of action of around 2 minutes and lasts for around 25–40 minutes, although this is dose dependent. It does not generally produce histamine release and lacks cardiovascular effects (BNF 2012).

Analgesics

A variety of analgesics are used in anaesthesia, the majority of which are opioids (Figure 13.4). **Alfentanil** and **Fentanyl** are opioid analgesics that are administered at the induction of anaesthesia and are particularly used during short procedures (BNF 2012). **Remifentanil** is an opioid analgesia that can supplement anaesthesia during induction. It should not be administered by intravenous injection intraoperatively; however, it is well suited to continuous infusion. **Morphine**, **pethidine** and **diamorphine** are other opioid drugs often used during anaesthesia and postoperatively.

14 Perioperative fluid management

Figure 14.1 Compartmental distribution of total body water in a 70 kg male

Total body water = approximately 42 litres

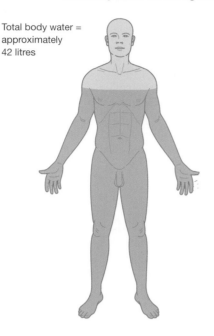

Figure 14.2 Osmosis

Osmosis is the movement of fluid across a membrane into an area where there is a high concentration of solutes. Osmotic pressure is pressure that is applied to the chamber with the highest ratio of solutes, in order to prevent fluid moving from the chamber with the lowest level of solutes to the chamber with the highest number of solutes.

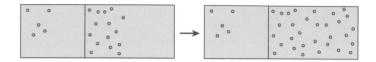

Figure 14.3 Crystalloids

Samples of crystalloid solutions

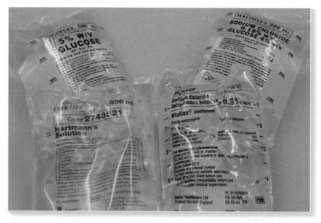

Figure 14.4 Colloids

Samples of colloid solutions

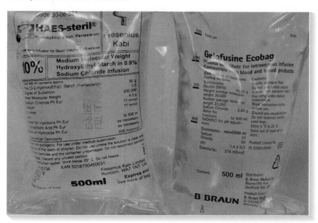

Figure 14.5 Intravenous cannula inserted in hand ready for anaesthetic drugs or intravenous fluids

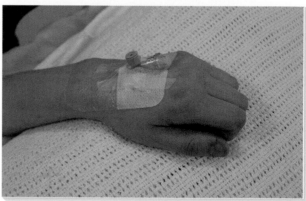

Source: All photos from Aintree University Hospital, Liverpool.

Perioperative Practice at a Glance, First Edition. Paul Wicker. © 2015 John Wiley & Sons, Ltd. Published 2015 by John Wiley & Sons, Ltd.

Intraoperative fluid management includes supplying the patient with the basic fluid requirements throughout the period of surgery, replacing preoperative fluid deficits caused by fasting, and replacing intraoperative fluid losses caused by blood loss, fluid redistribution and evaporation (Figure 14.5). Selection of appropriate fluids depends on the surgical procedure and the expected blood loss. Normally 0.9% sodium chloride and/or 5% dextrose are used when the patient undergoes minimal fluid loss; however, Hartmann's solution (compound sodium lactate) may be used when fluid losses are high.

Maintaining normal intravascular volume is important to achieve the best perioperative outcomes. The main goal of perioperative fluid management is therefore to create a balance between providing too little fluid and fluid overload. If fluids are restricted, then hypotension, increased postoperative nausea, inadequate organ perfusion and impaired tissue oxygenation can occur (Clancy et al. 2002). On the other hand, infusing the patient with too much fluid can lead to interstitial oedema, poor wound healing, delayed gastric emptying, prolonged resumption of bowel function and heart failure (Bamboat & Bordeianou 2009).

Intraoperative patients have no control over their water balance and therefore it is essential that anaesthetists, and practitioners, are aware of the need to control water balance appropriately. Intravascular volume needs to be assessed accurately throughout the patient's surgery, and fluids or electrolyte deficits needs to be replaced as required. Failure to maintain appropriate fluid levels may result in severe problems or even death. The main objectives of fluid management are therefore to maintain good tissue perfusion, ensure adequate oxygen delivery, maintain normal electrolyte concentration and maintain normoglycaemia and pH of the blood (Clancy et al. 2002). The overall goal is thus to maintain the effective circulatory volume while avoiding interstitial fluid overload whenever possible (Wicker 2010).

A human body weighing around 70 kg contains approximately 42 litres of fluid: 28 litres are intracellular fluid (ICF), 11 litres are extracellular fluid (ECF) and 3 litres are plasma (Figure 14.1). Fluid passes between intracellular (ICC) and extracellular (ECC) compartments by osmosis (Figure 14.2). Solutes, such as NA^+, K^+ and HcO_3^-, tend to stay within each of the compartments, and ICC tend to contain a greater quantity of solutes than ECC (English et al. 2013).

Perioperative fluid management is managed by providing crystalloid solutions to support interstitial fluid volume (within cells) and colloids to provide intravascular volume (plasma and red blood cells; Wicker 2010). When sodium chloride (normal saline) is given, the sodium is prevented from gaining access to the ICF by the sodium pumps in the cells. As this results in maintaining isotonic solutions, water is not exchanged between ICF and ECF. However, if water only is infused, usually in the form of dextrose 5%, then it enters both the ICF and the ECF, expanding the total body water (TBW).

Crystalloids (e.g. compound sodium lactate and normal saline; Figure 14.3) are true solutions that contain no particulates, and they expand intravenous circulation (IVC) adequately and generate a small increase in plasma volume. Crystalloids do leave the IVC faster than colloids, reducing by about 50% in around 30 minutes. Crystalloids, however, are just as effective as colloids in restoring intravascular volume if they are given in sufficient quantities; that is, around three or four times the volume needed when using colloids (Clancy et al. 2002).

Effects of crystalloids
Hartmann's solution
This is an isotonic solution that has little effect on ICF, although its effects increase depending on the volume of solution infused. The lactate is converted by the body into bicarbonate and it also tends to lower serum Na^+.

Normal saline (NS)
This solution is normally at a concentration of 0.9%. Large volumes of NS can produce hyperchloremic acidosis due to the high sodium and chlorine content (approximately 154 mEq/L). Plasma bicarbonate decreases as chloride concentration increases. Its preferred use is when the patient is undergoing hypochloremic metabolic acidosis. Hyperchloremia can result in renal vasoconstriction, decrease in glomerular filtration rate, suppression of renin activity and lowered blood pressure (Quilley et al. 1993).

5% dextrose
Normally the glucose is metabolised in the body, leaving pure water. This solution helps to maintain fluids in patients on sodium restriction.

Hypertonic saline (2%, 3% and 7.5%)
Small volumes are normally used for reducing intracranial pressure. This solution increases plasma volume by extracting fluid (via osmosis) from the interstitial fluid volume (IFV) and ICF (Clancy et al. 2002).

Effects of colloids
Colloids (Figure 14.4) contain particles suspended in fluid, rather than being a solution that does not contain particles. Examples of colloids include blood-derived albumins, dextrans, gelatins and starches (English et al. 2013). Colloids normally have a high molecular weight and are therefore unable to pass through semi-permeable membranes, so they remain confined in the intravascular compartments. Colloids also are not able to correct water and electrolyte deficiencies (Clancy et al. 2002). Colloids, often Gelofusine, are therefore the most obvious choice to expand intravascular fluids, since most of the colloids stay in the IVC for up to six hours. Less than 1–1.5 litres per day of colloids is therefore normally required, and initial resuscitation is rapid.

Blood and blood byproducts
Blood and blood byproducts are also used to replace a loss of fluids in the body. During surgery, loss of blood can be a major issue. These blood products include whole blood, packed red blood cells, leukocyte-depleted blood, fresh frozen plasma, platelets and other products (Clancy et al. 2002). Normally, crystalloid or colloid solutions replace minimal blood loss, as long as there is a low risk of anaemia, which is less than 7–8 gm/dl of haemoglobin. If haemoglobin drops below 7 gm/dl, or blood loss is greater than approximately 15% of blood volume, then transfusion of blood or packed red blood cells is required. The average blood volume in adults is 75 ml/kg in males and 65 ml/kg in females.

15 Monitoring the patient

Figure 15.1 CARESCAPE Monitor B850

The CARESCAPE Monitor B850 can be used for patients both preoperatively and postoperatively. The monitor is a high-acuity monitor that can help practitioners manage their patients by providing a dependable level of data continuity and integration across care areas

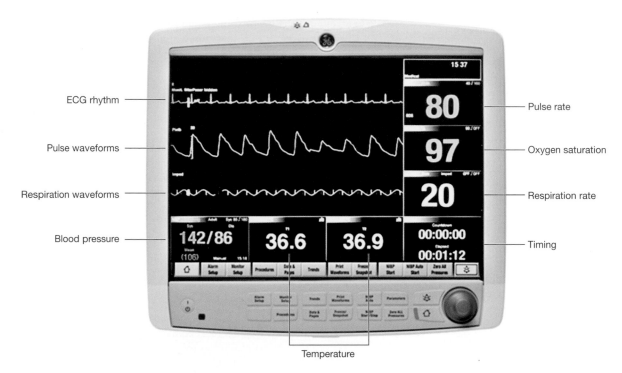

ECG rhythm

Pulse waveforms

Respiration waveforms

Blood pressure

Pulse rate

Oxygen saturation

Respiration rate

Timing

Temperature

Source: GE Healthcare. Reproduced with permission of GE Healthcare.

The CARESCAPE Monitor B850® system
(http://www3.gehealthcare.com/en/Products/Categories/Patient_Monitoring/Patient_Monitors/CARESCAPE_Monitor_B850)
is indicated for monitoring the status of:
• Haemodynamics, including ECG, ST segment, arrhythmia detection, ECG diagnostic analysis and measurement, invasive pressure, non-invasive blood pressure, pulse oximetry, cardiac output, temperature, impedance respiration and SvO2 (mixed venous oxygen saturation)
• Airway gases: Fi/Et CO_2, O_2, N_2O and anaesthetic agent
• Spirometry
• Gas exchange: O_2 consumption (VO_2), CO_2 production (VCO_2), energy expenditure (EE) and respiratory quotient (RQ)
• Neurophysiological function, including electroencephalography (EEG), entropy, bispectral index (BIS) and neuromuscular transmission (NMT) monitoring

Perioperative Practice at a Glance, First Edition. Paul Wicker. © 2015 John Wiley & Sons, Ltd. Published 2015 by John Wiley & Sons, Ltd.

onitoring of patients may not prevent all perioperative adverse incidents, but it does reduce the risks by detecting the consequences of errors, and by giving early warning that the condition of a patient is deteriorating (AAGBI 2007). Monitoring the patient is therefore one of the most important tasks during anaesthesia in order to assess the patient's physiological status during surgery and anaesthesia. Monitoring must also be used alongside careful clinical observation by the anaesthetist and the practitioner, as there may be occasions when the equipment does not detect unfavourable clinical developments (Australian and New Zealand College of Anaesthetists 2013). The anaesthesia team is responsible for recording the results on the patient's notes and in the care plan. This provides a record of the patient's status during surgery, which may be useful during and after the procedure. Monitors are therefore employed to provide continuous assessment of the patient's physiological status and the depth of anaesthesia (Figure 15.1; O'Neill 2010).

Some of the monitors used include electrocardiogram, pulse oximeters, nasopharynx temperature probe, vapour analyser, capnography and non-invasive blood pressure monitor (AAGBI 2007). When clinically indicated, several other devices are also used and need to be understood in order to ensure that they are fitted correctly and provide appropriate results, for example electroencephalogram, central venous pressure, transoesophageal echocardiogram, cardiac output monitor, neuromuscular function monitor and respiratory monitor.

Electrocardiogram (ECG)

The ECG monitor measures and records the electrical activity of the heart, which indicates normal or abnormal cardiac rhythms, providing the anaesthetic team with early warnings of cardiac problems. Normal sinus rhythm is initiated by the sinus node, which contracts the right and left atrial muscles followed by the ventricles. Contraction of cardiac muscles is called systole (O'Neill 2010). The atria and ventricles contract at different times, leading to a sequence of blood leaving the atria to enter the ventricles, followed by blood leaving the ventricles to enter the pulmonary artery and the aorta. This sequence is recorded on the ECG as a PQRST wave. Normal sinus rhythm in adults is around 60–80 beats per minute, although babies and children may have heart rates as high as between 100 and 150 beats per minute (AAGBI 2007). Abnormal cardiac rhythms include tachycardia, supraventricular tachycardia, atrial flutter, sinus bradycardia, atrioventricular block, atrial fibrillation and asytole.

Pulse oximeters

A pulse oximeter measures the saturation of oxygen in the patient's blood. Normal oxygen saturation is between 94% and 100%; anything less than 94% is seen as causing problems for the patient. The pulse oximeter is normally attached to a finger, earlobe or toe. The light source in the probe passes through the tissue and the patient's oxygen concentration is measured via the absorption of the light, and then recorded on the monitoring screen (O'Neill 2010). The light is detected by light sensors and is altered by the levels of oxyhaemoglobin and deoxyhaemoglobin. The pulse oximeter should be regularly checked to ensure that it is correctly placed on the extremity and also that circulation at that point is not impaired.

Temperature probes

The patient's temperature must be recorded prior to anaesthesia, because having a temperature of less than 36 °C puts the patient at risk of hypothermia, and therefore the surgery and anaesthesia should not commence. For example, the patient's body temperature can fall one or two degrees because of the lack of shivering and peripheral vasodilation while under anaesthesia (O'Neill 2010). The patient's temperature is normally monitored every 30 minutes throughout surgery to ensure that it is kept within normal limits, especially during long procedures and when warming devices are being used. Heat production is also reduced during anaesthesia as anaesthetic agents reduce metabolic rate, relax muscles and prevent behavioural responses to heat loss. The patient's temperature can furthermore be altered by exposure of internal organs, such as abdominal contents, and the use of cold saline solutions or washouts.

Vapour analyser

Vapour analysers are monitored by anaesthetists during anaesthesia. The purpose of such a device is to monitor the concentration of volatile anaesthetics in the gas flow using MAC values. The monitor can record the vapourising agent and the percentage of volatile anaesthetic in the gas on the monitor. Vapour analysers are invaluable for assessing the correct concentration of an inhalation agent. However, they do not always detect all possible contaminants (Strachan & Richmond 1997).

Capnography

A capnograph measures and records end tidal CO_2, which is a direct measurement of the ventilation of the lungs. Correct or appropriate levels of CO_2 help to confirm that the endotracheal tube is placed correctly and that the patient is receiving the appropriate level of oxygen (O'Neill 2010). The CO_2 sampling tube connects to the far end of the breathing circuit, thereby detecting the CO_2 expired by the patient. The other end of the sampling tube connects to the monitor. The levels of carbon dioxide are recorded on the monitor as waveforms. The rise or fall of CO_2 levels recorded by the capnograph alerts the anaesthetic team to issues such as faults in the breathing circuit or ventilation system ($\downarrow CO_2$), hypotension ($\downarrow CO_2$), malignant hypothermia ($\uparrow CO_2$) and reinhalation of gases by the patient during ventilation ($\uparrow CO_2$; AAGBI 2007).

Non-invasive blood pressure (NIBP) measurement

NIBP is measured using a blood pressure cuff, which is fastened around the arm or leg. The air tube is then attached to the monitor, which inflates and deflates the cuff according to time settings. The blood pressure reading is displayed on the monitor and consistently registers systolic, mean and diastolic pressures. Invasive blood pressure monitoring equipment is also used to provide a continuous record of blood pressure. This normally works by connecting a monitor to a transducer, which in turn is connected to an intra-arterial line.

16 General anaesthesia

Figure 16.1 Anaesthetic drugs cupboard in anaesthetic room

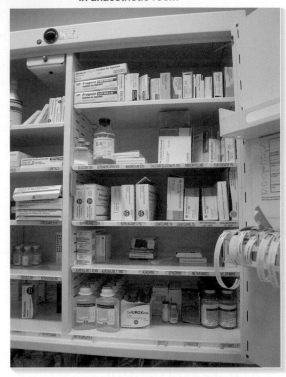

Figure 16.2 Anaesthetic drugs prepared for anaesthetic, including Propofol, muscle relaxants and analgesics

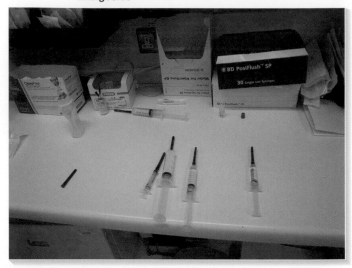

Figure 16.3 Patient anaesthetised in the anaesthetic room

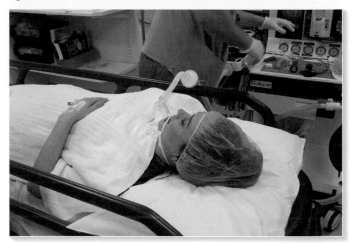

Source: All photos from Aintree University Hospital, Liverpool.

Perioperative Practice at a Glance, First Edition. Paul Wicker. © 2015 John Wiley & Sons, Ltd. Published 2015 by John Wiley & Sons, Ltd.

General anaesthetics (GA) are drugs that produce reversible loss of all sensations and consciousness and depress the central nervous system (CNS) to a sufficient degree to permit surgery to occur (Figure 16.1). The 'triad of anaesthesia' highlights the need for unconsciousness, analgesia and muscle relaxation.

Signs and stages of anaesthesia (Guedel's signs)

GA cause a descending depression of the CNS: the higher functions are lost first and progressively lower areas of the brain are involved. The vital centres located in the medulla are paralysed as the depth of anaesthesia increases. In 1920, Guedel (Larson 2008) described four stages of anaesthesia, which, although updated, are still applicable today (Hughes & Mardell 2012). The first stage is **analgesia**, which starts from the beginning of anaesthetic inhalation and lasts up to loss of consciousness. Pain is progressively abolished during this stage. The second stage is **excitement**, when the patient may experience delirium, become restless and their heart rate and BP may rise, which is unlikely to occur in modern anaesthesia. The third stage is **surgical anaesthesia**, when the patient becomes unconscious, breathing is regular and the skeletal muscles relax, allowing surgery to start (Figure 16.2). The fourth stage is **medullary paralysis**, which results in cessation of breathing, failure of circulation and possibly death. This stage should never be reached in general anaesthesia.

Induction, maintenance and extubation

Patients may be premedicated on the ward before anaesthesia using drugs such as opiates or sedatives, to allay anxiety and apprehension prior to anaesthesia. Anti-anxiety drugs also include benzodiazepines like diazepam, midazolam or lorazepam, which are popular because they produce tranquillity and smooth induction, with little respiratory depression or postoperative vomiting (Goodman & Spry 2014).

Following preparation of the patient in the anaesthetic room, the patient is induced with an intravenous induction agent after adequate preoxygenation (Figure 16.3). Intravenous anaesthetic induction agents are drugs that are used for induction of anaesthesia and on injection produce rapid loss of consciousness. Thiopentone sodium and propofol are frequently used and have a rapid onset and short duration of action. Muscle relaxants, such as suxamethonium or rocuronium, are given to facilitate laryngoscopy and intubation. Anticholinergics such as atropine or hyoscine may also be administered, primarily to reduce salivary and bronchial secretions, although their main use now is to prevent vagal bradycardia, hypotension and laryngospasm, which is precipitated by respiratory secretions (Goodman & Spry 2014).

Anaesthesia is then usually maintained by an inhalational agent, analgesics and non-depolarising muscle relaxants such as atracurium or pancuronium. Inhalational agents refer to the delivery of gases or vapours (including O_2) to the respiratory system to produce anaesthesia (Hughes & Mardell 2012). Nitrous oxide (N_2O) is a weak anaesthetic but a powerful analgesic, and therefore needs other agents for appropriate surgical anaesthesia. Isoflurane depresses the respiratory drive and ventilatory responses, and is an excellent muscle relaxant that potentiates the effects of neuromuscular blockers. Sevoflurane and desflurane produce rapid induction and emergence from anaesthesia with minimal systemic effects, including mild respiratory and cardiac suppression.

Anaesthesia is maintained with an N_2O and O_2 mixture along with an inhalational anaesthetic agent and other anaesthetic drugs. Neostigmine is used to reverse muscle paralysis during extubation.

Administration of anaesthetic agents

Different techniques are used according to the facilities available, agents used, condition of the patient, and type and duration of operation. Using an anaesthetic machine, the gases are delivered to the patient through a tightly fitting face mask or endotracheal tube. Respiration can be controlled and assisted by the anaesthetist. Using an open system, the exhaled gases are allowed to escape through a valve and fresh anaesthetic mixture at a high flow rate is drawn in each time the patient breathes (Goodman & Spry 2014). Using a closed system, the patient rebreathes the exhaled gas mixture after it has circulated through soda lime, which absorbs CO_2. The flow rates are low, which is useful for expensive agents such as desflurane; however, determination of inhaled anaesthetic concentration is difficult. An alternative is to use a semi-closed system where partial rebreathing is allowed through a partially closed valve (Goodman & Spry 2014).

Total intravenous anaesthesia (TIVA)

Total intravenous anaesthesia is a technique of general anaesthesia that uses a combination of agents given intravenously in the absence of all inhalational agents, including nitrous oxide. Propofol was introduced into clinical practice in 1986 and has become widely used as a component of TIVA. TIVA has grown in popularity in recent times because the pharmacokinetic and pharmacodynamic properties of modern drugs such as propofol and the newer synthetic, short-acting opioids make them very suitable for administration by continuous infusion (Hughes & Mardell 2012). Furthermore, the development of enhanced delivery systems that can control TIVA are as straightforward and user friendly as conventional inhalational techniques. The result is an easy-to-use modern system of providing anaesthesia, which allows rapid, precise and independent control of amnesia, hypnosis and analgesia (EBME 2013)

Complications of general anaesthesia

During anaesthesia complications can include respiratory depression and hypercarbia, salivation, respiratory secretions, cardiac arrhythmias and asystole, fall in BP, aspiration of gastric contents leading to acid pneumonitis, laryngospasm and asphyxia, delirium and convulsions. After anaesthesia, patients can suffer from nausea and vomiting, persistent sedation and impaired psychomotor function, pneumonia, atelectasis, organ toxicities including liver and kidney damage, nerve palsies due to faulty positioning, and emergence delirium. Postoperative nausea and vomiting can be prevented by using anti-emetics such as metoclopramide, ondansetron and granisetron. By enhancing gastric emptying, they reduce the chances of reflux and its aspiration. Combined use of metoclopramide and H2 blockers (which block the histamine H2 receptors in the stomach, decreasing the production of acid by these cells) is more effective.

17 Local anaesthesia

Figure 17.1   Local anaesthetic being injected prior to insertion of an intravenous cannula

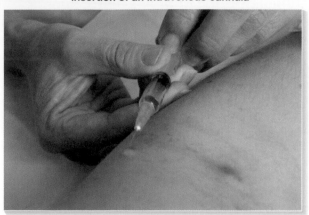

Figure 17.2   Local anaesthetic injected into a knee

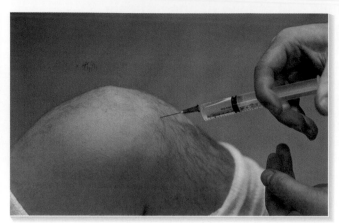

Figure 17.3   EMLA

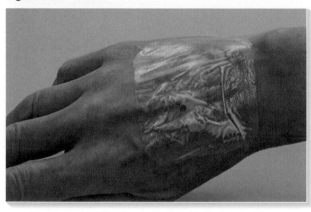

EMLA is an acronym for eutectic mixture of local anaesthetics. It contains lignocaine 2.5% and prilocaine 2.5% in a cream. It takes 40 minutes to work effectively. An occlusive dressing is placed on top to prevent loss or removal of the EMLA cream

Source: All photos from Aintree University Hospital, Liverpool.

A local anaesthetic (LA) is a drug that causes reversible local anaesthesia and a loss of nociception. When it is used on specific nerve pathways (as a nerve block), effects such as analgesia (loss of pain sensation) and paralysis (loss of muscle power) can be achieved.

Local anaesthetic drugs temporarily block impulse conduction along nerve axons. They act by blockading sodium channels so that the threshold for excitation increases, impulse conduction slows down, the rate of rise of the action potential declines, and the ability to generate an action potential is abolished or cancelled. When the influx of sodium is interrupted, an action potential cannot arise and signal conduction is inhibited. Local anaesthetics block conduction in the following order: small myelinated axons (e.g. those carrying nociceptive impulses), non-myelinated axons and then large myelinated axons. Thus, a differential block can be achieved, in other words pain sensation is blocked more readily than other sensory modalities. On occasion, patients may suffer from local anaesthetic toxicity.

Clinical use of local anaesthetics

There are three modes of LA administration: surface, infiltration and nerve blockade (O'Neill 2010). Surface anaesthesia is when there is direct application of the drug on the surface, such as skin and wounds (Figure 17.1). Infiltration anaesthesia occurs when LA is injected into subcutaneous tissue in order to paralyse nerve endings during minor surgical and dental procedures. A nerve block occurs when LA is injected in the vicinity of major nerves, and is used for surgical, dental and diagnostic procedures and for pain management (Hopley & Van Schalkwyk 2006).

Local anaesthetics belong to one of two classes: aminoamides and aminoesters. Synthetic local anaesthetics are structurally related to cocaine, but they differ from cocaine mainly in that they do not produce hypertension or local vasoconstriction, with the exception of ropivacaine and mepivacaine, which do produce low level vasoconstriction. Aminoesters include agents such as benzocaine, chloroprocaine, dimethocaine, novocaine and amethocaine. Aminoamides include bupivacaine, dibucaine, levobupivacaine, lidocaine, mepivacaine, prilocaine and ropivacaine. Lidocaine is one of the most popular drugs, as it is one of the fastest-acting local anaesthetics listed above (Hopley & Van Schalkwyk 2006).

Local anaesthetics provide a reversible regional loss of sensation leading to the reduction of pain, thereby facilitating surgical procedures. Delivery techniques include topical anaesthesia, infiltrative anaesthesia, ring blocks and peripheral nerve blocks. Local anaesthetics are easy to administer and are safer than general or systemic anaesthetics, therefore they are used whenever applicable (O'Neill 2010).

Topical anaesthetics

Administration of topical anaesthetics to control pain associated with procedures such as laceration repair may avoid the need for local anaesthesia injections and associated pain from the injections. Many dosage forms exist, such as gels, sprays, creams, ointments and patches, which provide the clinician with choices for application under various circumstances. Topical anaesthetics are used for various skin and mucous membrane conditions, for example pruritus and pain due to minor burns, skin eruptions (e.g. varicella, sunburn, poison ivy, insect bites) and local analgesia on intact skin (Coventry 2007). With the exception of lignocaine–prilocaine in combination (EMLA; Figure 17.3), topical anaesthetics are poorly absorbed through intact skin. EMLA has also been applied to children to minimise discomfort prior to injections or starting an intravenous line (Gavin 2008). EMLA should be removed after it has been used to prevent skin damage or irritation.

Infiltrative local anaesthetics

Patient comfort is essential during the administration of local anaesthetic agents. Infiltration anaesthesia is accomplished by administering the local anaesthetic solution intradermally, subcutaneously, or submucosally across the nerve pathway that supplies the area of the body that requires anaesthesia. A common administrative technique is to inject the local anaesthetic subcutaneously in a circular pattern around the operative site, which is often referred to as a 'field block' technique (O'Neill 2010). When injected, local anaesthetics reversibly block nerve conduction near their site of administration, thereby producing temporary loss of sensation in a limited area. Lower concentrations of local anaesthetics are typically used for infiltration anaesthesia (Hopley & Van Schalkwyk 2006). Reduced dosage is required for patients who are debilitated or acutely ill, who are either very young or very old, and in patients with liver disease, arteriosclerosis or occlusive arterial disease (Gavin 2008). A common use for injected anaesthetics includes subcutaneous infiltration for IV placement, superficial biopsies or suturing; submucosal infiltration for dental procedures or laceration repairs; wound infiltration for postoperative pain control at an incision site; intra-articular injections (Figure 17.2) for orthopaedic postsurgical pain control or arthritic joint pain control; and infiltrative nerve blocks to reduce pain in ankles, the scalp or digits (Coventry 2007).

Adverse effects are usually caused by high plasma concentrations of a local anaesthetic drug that result from inadvertent intravascular injection, excessive dose or rate of injection, delayed drug clearance or administration into vascular tissue. Possible adverse effects caused by high plasma concentration may include seizures as a result of CNS stimulation or respiratory arrest caused by CNS depression; bradycardia, arrhythmias, hypotension, cardiovascular collapse and cardiac arrest caused by heart depression, or hypertension, tachycardia and angina caused by local anaesthetics that contain epinephrine; other adverse effects can include transient burning sensation, skin discoloration, swelling, neuritis, tissue necrosis and sloughing (Gavin 2008; O'Neill 2010). Allergic reaction to local anaesthetics is rare and accounts for less than 1% of all reactions to local anaesthetics. Allergic reactions may be attributed to other factors such as acute toxicity (e.g. inadvertent intravascular injection that causes high plasma levels), psychomotor reactions (e.g. patient is anxious or apprehensive), pharmacological properties of local anaesthetics, concurrent drug therapy (e.g. tachycardia caused by epinephrine) or preservatives such as paraben or sulfites, which may be present in multidose vials.

18 Regional anaesthesia

Figure 18.1 Vertebral column anatomy

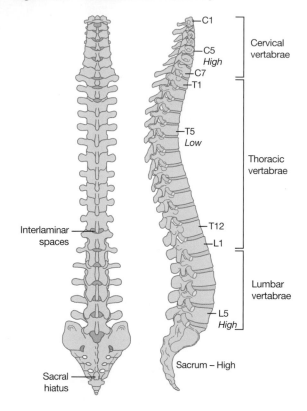

C1

C5
High

C7

T1

T5
Low

T12

L1

L5
High

Cervical
vertabrae

Thoracic
vertabrae

Lumbar
vertabrae

Sacrum – High

Interlaminar
spaces

Sacral
hiatus

Figure 18.2 Vertebral column anatomy detail

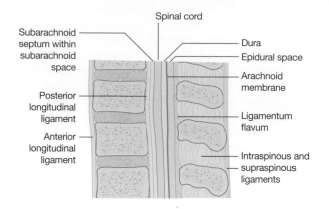

Spinal cord

Subarachnoid
septum within
subarachnoid
space

Posterior
longitudinal
ligament

Anterior
longitudinal
ligament

Dura

Epidural space

Arachnoid
membrane

Ligamentum
flavum

Intraspinous and
supraspinous
ligaments

Figure 18.4 Epidural injection

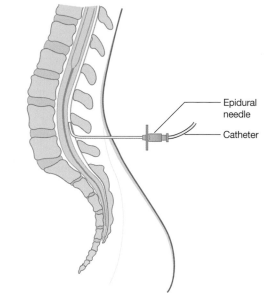

Epidural
needle

Catheter

Figure 18.3 Caudal epidural block

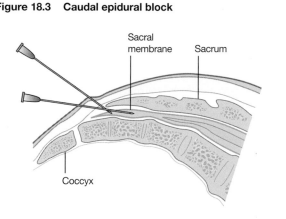

Sacral
membrane

Sacrum

Coccyx

Perioperative Practice at a Glance, First Edition. Paul Wicker. © 2015 John Wiley & Sons, Ltd. Published 2015 by John Wiley & Sons, Ltd.

Regional anaesthesia is used on large parts of the body, such as the back, arm, leg or the lower half of the body. This differs from local anaesthesia, which is used on small parts of the body such as a tooth or an area of skin. Regional anaesthetic techniques can be used centrally or peripherally. The central techniques can include epidural and spinal anaesthesia. The peripheral techniques can include brachial plexus blocks and nerve blocks, for example at the ankle or axilla (Burkard *et al.* 2005). Regional anaesthesia may be performed as a single injection, normally lidocaine or bupivacaine, via a syringe or as a continuous infusion via a catheter, through which medication is given over a prolonged period providing a continuous peripheral nerve block. Regional anaesthesia can also be induced by injecting local anaesthetics directly into the veins of a limb, following the occlusion of the circulation by using a tourniquet. This is called an intravenous regional technique (for example a Bier's block). The three areas covered in this chapter include epidural, spinal and intravenous regional techniques.

Anatomy of the spine

The spine has 33 vertebrae in total, including 7 cervical, 12 thoracic, 5 lumbar, 5 sacral and 4 coccygeal vertebrae, with the high points between C5 and L5 and the low points between T5 and S2. The spinal cord starts at the foramen magnum and ends at L1. The cauda equina are a nerve group at the lower dural sac. The sagittal sections are composed of the outermost layer, being the supraspinous ligament, the middle layer being the intraspinous ligament and the innermost layer being the ligamentum flavum. Between each of the spinous processes are the supraspinous and intraspinous ligaments. From the inside outwards, the spinal cord is covered by the pia mater, the subarachnoid space, the arachnoid mater and then the dura mater, external to which is the epidural space, which is surrounded by the ligamentum flavum.

Effects of local anaesthetics

The factors affecting the distribution of the anaesthetics in the spine include the site of injection, the patient's anatomy, the volume of the cerebrospinal fluid (CSF), characteristics of the local anaesthetic and the dose and volume used. The uptake of the local anaesthetic occurs by diffusion and the elimination of the anaesthetic determines the duration of the block, for example vasoconstriction can decrease the rate of elimination and make the block last longer (Hadzic 2007). Cardiovascular effects can become apparent if sympathetic preganglionic neurones are blocked, leading to a reduction in venous return, stroke volume, cardiac output and blood pressure. These effects can be reduced by increasing cardiac preload by infusing a minimum of 1 litre of a crystalloid solution, or by giving ephedrine to reduce hypotension. High spinal anaesthesia can lead to paralysis of abdominal and intercostal muscles leading to coughing and limited clearing of airway secretions, as well as apnoea caused by hypoperfusion of the respiratory centre (Hadzic 2007).

Spinal technique

In preparation for spinal anaesthesia (Figures 18.1 and 18.2), the patient should be monitored using an ECG, non-invasive blood pressure and pulse oximeter. Patients are normally positioned in a lateral or sitting position; however, they can also be prone (Burkard *et al.* 2005). Spinal needles are used to deliver anaesthetic drugs. They usually have a sharp and pointed cutting edge and a hollow throughout the length of the needle, sometimes with a hole along the side of the needle (O'Neill 2010). Using the midline approach, the needle progressively penetrates the skin, subcutaneous tissue, supraspinous ligament, interspinous ligament, ligamentum flavum, epidural space, dura mater and finally the arachnoid mater and into the subarachnoid space. The local anaesthetic spreads to the cauda equina and nerve roots, and may defuse to the spinal cord. Contraindications for spinal surgery include issues such as infection, coagulopathy, hypovolaemia or increased intracranial pressure (Hadzic 2007). Complications can include back pain, headache and failed block.

Epidural technique

Epidural anaesthesia (Figures 18.3 and 18.4) is commonly used because of its versatility, and can be used at any part of the spine from the neck downwards. It is most often used for surgery on the lower limbs, perineum, abdomen, thorax and pelvis (Burkard *et al.* 2005). The most common point of injection for an epidural anaesthetic is the midline of the lumbar vertebrae for surgery on lower limbs, or the thoracic region for surgery on the abdomen. The needle is inserted as far as the epidural space, and an epidural catheter is then inserted and the needle removed (Wedel & Horlocker 2005). The epidural space lies between the vertebral ligaments and the dura mater and contains fatty areolar tissue. The anaesthetic agent spreads through the areolar tissue towards the nerve roots and spinal cord. The extent of the sensory blockade can be assessed by a 'pin prick' using a needle, cold ether spray or ice. Complications of epidural anaesthetics include penetration of a blood vessel, hypotension, headache, back pain and infection (Hadzic 2007).

Intravenous regional techniques

Bier's block is one of the most common uses of intravenous regional techniques. Usually the Bier's block is used for open surgery or closed reductions of the hand or lower arm (O'Neill 2010). Because of the possible complications caused by the tourniquet, time is limited to a maximum of 90 minutes. This procedure should not be used for crush injuries or in small children. An intravenous catheter is inserted in the limb as distally as possible. A double tourniquet is then placed on the limb, the limb is exsanguinated and the proximal cuff is then inflated. Lignocaine or prilocaine is injected and the catheter is removed (Rosenberg & Heavner 1985). The tourniquet may be totally deflated after around 25 minutes, as the local anaesthetic will have been absorbed by the tissues in the arm. Prior to 25 minutes, systemic toxicity may occur if the cuff is deflated, allowing the local anaesthetic to circulate around the body.

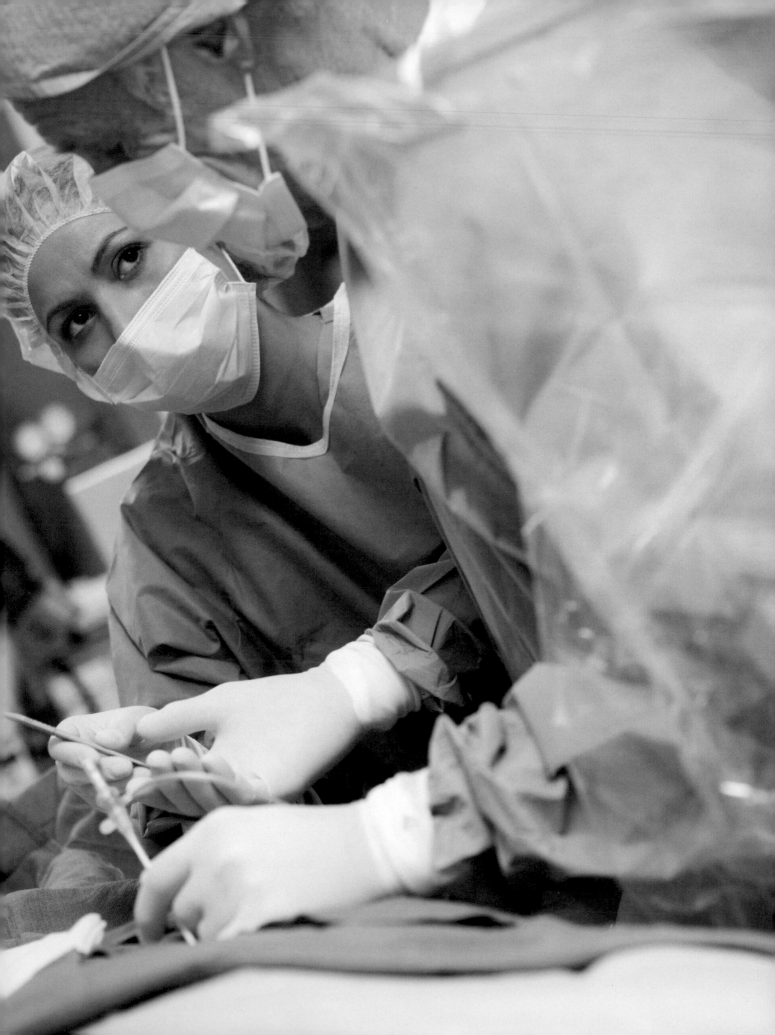

Surgery

Part 3

Chapters

19 Roles of the circulating and scrub team 42
20 Basic surgical instruments 44
21 Surgical scrubbing 46
22 Surgical positioning 48
23 Maintaining the sterile field 50
24 Sterilisation and disinfection 52
25 Swab and instrument counts 54
26 Working with electrosurgery 56
27 Tourniquet management 58
28 Wounds and dressings 60

19 Roles of the circulating and scrub team

Figure 19.1 The circulating and scrub team

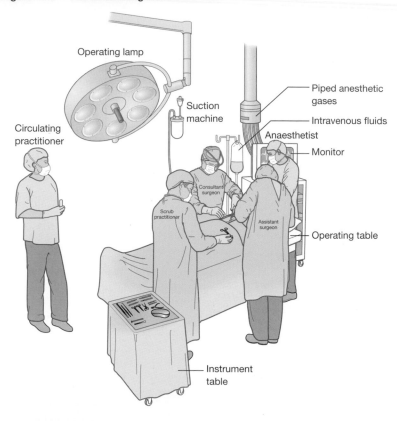

- Operating lamp
- Suction machine
- Piped anesthetic gases
- Intravenous fluids
- Anaesthetist
- Monitor
- Circulating practitioner
- Consultant surgeon
- Scrub practitioner
- Assistant surgeon
- Operating table
- Instrument table

Figure 19.2 Practitioners cleaning operating room following surgery and preparing for the next patient's arrival

(a)
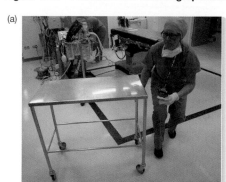

(b)
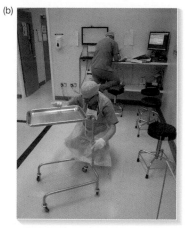

(c)
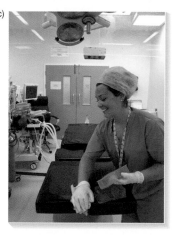

(d)
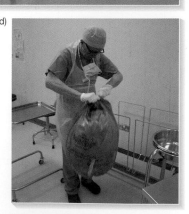

Source: All photos from Aintree University Hospital, Liverpool.

Perioperative Practice at a Glance, First Edition. Paul Wicker. © 2015 John Wiley & Sons, Ltd. Published 2015 by John Wiley & Sons, Ltd.

Scrub practitioners train either as preregistration operating department practitioners (ODPs) or as postregistration nurses. ODP training is now increasing in popularity, as the training programmes are designed specifically to train perioperative practitioners in all three roles in the operating department: anaesthesia, surgery and recovery. Scrub practitioners must have a thorough knowledge of operating room procedures, including the instruments needed for specific surgery, and must be able to stay calm and clear-headed even under pressure. Communication skills are essential for practitioners to help in their primary duties of working with surgeons and assisting them during the surgery (Wicker & Nightingale 2010). Perioperative practitioners provide patient care before, during and after surgical procedures. They are registered, with specialised surgical expertise, and can serve in the surgical team as either scrub or circulating practitioners. Scrubbing in to work directly with the surgeon is the more exciting of the two roles, but circulating practitioners are also vital to the surgical team (Figure 19.1).

Circulating practitioners

It is important that practitioners create and maintain a clean and sterile environment in preparation for treating patients. Having a clean and safe environment will promote health for staff and affect the health of patients positively (Gruendemann & Fernsebner 1995). Educating a patient is one of the most important aspects of perioperative care. It is important that perioperative practitioners support and care for patients and educate them about their treatment and health before and after surgery.

Before a surgical procedure gets underway, the circulating practitioner is responsible for setting up the operating room correctly (Phillips 2007). This includes checking its inventory of disposables, such as pads and sponges, and sterilised instruments from the autoclave. The circulating and scrub practitioners set up the surgical area, laying out instruments and supplies according to the surgeon's preferences. The circulating practitioners also check all equipment needed during the procedure to verify that it is functioning normally. When the patient arrives in the OR, the circulating practitioner usually verifies the patient's identity and necessary consent forms and then reviews the site and nature of the procedure with the surgeon (Phillips 2007).

During the surgical procedure, circulating practitioners remain outside the sterile field. Circulating practitioners also work to promote the cleanliness and sterility of the operating room and tell operating room staff of anything that may cause contamination. They are also responsible for opening sterile objects, so that the surgical team may easily access the sterile equipment without becoming contaminated (Phillips 2007). The circulating practitioners and other members of the surgical team position the patient correctly on the operating table. The circulating practitioner connects any necessary equipment, such as suction and diathermy, and liaises with the surgeon about their needs. During the operation, the circulating practitioner provides the surgical team with sterile fluids and medications as needed and renews the surgical team's supplies if they require extra disposables or instruments. Each member of the surgical team has specific personal responsibilities, and maintaining an oversight of the patient's condition is one of the circulating practitioner's responsibilities (Wicker & Nightingale 2010).

Perioperative practitioners also play a role in patient care before and after procedures. Before surgery, a practitioner draws up the patient's plan of care and spends time with them to properly document and record any allergies or other health-related issues. After surgery, the circulating practitioner helps the scrub nurse and other staff to clean the room and prepare it for the next procedure (Figure 19.2; Wicker & Nightingale 2010).

Scrub practitioners

The role of scrub practitioners is to support and assist surgeons during the surgical procedure, to ensure the best, safest and most effective care for the patient (Smith 2005). To do this they must have knowledge of anatomy and physiology, surgery, and the instruments and equipment needed for the procedure. An experienced scrub practitioner supports the surgeon in undertaking a smooth and efficient procedure, and can anticipate what is needed to prepare efficiently and prevent waste.

Before surgery

Scrub practitioners' duties begin well before the start of the operation. They ensure that the operating room is clean and ready to be set up, and then prepare the instruments and equipment for surgery. They count all items used in surgery, and preserve the sterile environment by scrubbing hands and arms with Betadine® or chlorhexidine and putting on sterile garments, including a gown, gloves and face mask (Gruendemann & Fernsebner 1995).

During surgery

During the operation, one of the scrub practitioner's primary duties is selecting and passing items such as instruments, swabs and sponges to the surgeon, as well as supporting the surgeon and ensuring patient safety (Smith 2005). Practitioners must understand the surgical procedure and the patient's anatomy, and know which instruments are used for specific procedures and when they are needed, so that they can hand them to the surgeon quickly (Phillips 2007). The scrub practitioner must also watch for hand signals to be aware when the surgeon is ready for the next instrument or when the surgeon has finished using an instrument and is ready to hand it back to the scrub practitioner, who cleans the instruments after use and places each instrument back in its place on the table. When necessary, the scrub practitioner requests more instruments or supplies from the circulating team members.

After surgery

Towards the end of the operation and once surgery is finished, scrub practitioners count all instruments, sponges and other tools and inform the surgeon of the count. They then remove instruments and equipment from the operating area, help apply dressing to the surgical site and usually transport the patient to the recovery area (Wicker & Nightingale 2010). They also complete any necessary documentation about the surgery or the patient's transfer to recovery.

20 Basic surgical instruments

Figure 20.1 An array of surgical instruments including: needle holders, retractors, scissors, tissues forceps, curettes, towel clips, bone holders, suction devices etc.

(a)

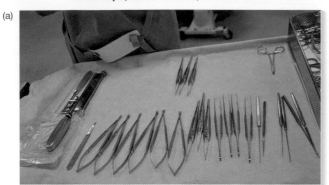

(b)

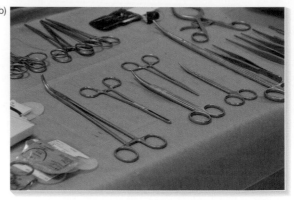

(c)

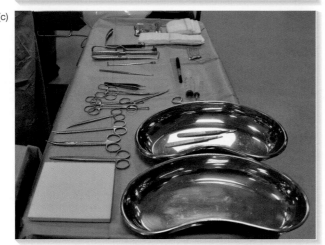

Source: Medical Illustration, University Hospital of South Manchester.
Copyright: UHSM Academy.

Figure 20.2 Instrument trays being set up for gynaecological surgery

(c)

(b)

(a)

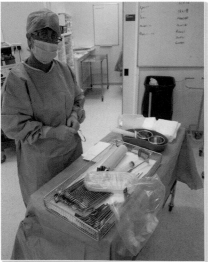

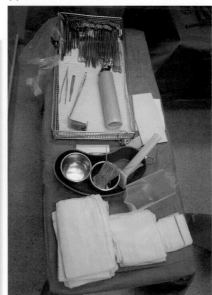

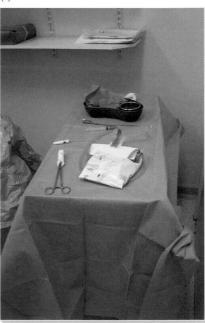

Source: Liverpool Women's Hospital.

There are literally thousands of surgical instruments, so this chapter will cover the basic surgical instruments used in most surgical procedures (Figure 20.1). Instruments are classified according to their purpose, including actions such as cutting and dissecting, grasping and holding, clamping and occluding, exposing and retracting, suturing and stapling, suctioning and aspirating, micro instrumentation and powered surgical instruments. The scrub practitioner is responsible for counting all instruments before and after the surgery, careful handling of instruments, protecting sharp ends of instruments and laying them out on the trolley in preparation for surgery (Figure 20.2). The scrub practitioner should know the names of the instruments, their intended purpose and when the surgeon requires them, and how to pass them to the surgeon in a safe and effective manner. Scrub practitioners also need to clean instruments during surgery and pack them safely after surgery finishes to maintain their working condition.

Types of instruments
Cutting and dissecting
Surgeons normally carry out cutting and dissecting with scalpels as a first step in surgery. The most common scalpels are numbers 10, 11, 15, 20 and 23. Scalpel blades attach to Bard Parker handles and are either handed to the surgeon in a kidney dish or placed in their hand. The practitioner holds the handle between the thumb and forefinger, with the blade under the practitioner's palm, and then places it in the surgeon's hand, handle first. The number 10 and 20 blades are those most commonly used for cutting almost everything including skin, fat, muscles and nerves (Phillips 2007). Vascular surgeons often use a number 11 blade, and plastic and paediatric surgeons often use a number 15 blade. Surgeons also use scissors for cutting tissues, including curved and straight Mayo scissors that are able to cut tough tissues, for example ligaments, and curved Metzenbaum scissors that cut delicate tissues (Whalan 2006). Suture scissors are used to cut sutures or items such as tapes, dressings or swabs.

Grasping and holding
Toothed forceps, for example Lanes tissue forceps, are useful for holding tough tissues such as skin, ligaments or muscles. Non-toothed forceps can hold delicate tissues, such as blood vessels and nerves, which may rip easily (Whalan 2006). Allis forceps and Babcock forceps are held in the same way as scissors, but the ends have broad metallic prongs that can grip on to tissues such as skin or visceral organs without too much pressure. Babcock forceps are designed to hold on to bowel tissues, whereas Allis forceps are designed to hold on to skin flaps, the peritoneum or small blood vessels. Orthopaedic surgeons use bone holders to hold or manipulate bones.

Clamping and occluding
Artery forceps clamp blood vessels so that surgeons can cut and tie them without the loss of blood (Whalan 2006). Surgeons also use them to hold and manipulate tissues. Artery forceps include mosquito forceps (very small), Dunhill, Spencer Wells or Criles forceps (medium) and Mayo forceps, which are large. Kocher's forceps are similar to Mayo's forceps but contain a tooth at the tip of the blades that can grab on to tissues and hold them tightly (Phillips 2007). Surgeons use non-crushing intestinal clamps to close the ends of the intestine after it has been cut or dissected. Vascular clamps of various sizes from very small to very large are similar and are also non-crushing.

Exposing and retracting
Many types of retractor exist. The Balfour retractor is large and is used during a laparotomy to hold open the abdominal wall so that the surgeon can see the organs inside (Gruendemann & Fernsebner 1995). The Langenbeck retractor, which is L shaped, is used to hold wounds open by hand. The Farabeuf retractor has a long, flat blade with L-shaped bends on each end, which hold and retract deep tissues. The Travers and Weitlaner retractors are self-retaining retractors that lock into position and hold wounds open while grasping on to the tissue edges with curved prongs. Surgeons also use various hooks to retract skin edges, such as skin hooks and bone hooks (Phillips 2007). The Senn and cat's paw retractors are small and help to retract skin in minor surgery.

Suturing and stapling
Sutures are attached to needle holders. The tips often have tungsten carbide jaws with cross-hatched serrations to hold the needle firmly to eliminate twisting or turning of the needle and to prevent damaging it (Phillips 2007). Mayo's needle holders are commonly used as they are simple and sturdy instruments. Bowel staplers are used for anastomosing ends of the bowel. Skin staples are also single use and are in the shape of a 'gun'. The surgeon presses the skin stapler on the skin and then presses the 'trigger' to release the staple into the skin.

Suctioning and aspirating
Suction devices remove blood and fluids to give a clear view of the surgical field and they help to monitor blood loss. They are often used in intermediate or major operations, for example in a laparotomy, where fluid is poured into the abdomen to clean the abdominal contents following surgery (Phillips 2007). There are various types, sizes and shapes of suction device used, including Yankaur suckers, which are employed mostly for superficial wound suctioning and for suction of the mouth and throat. The Frazier sucker is small and is used in neurosurgery, spinal, max-fax or minor orthopaedic surgery, where there is little fluid. The Poole abdominal suction device is long, with suction holes along its length, and is used for removing large amounts of fluid.

Microinstrumentation
Very small instruments are used for fine and detailed microsurgery, often while viewing through a microscope. A typical example is while operating on an eye. These instruments include micro forceps, fine tying forceps, capsulotomy scissors, tenotomy scissors and curved needle holders.

Powered surgical instruments
There is a vast array of electrically powered instruments, the most common of which are drills, burrs, saws, reamers and abraders. These are often used in orthopaedics for several uses, including cutting bone, drilling holes for screws and reaming the inside of bone shafts to enable the insertion of nails.

21 Surgical scrubbing

Figure 21.1 Scrub procedures

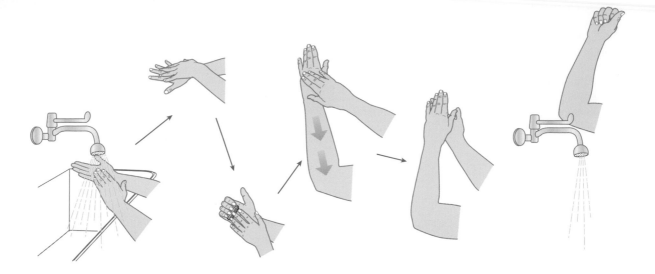

Figure 21.2 Using scrub solution to wash hands and arms

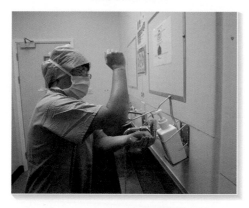

Figure 21.3 Rinsing hands and arms at end of scrubbing

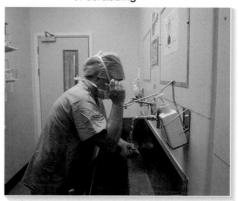

Figure 21.4 Drying hands and arms carefully to prevent contamination

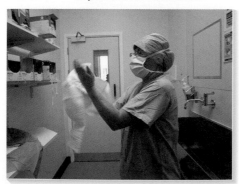

Figure 21.5 Donning gloves and gown ready for surgery

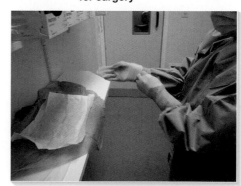

Source: Liverpool Women's Hospital.

Hand washing has been an important part of preventing infection for at least 150 years. Hungarian physician Ignaz Semmelweis identified its significance in 1847 (Horton 1995). The reason is that microorganisms live both on the skin and in the skin, and during surgery these can lead to surgical site infections. Perioperative practitioners therefore need to understand the requirement for correct and appropriate hand washing, using the best solutions available and in the correct circumstances and situations. When scrubbing for surgery, correct hand-washing techniques are still more important, given that open wounds are even more susceptible to contamination.

Solutions used for surgical scrubbing include Betadine (containing povidone iodine) and Hibiscrub® (containing chlorhexidine). Betadine, a mixture of povidone iodine and detergent, is a skin cleaner and disinfectant hand wash and is used for cleansing hands prior to surgery and other aseptic procedures. Hibiscrub is an antiseptic that is effective on both Gram-positive and Gram-negative bacteria. It has both bactericidal and bacteriostatic mechanisms of action and is also useful against fungi and viruses. Sometimes alcohol hand-rubbing solutions may be used between surgical cases when hands are not dirty or contaminated, after the removal of sterile gloves (Chow et al. 2012; WHO 2006). Other hand-washing agents that can be used for surgery include iodophors, triclosan and plain soap (WHO 2006).

In practice settings, education, audits, guidelines and protocols for standardised surgical scrubbing procedures (Figure 21.1) should be established for new and existing staff alongside infection control teams.

Surgical scrub procedure

1 Remove all jewellery, check that your mask and hat are in position and your hair is covered. Ensure that the gown pack is open and ready, select correct glove size and type. Check time on clock – estimated time for surgical scrub is usually 5 minutes.

2 Regulate the flow and temperature of the water so that it is not too hot or the flow too strong.

3 Open the package containing the brush and lay the brush on the back of the scrub sink in its packet.

4 Dispense scrub solution (e.g. Betadine or Hibiscrub) and wet hands and arms up to the elbow for an initial prescrub wash (Figure 21.2). Use several drops of scrub solution. Work up a heavy lather, and then wash the hands and arms to 2 inches above the elbow.

5 Rinse hands and arms thoroughly, raising the hands to allow the water to run from the hands to the elbows, letting the water drip from the elbows into the scrub sink. Cover hands and arms with detergent, once more to 2 inches above the elbow.

6 Take the file (normally presented with the brush) and clean the spaces under the fingernails of both hands under running water if needed, then discard the file.

7 Take the brush and scrub the spaces under the fingernails of the right and left hands, for around 30 seconds each. Keep hands and arms above the elbow and arms away from the body. Do not use the brush to scrub the hands or arms, as this may damage the skin or release bacteria (WHO 2006).

8 Discard the brush and rinse the hands and arms under the tap, allowing water to run from hands to elbows.

9 Dispense scrub solution once more and wash hands using the 7 steps of the modified Ayliffe technique (Ayliffe et al. 1978) as follows:

- Rub palm to palm
- Rub palm with fingers interlaced
- Rub back of both hands, with fingers interlocked
- Rub backs of fingers, interlocked
- Rub thumbs
- Rub both palms with fingertips
- Rub wrists with opposite hand

10 Using circular strokes on all four sides of the arm, move up the forearm using your hand, ending at mid-forearm, using extra scrub solution as required.

11 Repeat for the other arm.

12 Rinse hands and arms from fingertips to above the elbow in one slow, careful movement, keep hands above the elbow. Repeat for the other side (Figure 21.3).

13 Allow the water to drip from your elbows before leaving the scrub sink.

14 Slightly bend forward, pick up the hand towel from the top of the gown pack and step back from the table, take hold of the towel and open it. Do not allow the towel to touch any unsterile part of your body (Figure 21.4).

15 Hold the towel with one of your hands and dry your other hand and arm with a rotating motion. Work from your fingertips to the elbow without returning to previous parts of the arm or hand.

16 Use the second towel to dry the other arm in the same fashion.

17 Dry the hands, forearm and arms thoroughly to prevent difficulty with donning gloves and gowns. Discard towels into the waste receptacle.

18 Prepare to don the surgical gown and gloves (Figure 21.5).

Side effects of surgical scrubbing

The main side effects of surgical hand scrubbing are allergies, dermatitis and skin irritation, normally caused by chlorhexidine or other scrub solutions. Tap water can also contain bacteria such as Pseudomonas spp. or Pseudomonas aeriginosa, which are linked to infections in operating theatres, wards and intensive care units (ICU). A way of preventing this from happening is to use a waterless alcohol-based hand rub, normally containing isopropyl alcohol 70%, chlorhexidine and an emollient, after drying the hands and arms (WHO 2006).

Some hand hygiene practices can also increase the risk of skin irritation. Wearing gloves while hands are still wet from either washing or applying alcohol increases the risk of skin irritation. All products have a potential risk, so providing an alternative for use by individuals with sensitivity or reactions to the hand hygiene product available may help to reduce problems.

22 Surgical positioning

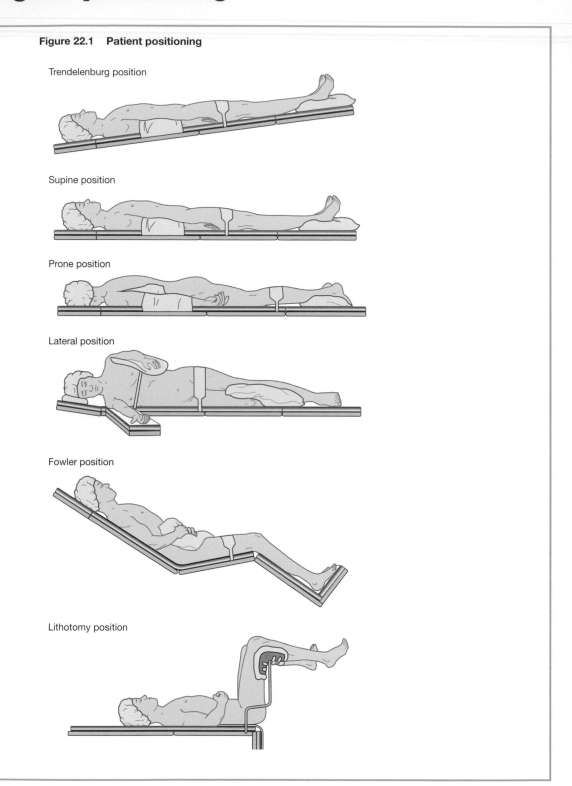

Figure 22.1   Patient positioning

Trendelenburg position

Supine position

Prone position

Lateral position

Fowler position

Lithotomy position

The main objectives of surgical positioning are to optimise the position of the surgical site, to assist the surgical procedure, to minimise the risk of adverse physiological effects, such as nerve damage or pressure sores, to assist the monitoring of the patient's physiology, and to ensure safety and secure attachment of the patient to the table. The anaesthetist and surgeon work together to ensure that the patient is in the best position – for surgery and for the patient's well-being.

Safety measures during positioning include first identifying the patient and confirming the site of surgery. The patient also has to be assessed for their flexibility. For example, putting a patient in the lithotomy position when they have a fractured hip would not be acceptable. Locking the operating table and bed is important when moving the patient from one to the other, to prevent the patient from falling (Phillips 2007). The anaesthetist is responsible for ensuring that the patient's head is protected during positioning, to prevent neck pain or damage, and to prevent the endotracheal tube from being dislodged. Crossing the ankles is also dangerous, as it may lead to deep venous thrombosis. It is important to consider the patient's anatomy and physiology during positioning, for example the risks of compromising the respiratory system, circulation, nerves, muscles and soft tissue.

Equipment requirements for positioning

The operating table is the primary piece of equipment used for positioning the patient. Operating tables come with various fittings that practitioners use to site the patient in various positions. Practitioners attach the patient to the table with restraint straps to prevent the patient from falling (Pirie 2010). Other common devices include gel pads, head rests, head rings, shoulder braces or supports and body restraint straps (Wicker & Nightingale 2010). The operating table is also able to bend so that patients can sit up, the lower end of the table can bend to allow the knees to flex, and removing parts of the table enables the fitting of other devices.

The anaesthesia screen forms a barrier between the surgery and the patient's head, isolating the anaesthetist from the surgery. There is a bar over the patient's head, which the surgeon drapes with the covering sheet and/or the surgical drapes to form a screen.

Arm boards are common and are needed for almost all surgical patients (Wicker & Nightingale 2010). Practitioners extend the arm outwards from the table, but they do this carefully to prevent brachial plexus damage. The arm is then secured to the arm board by a strap, and cushions or gel pads may be placed under the arm to protect it from damage.

Stirrups are used for anal, perineal or gynaecological surgery, to expose the areas needed for surgery. A single knee may be raised on one stirrup during arthroscopy to bend the knee and give access to the knee joint.

Surgical positions

The supine (dorsal) position is used for most types of surgery: the patient lies flat on their back with their arms at the side or extended on arm boards (Pirie 2010). Back ache and neck ache may result from this position, especially if surgery takes a long time. Placing a support under the lumbar region to support the curve of the spine can reduce back ache. The Trendelenburg position involves tipping the supine body, head downwards, at an angle of 20° or less (Pirie 2010). This position may be used during the repair of inguinal hernias. Reverse Trendelenburg is a head-up position that may be employed for surgery to the head. In both cases, securing the patient to the table is essential to prevent slippage.

The prone position is where the patient lies flat on the operating table, face downwards (Phillips 2007). Practitioners can place pillows under the patient's shoulders, hips and feet to facilitate breathing and reduce the strain on the body. Using a cut-out pillow (or head ring) to support the head allows the head to face downwards rather than sideways. The patient must be strapped to the table securely to prevent their arms or legs falling off the table.

The lateral position is used when patients need to lie on their side with their back slightly bent. In this position, the patient is strapped to the table and supports put in place to preserve the position. The position for kidney surgery is also lateral, but the patient is placed in a straight position, and the table is bent in line with the hips to open up the side for access to the kidney.

Gynaecologists use the lithotomy position for procedures such as vaginal surgery, and it is also employed in general surgery for lower bowel surgery. This position may cause pressure on nerves, muscles and joints, leading to postoperative pain and perhaps damage. Practitioners raise the patient's knees simultaneously, abduct the legs and then place them in the stirrups attached to poles connected to the table (Phillips 2007). The feet and legs are attached to the stirrups using a crepe bandage or straps. The practitioner then removes the end of the table to give access to the perineal area. Cushions, pillows or gel pads can also help to prevent damage to the legs.

The jackknife position is adopted by placing the patient prone with their arms on arm boards placed upwards towards their head. The patient's head is supported by using a foam cut-out pillow, allowing the head to face downwards towards the operating table. The operating table is then angled so that the patient bends forward at the waist by around 90°. This position is used mostly for sacral, perianal and perineal surgery, and also for occipital or posterolateral cranial surgery. The position has to be adopted carefully and the patient carefully monitored during the surgery to avoid any injuries.

Several other surgical positions exist, but in all cases the patient has to be positioned carefully and securely to ensure that no harm is caused by unnatural positioning.

23 Maintaining the sterile field

Figure 23.1 Sterile and unsterile members of the team and the sterile field

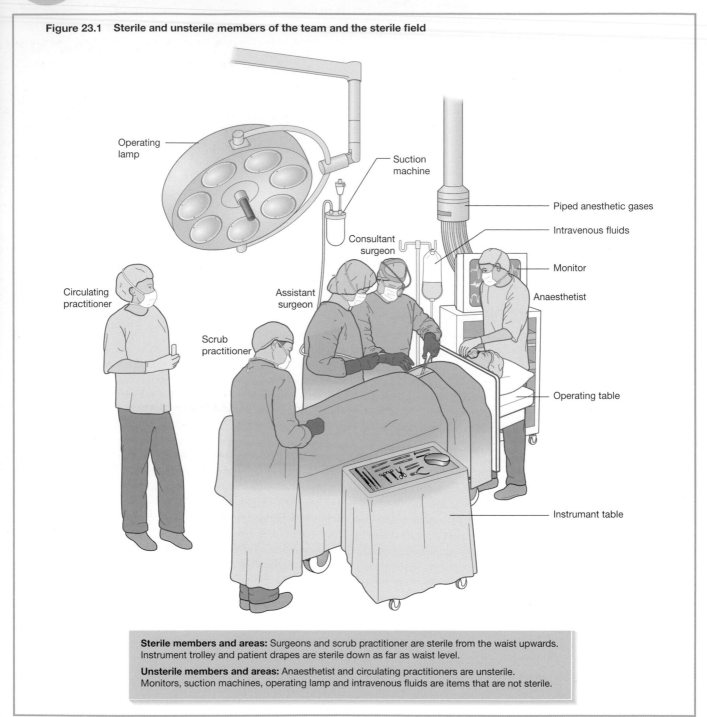

Sterile members and areas: Surgeons and scrub practitioner are sterile from the waist upwards. Instrument trolley and patient drapes are sterile down as far as waist level.

Unsterile members and areas: Anaesthetist and circulating practitioners are unsterile. Monitors, suction machines, operating lamp and intravenous fluids are items that are not sterile.

Surgical asepsis during surgical operations relies on procedures that ensure that an area of the body or sterile object is free from microorganisms or contamination from either blood or body fluids, or contamination from unsterile objects. The sterile field is usually considered to be the site around the surgery. However, it also includes other items or areas such as a sterile tray, an open gown pack, or the inside of a sterile wrap containing an instrument or item being handed to the scrub practitioner (Manley & Bellman 2013). Contamination of any part of the surgical sterile field may result in surgical site infections, leading to increased morbidity or mortality.

Sterile procedures

The scrub practitioner should keep the sterile surgical field clean, dry and uncluttered, to prevent contamination (Meara & Reive 2013). The surgical team should always hold sterile items above their waist, in their vision and in front of their body, not to the side or behind another member of the team. Non-sterile members of the theatre team should keep away from the sterile fields as much as possible. However, circulating practitioners will approach the instrument tray to hand over items such as extra instruments, swabs or packs. They need to do this carefully, without contaminating either the item being handed over or the instrument tray itself.

There are three possible ways of handing over an item to a scrub practitioner: using the drop technique, the 'mitten' technique or by wearing sterile gloves (Meara & Reive 2013). The drop technique involves opening a sterile package, with the sealed edge pointed towards the scrub practitioner. The practitioner can then drop the internal package into a bowl or dish. The 'mitten' technique involves wrapping the outside layers of the package around the hands of the circulating practitioner and handing the package to the scrub practitioner. This procedure is often used for large or irregular-shaped items such as bowls, drapes or heavy equipment. Items can also be opened outside the sterile field by first opening the outside wrap on a bench or table. The circulating practitioner dons sterile gloves using a sterile technique, and the sterile item is picked up and given to the surgical team or placed on the instrument tray. This procedure would only be undertaken in special circumstances when large or cumbersome objects needed to be given to the surgical team after surgery had started.

Preparing a sterile tray

The circulating practitioner places the sterile instrument tray on a trolley and opens the outer covers. The sterile inside wrappers are then opened by the scrub practitioner. Once opened, it is essential that the tray remain sterile, therefore there are several actions that need to be undertaken during the surgical procedure (Rothrock 2011). Contaminated items, such as non-sterile bottles, instrument covers and unopened items, need to stay off the tray. Pouring any solution into a bowl must be done without touching the bowl or by holding the bottle, which is unsterile on the outside, over the tray. It is essential that visitors to the operating room, new students or untrained staff are fully aware that they cannot touch anything on the sterile tray and need to keep their bodies a safe distance away from the tray. The scrub practitioner receives all surgical items, instruments or pieces of equipment before the start of surgery. Finally, if contamination occurs, then the instrument tray may need to be discarded and a new tray provided (Manley & Bellman 2013).

Surgical draping

Surgical drapes cover the patient and the operating table, and create a sterile field around the site of surgery (Meara & Reive 2013). Drapes help to reduce the passage of microorganisms between the wound and other parts of the patient's body, and between sterile and non-sterile areas. The best draping materials are resistant to blood and fluids, lint free, warming for the patient and non-flammable. Drapes are now usually single use and made of paper and a plastic film to prevent leakage of fluids. Drapes also cover other items such as instrument trolleys, basins and Mayo stands. Plastic incisional drapes are made of impermeable polyvinyl sheeting. These are normally used as vertical isolation drapes in orthopaedic surgery, including for example dynamic hip screw insertion or plating of the femur. The area of the drape around the surgical site is adherent to the skin and the incision is made directly through this part of the drape.

The standard draping procedure involves the scrub practitioner handing the drapes over to the surgeon and assisting with their application from the sterile area to the unsterile areas (Rothrock 2011). The drape should be unfolded and allowed to drop into position. Edges of the drapes falling below the waist or level of the table should not be touched again, as those edges may be unsterile. One way of applying drapes would be to use four small drapes to surround the area where the surgery is taking place, two large drapes to cover the patient top and bottom, and then a plastic adherent drape to cover the wound area, for example an Opsite® drape. Sometimes a single drape can be used to cover the entire patient, with a hole in the drape to expose the site of surgery, which is then covered with a plastic adherent drape. Various other types of sheets are also used for draping patients, including fenestrated and split sheets, which are used for areas of the body such as abdomen, chest, backs, limbs, head or neck. Lithotomy drapes are employed for surgery on the perineum, genitalia, cystoscopy, haemorrhoidectomies and vaginal procedures. The drape consists of a fenestrated sheet (with the hole in the sheet around the perineum) and two triangular leggings. In all surgical situations it is important that only sterile drapes are used. If they become contaminated during placement, then they must be discarded and new drapes used.

24 Sterilisation and disinfection

Figure 24.1   Procedures for disinfection and sterilisation

Disinfection

> **Intermediate-level disinfection**
>
> Alcohol solutions, for example ethyl or isopropyl alcohol
> Phenolic and iodophor-based detergent solutions
> Ozone, a powerful oxidant that can oxidise and destroy
> microorganisms, compatible with items such as stainless
> steel, aluminum, ceramics, glass, Teflon and polyethylene
> Filters, used to isolate microorganisms from the equipment
> Boiling in water for 20 minutes, normally using metal
> instruments, only in the absence of sterilisers or
> sterilisation chemicals

> **Low-level disinfection**
>
> Alcohol solutions, for example ethyl or isopropyl alcohol
> Sodium hypochlorite
> Detergent solutions containing germicidal solutions such
> as phenol, aldehydes, alcohol, iodophor, ammonium or
> heavy metals
> Microwave generators for disinfection of products that are
> compatible with this

Sterilisation

> **Low-level sterilisation**
>
> Glutaraldehyde solutions for short periods of time
> Solutions and gases containing chlorine dioxide
> Paracetic acid solutions, which are also sporicidal
> Hydrogen peroxide at 6%–30% concentration, either as a
> solution or a vapour
> Pasteurisation using sodium hypochlorite and/or water at a
> minimum of 70 °C for a minimum of 30 minutes
> Formaldehyde solutions or steam

> **High-level sterilisation**
>
> Heat sterilisation using either steam or hot air
> Ethylene oxide gas
> Glutaraldehyde solution for a long period
> Ionising and non-ionising radiation such as ultraviolet light,
> X rays and gamma rays
> Incineration using flames
> Formaldehyde solutions or steam for up to 12 hours
> Gaseous chlorine dioxide, especially for healthcare products

Figure 24.2   Sterile instruments which are stored safely within two coverings to keep them sterile.

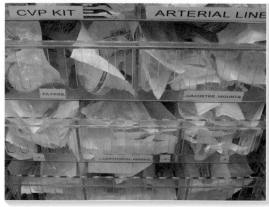

Source: Aintree University Hospital, Liverpool.

Perioperative Practice at a Glance, First Edition. Paul Wicker. © 2015 John Wiley & Sons, Ltd. Published 2015 by John Wiley & Sons, Ltd.

Microorganisms cause contamination, infection and decay of organic substances, therefore it is important that they are not present near sterile materials, devices or areas in the operating room. Disinfection and sterilisation are also essential for ensuring that medical and surgical instruments do not cause infections in patients (CHRSP 2008).

Cleaning refers to the removal of organic and inorganic material from objects and it is normally carried out manually, using water with detergents or enzymatic products (Meredith & Sjorgen 2008). Cleaning is an essential process before undertaking high-level disinfection and sterilisation, because inorganic and organic materials that remain on the surfaces of instruments can protect microbes that lie underneath. Sterilisation destroys or eliminates all forms of microbial life using physical or chemical methods (Meredith & Sjorgen 2008). Examples of methods of sterilisation include steam under pressure, dry heat, ethylene oxide gas, hydrogen peroxide, gas plasma and liquid chemicals (HICPAC 2008). Disinfection eliminates the majority of pathogenic microorganisms on inanimate objects, except for bacterial spores. In the operating room, objects are usually disinfected by liquid chemicals containing chloride or other chemical substances, water and perhaps detergents. Various factors can affect disinfection and sterilisation in a negative way, including prior cleaning of the object; dirty or soiled equipment; holes, hinges or crevices in the object; and the temperature and pH of the disinfection process (CHRSP 2008).

Methods of sterilisation

Sterilisation (Figure 24.1) takes place using physical methods, chemical agents or mechanical removable methods. Physical agents include dry and moist heat and ionising and non-ionising radiation. Chemical agents include gas and liquids, which can both sterilise and disinfect items depending on the chemicals used. Mechanical removal methods can also sterilise and disinfect using air and liquids through a process of filtration.

Physical agents

A physical method of sterilisation includes a hot-air oven. This kills microbes by oxidation, and operates between 50 °C and 300 °C. Under most circumstances the temperature is approximately 160 °C for one hour. The hot-air oven has insulation to keep the heat in and to conserve energy. These ovens sterilise instruments such as forceps, scalpels, scissors and glassware. Air circulates around the objects to ensure treatment on all sides of the objects.

Moist-heat sterilisation works via killing organisms by coagulating their proteins. This is carried out in various ways using temperatures below 100 °C, leading to pasteurisation; at 100 °C by boiling in water, using steam at normal atmospheric pressure; or using steam under pressure in an autoclave. Boiling kills bacterial pathogens, although the hepatitis virus can survive up to 30 minutes of boiling and endospores can survive up to 20 hours or more of boiling. An autoclave consists of a vertical or horizontal cylinder that has an opening at one end for placing in the materials to be sterilised

(Lines 2003). A pressure gauge shows the level of pressure and a safety valve is present to allow the escape of steam from the chamber if the pressure rises too much. Placing articles into a basket permits steam to permeate around them. Sterilisation takes a minimum of 15 minutes at an average temperature of 120 °C (HICPAC 2008).

Non-ionising radiation consists of electromagnetic rays with a longer wavelength than ultraviolet light. Items absorb the waves and become heated, which produces a similar effect as hot-air sterilisation. Non-ionising radiation is used for various items, including rapid mass sterilisation of prepacked syringes and catheters. Ionising radiation includes X rays, gamma rays and cosmic rays. These rays have a high penetrative power but do not cause items to rise in temperature, therefore they lead to cold sterilisation. Items sterilised in this way include plastic, syringes, catheters and metal foils.

Chemical agents

Chemical agents act by causing protein to coagulate, disrupting the cell membrane and affecting the physiology of the cell. Alcoholic agents such as ethanol or isopropyl alcohol are used at a concentration of around 60–90%. They have no action on spores, but can kill bacteria and viruses (CDPH 2013). Alcohol is used for situations such as disinfecting clinical thermometers and skin prior to venepuncture, and for cleaning rubber bungs on medicine bottles (Meredith & Sjorgen 2008). Formaldehyde and glutaraldehyde are less frequently used these days, but are still available. Formaldehyde is bactericidal (kills bacteria), sporicidal (kills spores) and can kill viruses. Uses of formaldehyde include preserving anatomical specimens, destroying spores in hair and wool and sterilising metal instruments. Glutaraldehyde is also effective against tubercle bacilli, fungi and viruses. Uses of glutaraldehyde include treating anaesthetic tubing, face masks, ET tubes, metal instruments and plastic tubing. Halogens include iodine and chlorine. Iodine is used in aqueous and alcoholic solutions for disinfecting the skin of hands while scrubbing, or prepping the skin of the patient before surgery (Lines 2003). It is bactericidal and can also damage spores. Chlorine is used in disinfectants and in water supplies. Phenols, such as Lysol and cresol, are also powerful microbicides and are commonly used as disinfectants (CDPH 2013). Ethylene oxide gas is used to sterilise instruments, equipment, sutures, glass and other items. It is colourless, highly penetrating and effective against bacteria, viruses and spores. There are also many other chemical agents used to disinfect or sterilise items.

Mechanical agents

Filtration helps to remove bacteria from heat-labile liquids such as sera, which are blood and body fluids, and antibiotics. Various filters are in use, including candle filters, asbestos filters, glass filters and membrane filters. Filters are employed for various reasons: for example, membrane filters are made of cellulose esters or other polymers and are used for sterilisation, sterility testing and preparation of solutions for parenteral use.

Cleaning, disinfection and sterilisation are therefore important considerations prior to patient surgery to help reduce the likelihood of intraoperative infection.

25 Swab and instrument counts

Figure 25.1 Practitioners completing the swab board following counting of swabs and instruments

Swab boards vary between hospitals although practitioners are always trained how to complete the boards according to hospital guidelines, rules and regulations.

(a)

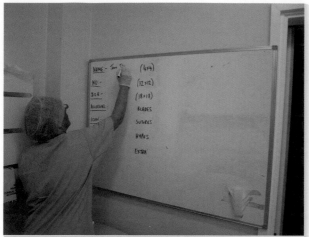

(b)

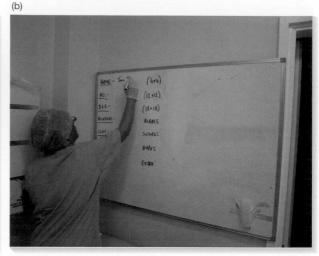

Source: (a) Liverpool Women's Hospital, (b) Aintree University Hospital, Liverpool.

Figure 25.2 Counting instruments following surgery, using an instrument count sheet

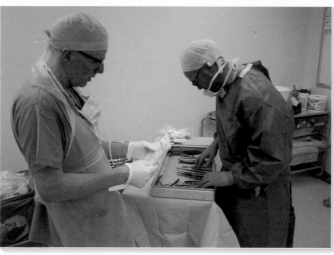

Source: Aintree University Hospital, Liverpool.

The Department of Health has classified the loss of swabs or instruments in a patient's body to be a 'never event' (Coates 2012). In other words, it should never happen. However, in reality it does. Gilmour (2012) highlighted, in a report from Pennsylvania in 2008, that incorrect counts of needles occurred 47% of the time, incorrect instrument counts 33% of the time and incorrect swab counts 20% of the time. During surgery, it can happen that swabs, instruments or needles are left inside the patient, dropped on the floor, mixed up with drapes or simply lost. These events occur because of human error, and it is therefore essential that practitioners carry out swab and instrument counts correctly, according to national guidelines and hospital policies (Bell 2012). It is accordingly important that both new and established theatre practitioners have access to the swab and instrument count (SIC) policy.

Rationale behind the swab and instrument count

The SIC ensures that nothing remains inside the patient's body. If something does, then that can result in illness or death, a longer recovery time, extended surgery times and infection (Gilmour 2005). Legal issues may also arise for the scrub practitioner and for the hospital. Theatre practitioners must communicate with the perioperative team and carry out the counts thoroughly and effectively to prevent the retention of swabs and instruments. Accountable items include swabs, packs, pledglets (small compressed pads), instruments, sutures, ties, needles, blades, clips (e.g. bulldog clips), patties and slings. The scrub practitioner is accountable for being aware of the location of all items used during surgery and for returning used items to the instrument tray.

Principles of the swab and instrument count

The scrub practitioner is responsible for starting the SIC with the circulating practitioner. The scrub and circulating practitioners carry out the count, and one of them must be experienced, qualified and registered. During a long surgical procedure the scrub practitioner is sometimes replaced by another scrub practitioner, who carries out a full SIC before the first scrub practitioner leaves the table (Smith 2005). Practitioners carry out a SIC before the surgery starts, during surgery if a cavity is closed (for example the bladder), before the start of wound closure and after surgery finishes. For major surgery there will therefore be a minimum of three counts, and for minor surgery (for example removing a sebaceous cyst) a minimum of two counts. Practitioners normally record SIC on whiteboards on the wall of the operating room (Figure 25.1). The board is used so that all staff can see the counts if required. The local hospital policy should detail how items such as swabs, needles, clips, patties and so on are recorded, and how items such as swabs are accounted for when discarded or taken away from the surgical procedure.

Practitioners carry out SIC routinely according to hospital policy, normally in the sequence of swabs, sharps, other items (such as sutures, slings or patties) and finally instruments and instrument trays (Figure 25.2; Gilmour 2012). Practitioners normally count items first at the site of surgery, then on the Mayo table and finally on the instrument trolley, thereby ensuring that items do not get counted twice. If a swab does get lost and cannot be found, then the patient should be X-rayed to detect the X-ray detectable marker on the swab. Surgical instruments or items occasionally drop off the operating table because of faulty placement or a knock. If this happens, they should be placed within sight of the scrub practitioner, perhaps in a bowl or near the swab board, to include them in the count. No items used during the procedure should be removed from the operating theatre until the final check is complete. If a SIC is incorrect, then the practitioner must inform the surgeon immediately.

Checking swabs and other items

Practitioners should carry out the swab check in the following way, and depending on hospital policy:

1 Before the start of the procedure, count all swabs and packs in bundles of five and record the count on the swab board.
2 Count and record other items, such as blades, sutures and needles, on the swab board.
3 Undertake counts before, during and after the procedure, and whenever an item becomes lost.
4 Discard any swabs with problems, such as missing X-ray strips or missing swabs from within packets, and remove them from the operating room before surgery starts.
5 During surgery, open individual swabs and packs and show to the circulating practitioner to verify that it is only one swab, not two swabs stuck together.
6 Count swabs and packs during the procedure and discard them into a swab disposal system. This may be a swab rack with plastic pockets, or a plastic bag that is tied up and placed in a basin.
7 Record swabs inserted into body cavities on the swab board.
8 Carry out an SIC when closing a cavity, closing the wound and once surgery is finished.
9 Verify and record correct swab checks using the Surgical Safety Checklist and the patient care plan.

Checking instruments

Practitioners use a checklist that is included within the instrument tray to check instruments:

1 All staff involved in the count must be able to identify the instruments.
2 Verify the instruments as being intact and working.
3 The checklist records instruments that are part of trays, although extra instruments may be included on the swab board.
4 Discard all single-use instruments following surgery.
5 Check and record all instruments at the start of the procedure and on completion of surgery.

26 Working with electrosurgery

Figure 26.1   Monopolar electrosurgery

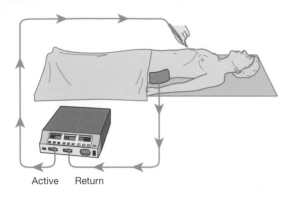

Active   Return

Figure 26.2   Bipolar electrosurgery

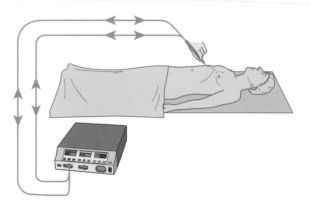

Figure 26.3   Surgical effects of electrosurgery

Dessication   Fulguration   Electrosurgical cutting   Blend

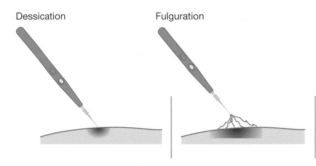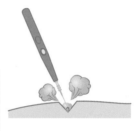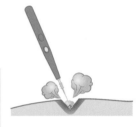

Figure 26.4   Electrosurgery used to cut tissues
The tip of the pencil is very thin which allows careful cutting of tissues and avoiding damage to other tissues.

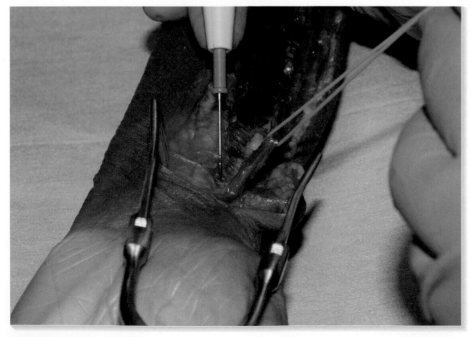

Source: Medical Illustration,
University Hospital of South Manchester.
Copyright: UHSM Academy.

Electrosurgery (diathermy) uses a high-frequency (2–3 MHz) alternating electrical current to heat tissues. High-frequency electrosurgical current does not stimulate muscles or nerves and therefore does not cause twitching, convulsions or fibrillation of the heart. Electrosurgery coagulates or cuts tissues quickly and easily. Almost every operating room in the world uses it, therefore most practitioners consider it safe to use. However, human error can still cause accidental harm to patients.

How does electrosurgery work?

A high-frequency monopolar current leaves the electrosurgical unit (ESU), travels down the cable and reaches the active electrode. The current then passes through the patient's tissues and on to the return electrode (also called the patient plate or indifferent electrode), which is large enough to minimise the heating effect under the plate. The current then returns via the cable to the ESU. The tip of the active electrode provides enough current density to create a high temperature at the point of entry of the current into the tissues. This high temperature produces an electrosurgical effect that controls haemorrhage by coagulation (desiccation or fulguration) or cuts tissues by causing cell disruption (Hainer 1991; Wicker 2000; Lee 2002; O'Riley 2010).

Electrosurgical current was originally connected to earth or ground. As the current could return to the mains circuit through any grounded appliance, this meant that patients often received burns in other areas. For example, if a patient was connected to ECG electrodes, then the current could return to the ESU via the ECG monitor, resulting in burns at the point of contact of the ECG electrodes. Most modern ESUs are now isolated; in other words, there is little or no contact between the electrosurgical current and the mains electric current (O'Riley 2010).

The three surgical effects of electrosurgery (Figure 26.3)

• **Desiccation** (COAG mode): Coagulation of tissue and/or blood. Using a low-power, low-voltage, intermittent waveform.
• **Fulguration** (COAG mode): Superficial necrosis of tissue. Using sparks, with a high-power, high-voltage intermittent waveform.
• **Cutting** (CUT or BLEND mode): Rapid heating of tissues over a small area causes a scalpel-like effect. Using a high-current, low-voltage constant waveform. BLEND mode also involves coagulation of blood and tissues (Figure 26.4).

Monopolar electrosurgery (Figure 26.1)

The monopolar circuit consists of the active electrode lead carrying current from the generator to the active electrode, which contacts tissues, causing coagulation or cutting. The electrosurgical current travels through the patient's body to the return electrode, which collects the current and returns it to the electrosurgical generator (Tucker 2000; Wicker 2000; Soon & Washington 2010; Wicker & O'Neill 2010; Valleylab 2013). Monopolar electrosurgery is often used for central areas of the body such as muscles, abdomen, legs and arms. It should not be used for peripheries such as fingers, ear lobes or penis, as it may cause vascular damage.

Bipolar electrosurgery (Figure 26.2)

The bipolar circuit consists of two leads that connect to the generator, and a pair of insulated forceps. The active lead carries the current towards the bipolar forceps; one tine of the forceps is the active electrode and the other tine is the return electrode.

The current only passes through the tissue between the two tines and returns to the generator via the return lead. A return electrode (i.e. patient plate) is not required to be attached to the patient (Hainer 1991). Bipolar electrosurgery is often used at low power and for sensitive areas of the body such as the brain, skin and eyes, as well as for peripheries such as fingers, earlobes or penis.

The return electrode

The patient return electrode returns the current safely to the generator because it has a large contact area with the patient's skin and permanent contact during the procedure (O'Riley 2010). Return electrodes are normally single-use, pre-gelled, dual-plate electrodes that employ a return electrode monitoring system (REM). When the electrosurgical generator detects problems arising with the plate it switches into standby mode, preventing the passage of electrosurgical current. However, some return electrodes are still single plates, which do not enable the REM system to work. Partial dislodging of the single-plate electrode can lead to serious burns underneath the plate.

Safety checks

It is important that rigorous safety checks, using hospital checklists or policies/procedures, are carried out before carrying out electrosurgery (Wicker 2000). These checks can include:

• Checking that all cables and electrodes are secure and working and that the insulation is intact.
• Store the active electrode in an insulated quiver to prevent accidental burns.
• Do not reuse single-use return electrodes.
• Place the return electrode on an area free from hair, skin lesions, wounds or scars, on a muscular area, close to the site of surgery.
• If the patient is moved during surgery, recheck the positioning of the return electrode.
• Ensure that the patient is not in contact with grounded metal objects.
• Check the skin before and after placing the return electrode.
• Dry alcoholic skin-preparation fluids before placing drapes over them, to prevent ignition of the fluid from electrosurgical sparks. Pooling of any fluids under the body can also lead to skin damage (Wicker 2000; O'Riley 2010).

Hazards of electrosurgery

These include:

• Accidental burns, caused by thermoelectric burns, chemical burns, fire or explosions (Prasad et al. 2006; O'Riley 2010; AFPP 2011; Valleylab 2013).
• Smoke inhalation. Electrosurgical smoke can contain allergens, toxins, and bacterial and viral particles (McCormick 2008; Watson 2010; Sanderson 2012).
• Interference with other electromedical devices causing activation of pacemakers, interference with ECG readings and artefacts on video screens.

Conclusion

Managers should train all practitioners to understand the electrosurgical equipment and use it properly, and anyone not trained should not try to use the equipment. **Remember**: The greatest defence against patient injury is a well-educated staff!

27 Tourniquet management

Figure 27.1
Attaching the velband

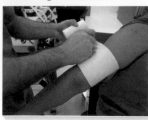

Figure 27.2
Wrapping the tourniquet

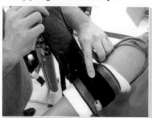

Figure 27.3
Fixing the tourniquet in place, and securing it

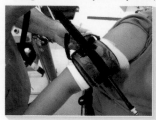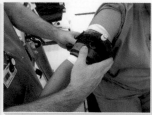

Figure 27.4   Attaching the tourniquet to the machine

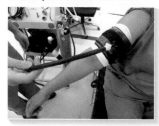

Figure 27.5   Applying the Rys-Davies Exsanguinator to remove blood from the arm. Following this the machine is switched on and the tourniquet inflates

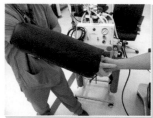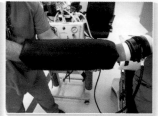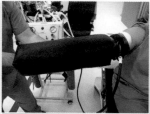

Figure 27.6   Applying an Eschmarch bandage

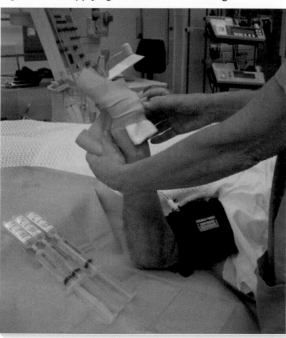

Figure 27.7   Tourniquet machine

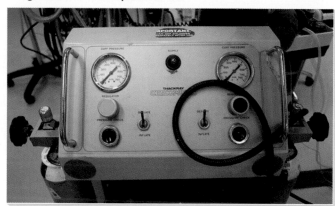

Source: All photos from Aintree University Hospital, Liverpool.

Tourniquets have been in use for centuries to control bleeding, especially during amputation (Wikipedia 2013). Various other types of tourniquet have been used over the years, and now patients are usually given automatic or non-automatic pneumatic tourniquets. The Esmarch bandage or a Rhys Davies exsanguinator (Rhys-Davies & Stotter 1985), an inflated elastic rubber cylinder that practitioners roll onto the limb, is used to exsanguinate limbs.

The purpose of employing tourniquets in the operating department is to facilitate surgery or anaesthesia. During anaesthesia, inflatable tourniquets prevent the spread of intravenous anaesthetic agents into arms and legs that have tourniquets attached. Non-inflatable tourniquets are made of rubber or elastic, which practitioners tie tightly around the limb; these are used for phlebotomy or insertion of cannulas. Surgery requires the use of inflatable tourniquets, for example to reduce fractures, arthroscopy of knees and peripheral joints, bone grafts, nerve injuries and tendon repairs (Sharma & Salhotra 2012). The tourniquet promotes a bloodless surgical field, enabling the surgeon to view the anatomy more easily (Richey 2007). Tourniquets also reduce blood loss, reduce the length of the operation and reduce complications caused by poor surgical vision. Tourniquets are not suitable for open fractures, crush injuries, wound infections, skin grafts or when the patient has severe hypertension (Richey 2007).

Applying the tourniquet

Friedrich von Esmarch promoted the use of a rubber bandage in 1873 (Wikipedia 2013), although he was not the first to use such a device (Klenerman 2003). The purpose of this device was to reduce blood loss during surgery. The modern Esmarch bandages are flat and up to 4 inches wide, and were designed by von Langenbeck (Klenerman 2003) based on Esmarch's original bandage. Surgeons use the Esmarch to exsanguinate a limb, and then remove it once the tourniquet is inflated. Side effects of the Esmarch bandage include nerve injury and underlying tissue damage caused by the bandage exerting high pressure (Sharma & Salhotra 2012).

A Velband® bandage or cotton padding is first wrapped around the limb above the wound and proximal to the body (Figure 27.1). The pneumatic cuff is then wrapped around the padding (Figure 27.2) and tied into position (Figure 27.3). The cotton padding prevents the cuff from damaging the skin. The cuff is then connected to the tourniquet machine (Figure 27.4), but not inflated. The limb is elevated and the Rhys Davies exsanguinator (Figure 27.5) or an Esmarch bandage (Figure 27.6) is applied from the periphery towards the cuff. Once the arm is exsanguinated, the cuff is then inflated and the exsanguinator removed. If the wound on the limb contains pus, necrotic tissue or infection, the practitioner cannot apply an exsanguinator as it may cause infective matter to be pushed into the tissues or upwards through blood vessels and the lymphatic system, leading to systemic infections. Therefore, elevating the limb helps to reduce the amount of blood in the circulation before applying the tourniquet.

Pneumatic tourniquets

Pneumatic tourniquets can be automatic or non-automatic, and can also have single or double cuffs (Wakai et al. 2001). Double cuffs are useful when the patient is undergoing regional anaesthesia, as the distal cuff is first inflated and the regional anaesthesia then applied. After that the practitioner inflates the proximal cuff over anaesthetised tissue, and then deflates the distal cuff. This leads to less pain under the tourniquet. Non-automatic (manual) cuffs involve the use of hand pressure to inflate them. Manual cuffs are used much less often now, as automatic cuffs are safer. When using automatic cuffs, the source of pressurised gas connects to the inflatable cuff, the cuff inflates to the required pressure and the exsanguinator is removed. The tourniquet machine (Figure 27.7) usually records and notes the pressure and the time, and has alarms to indicate changes in pressure and excessive time being spent inflated.

The surgeon will check the tourniquet width and position before surgery to ensure that it is in the correct position and not too close to the area of surgery. Anaesthetists should regularly remind the surgeon of the timing and pressure of the tourniquet, as prolonged use of tourniquets can lead to damage to skin, nerves and tissues. The normal pressure applied on the arm is systolic blood pressure plus 50–75 mmHg extra pressure. On legs it is normally systolic blood pressure plus 75–100 mmHg (Sharma & Salhotra 2012).

Side effects

Physiological changes can occur after applying the tourniquet. The cardiovascular system may be affected, resulting in a rise in circulating volume, systemic vascular resistance and central venous and systolic pressure (Sharma & Salhotra 2012). After applying the tourniquet for 30 minutes, diastolic blood pressure and heart rate may rise. Pain also increases because of pressure on the nerves and tissues, which can cause problems if the patient is not under a general anaesthetic. Other physiological issues include coagulation activation, catecholamine release and rises in body temperature. The nervous system may develop paraesthesia caused by high pressure, especially in the radial nerve or sciatic nerves, although permanent damage is rare. Muscle damage includes ischemia, mechanical damage and depletion of energy stores (Wakai et al. 2001). Skin pressure may result in friction burns or chemical burns, if chemicals leak underneath the cuff.

For these reasons, the maximum time allowed for tourniquets to be applied should be between 1 and 3 hours, with the optimum time 2 hours (Klenerman 2003). Minor physiological changes occur after 1 hour, but after longer periods permanent damage can occur. For example, muscles may be damaged after 4 hours and nerves after 8 hours. If surgery lasts longer than 2 hours, reperfusion should be considered for periods of up to 25 minutes to prevent permanent damage to tissues (Klenerman 2003).

28 Wounds and dressings

Figure 28.1 Applying Opsite © dressing to small wounds that have been sutured

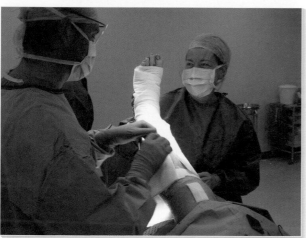

Figure 28.2 Covering an open wound with melolin dressings

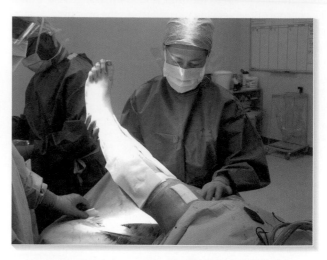

Figure 28.3 Wrapping soffban © wool around dressings to hold them in place

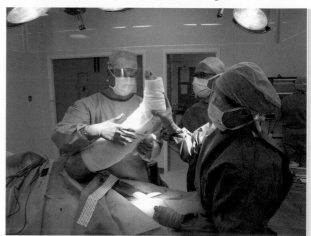

Figure 28.4 Applying a crepe bandage to the open leg wound to secure all dressings

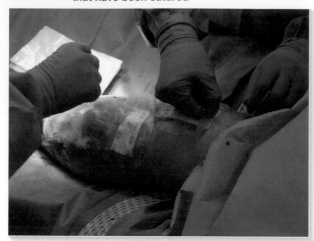

Source: All photos from Aintree University Hospital, Liverpool.

Any patient undergoing a surgical procedure is likely to need a dressing over the site of surgery. Surgical wounds vary and can include minor or major wounds, minimal-access surgery, trauma, small incisional cuts or excision of large areas of tissue. The purpose of wound dressings is to reduce the risk of infection and also to reduce pain, apply compression, immobilise injured areas, protect the wound and promote better healing. The wound needs to be assessed before applying the dressing to ensure that the most appropriate dressing is used.

Modes of healing

Primary intention healing involves closing and securing the wound using sutures, staples, steristrips (skin-closure strips) or glue. Healing occurs rapidly within about 10 days or so, assuming that no infection is present. Any leakage out of the wound after 2 days suggests that the wound is not healing or may be infected. **Secondary** intention healing is when a wound remains open and heals over time from the bottom of the wound upwards towards the skin (Rothrock 2010). Granulation and epithelial tissue fill the hole and eventually seal the wound. Secondary wound healing can occur following trauma where there is removal of a large area of tissue and the skin edges cannot be closed. **Tertiary** intention healing is when surgeons keep a wound open for up to 7 days, allowing exudate to drain out or infection to be treated. After that and once any problems have been resolved, the wound is closed using surgical techniques.

Infection of the wound is a major concern for surgeons, even though infection rates have fallen over the years because of better techniques and treatments (Rothrock 2010). *Staphylococcus aureus* is one of the most common causes of surgical infections, as it is part of patient's normal skin flora or can be passed from person to person, and therefore makes open wounds more likely to become infected. Another bacterium of importance is meticillin-resistant *Staphylococcus aureus* (MRSA), which is resistant to antibiotics and can lead to serious infection.

Types of dressings

Dressings protect open or closed wounds following surgery, and solve issues such as providing pain relief, debriding necrotic tissue, absorbing exudates and aiding in haemostasis. Dressings can be either adherent or non-adherent, and occlusive or non-occlusive. Occlusive dressings prevent the exchange of gases or water from the wound to the outer layer of the dressing (Pulman 2004). Adherent dressings are often made of gauze swabs, which are then held in place by, for example, sticky tape; semi-permeable thin, adhesive and transparent polyurethane film such as Opsite (Smith & Nephew, Figure 28.1); Tegaderm® (3 M); Soffban (Smith & Nephew), a soft natural viscose padding; and crepe bandages. As gauze adheres to tissue, removal of the dressing leads to debriding of the wound, removing necrotic or damaged tissues and foreign materials (Pulman 2004).

Opsite and Tegaderm are transparent, plastic-like adhesive film dressings that can cover wounds with a high level of exudate. Opsite allows the release of vapour, but not fluids, from the wound site, and prevents bacteria from accessing the site. A major advantage of this dressing is that practitioners can see the wound through the film, which can help in assessing whether the dressing needs to be removed. Removal of adherent dressings can also be painful, and adherence to tissues can lead to damage to underlying tissues and delayed wound healing (Pulman 2004).

Non-adherent dressings adhere to the tissues much less and reduce damage to tissues when removed. Occlusive or semi-occlusive dressings also prevent wound desiccation from happening, as fluids and vapours are not released from the dressing; this helps to encourage wound healing in a moist environment (Ignatavicius & Workman 2013).

Examples of semi-occlusive non-adherent dressings include Jelonet® or Tulle Gras® (Smith & Nephew) gauze, which are impregnated with paraffin or petrolatum. They are easy to remove from wound surfaces and tend not to damage tissues (Rothrock 2010). Non-adherent dry, thin perforated plastic film coating attached to an absorbent pad such as Melolin (Figure 28.2) or Melolite® (Smith & Nephew) are also non-adherent and absorb small amounts of exudate. Occlusive non-adherent dressings include hydrocolloid dressings such as Duoderm® (ConvaTec), hydrogels such as Intrasite® (Smith & Nephew) and foam dressings such as Allevyn® (Smith & Nephew). Hydrogels are effective at removing necrotic tissue from wounds because they absorb fluids that soak into the necrotic tissue, causing it to dissolve and be carried into the gel (Siddique *et al.* 2011). Foam dressings can also be used as secondary coverings for hydrogels in moderately exudative wounds (Siddique *et al.* 2011).

Bandages

Bandages are useful to hold dressings in place. However, they are also helpful in other ways, for example providing support for an injured limb, keeping dressings clean, reducing swelling and bleeding, and providing pain relief (Rothrock 2010). A bandage provides three layers of dressing: the dressing materials; cotton wool or synthetic material such as Soffban (Figure 28.3); and the bandage itself (Figure 28.4). Pressure bandages can also help to reduce swelling and minimise haemorrhage.

Complications

While dressings are essential for the protection of wounds, they can also cause problems. One of the most common problems is when they slip off the wound or move, for example around the limb, leading to discomfort or trauma if not recognised in time (Rothrock 2010). This can be caused by failing to tighten the bandage and fix it securely, or by adding too much padding underneath, allowing it to move around. Other complications include pressure sores, infection and hypoxic damage caused by extreme tightness of the bandage or covering. If there are signs of infection, swabs are taken and appropriate antibiotics given to the patient.

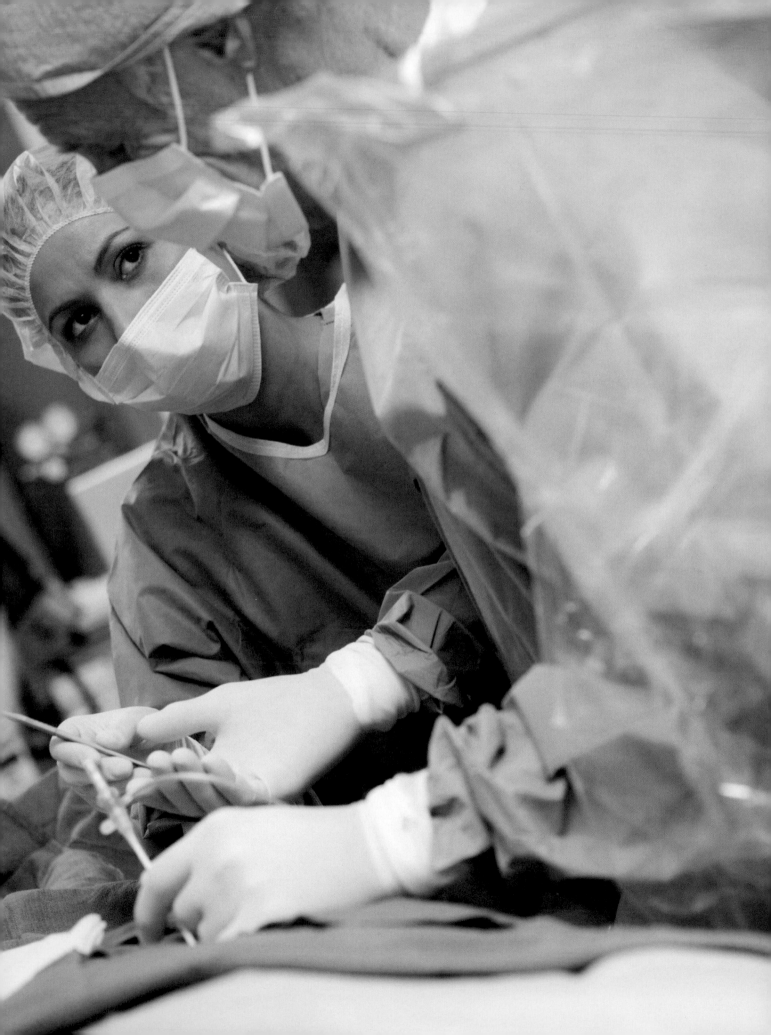

Recovery

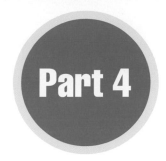

Part 4

Chapters

29 Introducing the recovery room   64
30 Patient handover   66
31 Postoperative patient care – Part 1   68
32 Postoperative patient care – Part 2   70
33 Monitoring in recovery   72
34 Maintaining the airway   74
35 Common postoperative problems   76
36 Managing postoperative pain   78
37 Managing postoperative nausea and vomiting   80

Introducing the recovery room

Figure 29.1 Patient being looked after in recovery by a recovery practitioner

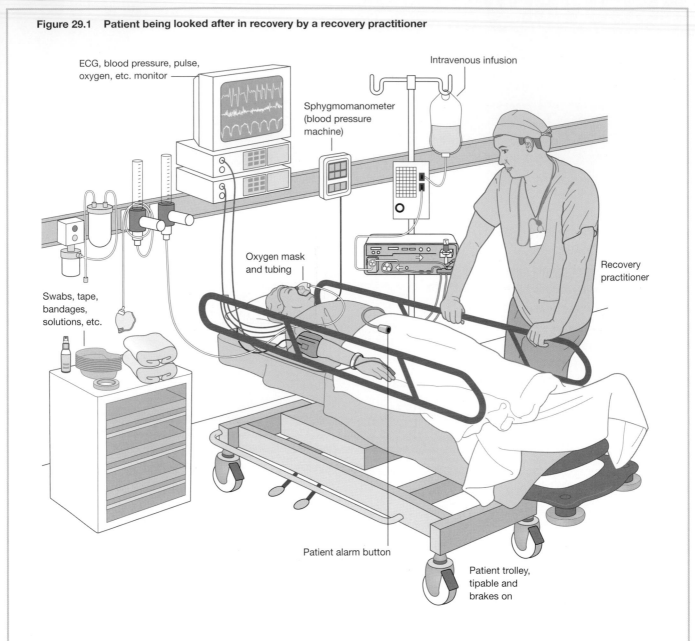

The recovery room, sometimes called the post-anaesthetic care unit (PACU), is part of the operating department. Recovery practitioners provide care for postoperative patients, detect and prevent complications, relieve patients' discomfort and closely monitor the patients' condition (Wicker & Cox 2010). On the patient's arrival, recovery practitioners check their condition regularly and stay at the bedside giving direct patient care (Hatfield and Tronson 2009). Essential equipment includes oxygen supplies, suction, ECG monitors, blood oxygen saturation (SpO_2) monitors, intubation equipment, cardiac arrest trolley and patient heating devices. When the patient recovers from anaesthesia and any problems have been resolved, practitioners arrange for their return to the ward. The recovery room usually supports patients for at least an hour, until they have recovered enough from the anaesthesia to be able to maintain their airway and to allow the effects of anaesthetic drugs to reduce.

To help the patient recover from the anaesthetic and surgery, the recovery room should be calm and relaxing, with a minimum amount of noise. Painting walls and ceilings in soft and pleasing colours helps to encourage relaxation. Indirect lighting is useful to prevent glare or harsh lights affecting patients as they wake up.

Caring for the postoperative patient

Recovery practitioners have special skills to care for a patient recovering from anaesthesia and surgery and must be able to carry out caring interventions to support and help the patient to recover (Wicker & Cox 2010). Airway maintenance is the primary role for practitioners, but observing wounds, drains, tubes and intravenous fluids, and reducing pain, are also important to preserve the patient's health. Ensuring that the patient's fluid balance is normal is vital because of blood loss during surgery, especially after lengthy surgery (Hatfield & Tronson 2009). Observing catheters and wound drainage tubes and preventing kinking or resolving blockages help to prevent problems caused by patients moving accidentally during the early stages of their recovery. It is also important to help the patient cough sputum up from the airways, and for them to take deep breaths several times regularly to ensure that their breathing and airways are clear. Dependent and lethargic patients, possibly following long anaesthesia and surgery or because they are elderly, are at risk of causing harm to themselves and therefore need constant supervision and monitoring (Smedley & Quine 2012).

The patient may need postoperative medicines during recovery, including anti-emetics, analgesics, antihypertensives and antibiotics (Wicker & Cox 2010). Safety measures may include keeping side rails raised; keeping the patient warm and comfortable; careful positioning of the patient to prevent discomfort and skin damage; ensuring that unconscious patients do not use a head pillow; and ensuring that a patient lying in the supine position has their head turned to one side so that secretions can drain from the mouth, as well as preventing the tongue from blocking the airway. Practitioners can prevent nosocomial infections by washing their hands, using soap and water, detergents or alcohol gel, both before and after working with each patient.

Patients who have undergone spinal anaesthesia

Patients who have been given spinal or epidural anaesthetics will be immovable for several hours. Practitioners should follow the patient's movements carefully and record any movements as they slowly recover. Spinal anaesthetics last longer than epidural anaesthetics. Spontaneous movements may lead to problems, such as the patient falling out of bed or damaging a limb. Therefore observing any patient movements after spinal anaesthesia is important until they start to recover. Spontaneous movements usually occur in the patient's toes and feet and then move up the legs. Feeling also returns after movement and as the anaesthetic wears off the patient begins to feel 'pins and needles' in their peripheries, slowly moving towards their body. Under normal circumstances, practitioners should keep patients supine for 6 to 8 hours to prevent spinal headache, which can occur if the patient sits up (Hatfield & Tronson 2009).

Patients who have undergone general anaesthesia

Maintaining the patient's airway is one of the most important tasks for the recovery practitioner. This will require knowledge and skills in managing an airway, the use of oxygen masks and Guedel airways, and resuscitation procedures. Practitioners must also observe and record the patient's level of consciousness until the patient fully recovers from the anaesthetic (Hatfield & Tronson 2009). This is needed because patients may lapse back into unconsciousness due to medication, and that can lead to airway and breathing problems. The patient can be categorised as **alert** (giving suitable responses to stimuli such as voices or pain), **drowsy** (half asleep and sluggish), **stupor** (lethargic and unresponsive, unaware of their surroundings) or **comatose** (unconscious and unresponsive to stimuli). To assess the level of consciousness, the practitioner should engage patients in a conversation to note their degree of orientation. Postoperative complications that need to be addressed can include issues such as nausea and vomiting, hypotension, pain, fluid imbalance, respiratory problems and cardiovascular problems (Hatfield & Tronson 2009; Smedley & Quine 2012).

Discharge from the recovery room

Once the patient has recovered from their anaesthetic, practitioners should tell them where they are and that practitioners are nearby and will help them as needed. It may also be advisable to tell the patient about the tasks the practitioner is going to be doing, for example checking the wound site or examining areas of the body. Once the patient has recovered, the ward staff will receive information before the patient leaves the recovery room. This includes the patient's name; type of surgery; mental alertness; recordings of vital signs; presence, type and functioning of drainage tubes, IV and so on; and the patient's general condition. All of this information is recorded on the patient's notes and then the patient can be transferred back to the ward.

(30) Patient handover

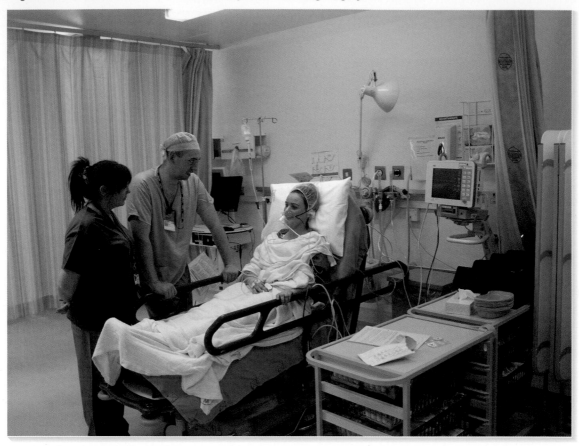

Source: Aintree University Hospital, Liverpool.

Admission into the recovery unit

An anaesthetist and a practitioner normally escort the patient from theatre into recovery. The recovery practitioner will ensure that the necessary equipment is readily available before the patient enters the recovery unit. This includes items such as an oxygen cylinder under the trolley for transporting the patient from theatre to recovery; an anaesthetic circuit for patients who have an endotracheal tube inserted; an oxygen mask for patients who are awake and extubated following surgery; and any other equipment needed to support the patient, for example monitors, intravenous infusion and medications (Wicker & Cox 2010). When the patient enters the recovery room, the recovery practitioner will receive a handover from the anaesthetist and the practitioner (Figure 30.1). The handover from the practitioner will include a description of the operative procedure carried out; the location of surgical drains, chest drains and IV cannulae; confirmation of a urinary catheter, nasogastric tube or any other tubes inserted into the patient; the method of skin closure used; the type of dressing used; and any problems that have developed during or following surgery, such as pressure sores, burns or damaged skin; information on care of the patient's belongings; and confirmation of the patient's records (Hughes & Mardell 2009). The handover from the anaesthetist will include the patient's name and the method of anaesthesia received; any relevant medical problems or past history; blood pressure, pulse and respiratory rate; analgesia administered during surgery and analgesia or medications prescribed for the patient while in recovery; types and quantities of intravenous fluid given during surgery and required in recovery; blood loss and urine output; quantity of oxygen required; and monitoring required while undergoing recovery (Hatfield & Tronson 2009). Before the anaesthetist leaves the patient to return to the operating room, the patient must be breathing and have a good oxygen saturation, stable blood pressure and normal pulse rate (Wicker & Cox 2010).

Initial assessment

On arrival in the recovery area, recovery practitioners check that unconscious patients are lying on their side with their head tilted backwards to keep the airway open, and that their blood pressure and pulse are at normal levels. The patient's oxygen supply is transferred from the oxygen cylinder to a pipeline supply, normally using a Hudson mask if the patient is already extubated. A simple Mapelson's C circuit (or Waters' circuit) may be used if the patient is still intubated. The anaesthetist will be responsible for removing the endotracheal tube or LMA if the recovery practitioner has not been trained to do so. Once the patient is assessed as breathing normally and is receiving adequate oxygen, they will be connected to standard monitoring (Hughes & Mardell 2009). Practitioners monitor patients for temperature, pulse rate and rhythm, ECG, blood pressure, oxygen saturation and respiratory rate, and inform the anaesthetist of any problems.

Assessing the patient using the ABCDE (airway, breathing, circulation, drugs/drips/drains/dressings, extras) approach is common practice (Hatfield & Tronson 2009; Younker 2008):

- The **airway** is assessed by checking breathing rate and watching the chest moving. Oxygen is normally administered at around 6 litres per minute and patient oxygenation will be monitored by the pulse oximeter. Suction can help to remove phlegm from the patient's mouth and pharynx, although this has to be undertaken carefully, under direct vision, in case it causes laryngospasm. If the patient is still unconscious, then the practitioner will insert an oral or nasal airway (Hughes & Mardell 2009).
- **Breathing** is assessed by feeling air flowing in and out of the mouth, and by listening to any abnormal sounds, such as rattles, crowing, gurgles, wheezes and stridor.
- **Circulation** is monitored by recording the blood pressure and pulse rate and rhythm. Intravenous fluids should be checked to ensure their flow rate, type of fluid, patency, and any problems with the location of the cannula. Wound dressings need to be monitored in case of excessive blood leakage, and drains and any other tubing should also be checked to ensure that they are flowing freely, and to measure the quantity of fluids exiting the wound.
- **Drugs** such as morphine are often given by the anaesthetist during surgery, and these may have an effect postoperatively on the patient's breathing and lucidity.
- **Extras** include, for example, air leaks, the patient's temperature, perfusion in the peripheries, blood glucose levels and wound condition.

While the ABCDE approach can be standardised for all patients, each patient nevertheless requires individualised care.

Documentation

Recording the patient's condition consistently, clearly and concisely while the patient is in the recovery room is important. The patient's records should contain information such as the time the patient entered the unit; recording of vital signs at regular intervals; any drugs that are given, including dosage and route; any untoward events; and any specific postoperative instructions. Before the patient leaves, the records also need to be signed and dated (Wicker & Cox 2010).

Discharge

Before returning to the ward, patients must meet appropriate criteria to ensure that they are safe and recovered from their anaesthetic. These criteria may include stable blood pressure, pulse rate and rhythm; being conscious and lucid; oxygen saturation at least 95%; any issues such as pain, nausea and vomiting resolved; the being clean, dry and warm; and all documentation being complete (Smith & Hardy 2007).

When the ward nurse arrives, the recovery practitioner will hand over all relevant information to ensure continuity of care to the patient, including the procedure that the patient has undergone; the type of wound closure and dressings; the anaesthetic and any drugs given, especially analgesics; location of drains, tubes or catheters; and postoperative instructions, including postoperative medications and the patient care delivered in the recovery room (Smith & Hardy 2007). Finally, the ward nurse will usually sign the record to agree to receive the handover of the patient.

31 Postoperative patient care – Part 1

Figure 31.1   Entering recovery

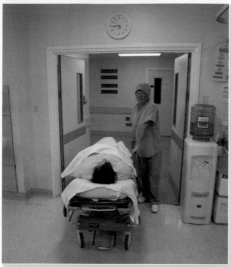

Respiration is influenced by:
• Pain
• Pulmonary oedema
• Opiates
• Airway obstruction

Observations required:
• Oxygen saturation
• Airway patency
• Chest movement
• Respiratory rate
• Blood pressure and pulse
• Skin colour

Box 31.2   Cardiovascular status

Cardiovascular status is influenced by:
• Pulmonary embolus
• Cardiac tamponade
• Tension pneumothorax
• Sepsis
• Anaphylaxis
• Adrenal insufficiency

Observations required:
• Blood pressure
• Peripheral oxygen saturation
• Pulse
• Respiration rate
• Temperature

Figure 31.3   Checking the patient's notes and surgical procedure

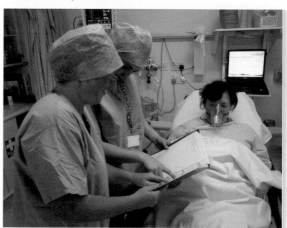

Figure 31.2   Patient feeling unwell

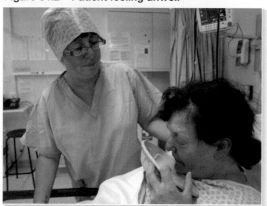

Source: All photos from Liverpool Women's Hospital.

Perioperative Practice at a Glance, First Edition. Paul Wicker. © 2015 John Wiley & Sons, Ltd. Published 2015 by John Wiley & Sons, Ltd.

Postoperative recovery observations include airway patency; respiratory status (rate and oxygen saturation); cardiovascular status (blood pressure and pulse); circulatory status (fluid balance and central venous pressure where available); temperature; haemorrhage/drainage volumes/vomiting/fluid balance; mental state; sweating/pallor; posture/facial expression; general condition, such as colour, orientation and responsiveness; and pain and discomfort (Figures 31.1, 31.2 and 31.3; Hatfield & Tronson 2009). The rationale behind these observations and interventions is to assess respiratory and cardiac function and the patient's general physical and psychological status, to maintain adequate ventilation and circulation, to identify and take action on any problems and to protect the patient from harm. Regular observations, compared against baseline observations taken preoperatively, help to assess the patient's condition following surgery and recovery from the anaesthetic and will accurately record the patient's progress. Practitioners observe patients by clinical monitoring and by general observation. The practitioner must have a sound knowledge and understanding of the patient's medical history, surgery and baseline vital signs. The ABCDE approach can assess the patient's Airway, Breathing, Circulation, Drugs/drips/dressings and Extras (Hatfield & Tronson 2009; see also Chapter 30). Recovery practitioners use record sheets or electronic forms that record observations clearly, and patient care plans that record other observations such as sweating, anxiety, vomiting, haemorrhage or fluid loss.

Respiratory status (Box 31.1)

Monitoring respiration is essential, as problems with respiration are one of the main causes of patient death during the immediate postoperative recovery. Respiratory status is also the first vital sign to be easily observed when the patient is deteriorating, either clinically or through general observation. Research studies, however, show that such monitoring is often omitted or respiration poorly assessed (NPSA 2007). Practitioners should regularly observe and record patency of the airway, breathing rate and depth, and any difficulties in breathing caused by respiratory depression or other causes. Practitioners always administer oxygen postoperatively until the patient is fully conscious and the effect of anaesthetic medications have reduced. Oxygen therapy helps to expel anaesthetic gases from the body, and is also required if the patient is under sedation from opiates. The anaesthetist prescribes oxygen therapy and lists the rate of administration and method of delivery.

Respiration is influenced by causes such as pain, pulmonary oedema, respiratory depression and airway obstruction. Changes in the patient's physiological state (for example cardiac problems) can also affect respiration. Pulse oximetry is used to monitor a patient's pulse and oxygen saturations. Patients receive oxygen therapy to maintain oxygen saturations above 95% and to prevent hypoxia or hypoxaemia (Anderson 2003). If oxygen saturation drops below 95% then the anaesthetist should be informed, as respiratory function will be compromised, resulting in inadequate tissue perfusion and hypoxia. Signs of respiratory complications can also be identified when the patient develops conditions such as disorientation, breathlessness, tachycardia, headaches and cyanosis.

Breathing and chest movements are normally symmetrical, regular and effortless. A normal breathing pattern in the postoperative patient is 12–20 breaths per minute. Above 24 breaths per minute, below 10 breaths per minute or apnoea needs further investigation and appropriate action (Anderson 2003). Opiates can cause a low respiratory rate, which may induce respiratory depression. To promote adequate ventilation postoperatively, it is advisable to monitor the patient's respiratory function closely, help the patient to turn from side to side, if possible, and assist with coughing. These measures will improve the patient's respiration and reduce the potential risk of pulmonary complications such as atelectasis (the collapse of a segment of the lung), bronchitis or pneumonia. While patients are still recovering from anaesthesia and in a semi-conscious state, they should be positioned in a lateral or semi-prone position without a pillow under their head, unless contraindicated by the surgery that they have undertaken. In the lateral position, the head can be hyperextended, taking care not to cause damage to the neck, which supports the easy passage of air into and out of the lungs and reduces the chance of the tongue falling back to block the airway. The lateral position also reduces the risk of aspiration should the patient vomit or have excessive mucous secretions, which can lead to atelectasis (Jevon & Ewens 2002).

Cardiovascular status (Box 31.2)

Monitoring haemodynamic stability is important because of the body's physiological response to stress and the risk of shock and haemorrhage based on the nature of the operation, as well as the method of pain control. Indicators of haemodynamic stability include blood pressure, peripheral oxygen saturation, pulse rate and rhythm, respiration rate and temperature. Measuring these indicators can be undertaken using electronic equipment or traditional manual equipment. Depending on their situation, patients may benefit from CVP monitoring in the ward environment to assess circulatory volume (Hatfield & Tronson 2009).

Hypovolaemic shock occurs when systolic blood pressure falls significantly, leading to inadequate tissue perfusion, cellular damage and possibly organ failure (NCEPOD 2001). Because the body compensates for fluid loss, patients can lose up to 30 per cent of their circulatory volume before systolic blood pressure measurements and heart rate are affected (Jevon & Ewens 2009). Poor tissue perfusion, however, can be an early indicator of hypovolaemic shock. Signs include restlessness or confusion because of cerebral hypoperfusion or hypoxia, tachycardia, hypotension, low urine output, increased temperature and cold peripheries. The reason for treating hypovolaemic shock is to restore adequate tissue perfusion. This may require blood transfusion or fluid resuscitation with crystalloid or colloid solutions, and increased oxygenation to maintain saturation above 95%.

Cardiogenic shock is another postoperative complication that results in the death of many acutely ill surgical patients (NCEPOD 2001). This may be caused by the failure of the myocardial 'pump' in response to surgery. During surgery the metabolic demands of the body increase and adrenaline (epinephrine) and noradrenaline (norepinephrine) are released as the heart rate increases. Tissues and cells of the body then need more oxygen, which places extra pressure on the myocardium, resulting in cardiac arrhythmia or myocardial infarction (Jevon & Ewens 2002). Treating cardiogenic shock requires close observation, appropriate levels of oxygen, and drug therapy such as digoxin to treat arrhythmias and improve contractility of the heart (Anderson 2003).

32 Postoperative patient care – Part 2

Figure 32.1 Example of a postoperative patient care plan

RECOVERY ROOM CARE

Key: ✓ = Yes   X = No   N/A = Not applicable   ★ = Indicates refer to recovery progress notes

Level of sedation score:-   0. Awake, Alert, Orientated   1. Drowsy, Asleep, Easy to rouse
   2. Drowsy/Difficult to rouse   3. Anaesthetised/Sedated, Unresponsive

Admission Time [ ]   Full hand over received [ ]

Immediate Care Assessment - on admission to recovery
UNDERTAKE A MEWS SCORE WITHIN APPROX, TEN MINUTES OF ADMISSION TO RECOVERY

AIRWAY SUPPORT

None [ ]   Oral [ ]   Nasal tube [ ]   ETT [ ]   LM [ ]   Trache [ ]   Jaw hold [ ]

BREATHING

Resps   Rate ....   Quality ....

O2

Litres [ ]   % [ ]   Humidified [ ]

Venti Mask [ ]   Ventilator [ ]   Nasal Specs [ ]   Breathing circuit [ ]   Temp [ ]   Sats SpO$_2$ [ ]

CIRCULATION

Arterial line   None [ ]   *in situ* [ ]   Site ....   Time removed ....
   BP ....   Pulse ....

Skin/   Flushed [ ]   Pale [ ]   Cyanosis [ ]   Pink [ ]   Other [ ]
Mucus
Membrane   Warm [ ]   Dry [ ]   Cool [ ]   Moist [ ]   Clammy [ ]

Sedation score ....

Intravenous Therapies in situ / site specify:-

Bladder Irrigation Present [ ]   Patent [ ]   **Colour**   Red [ ]   Pink [ ]   Clear [ ]
   Blood Clots [ ]

Comments:

Is a chest drain present? [ ]   **If yes, is it patent** [ ]

Source: Aintree University Hospital, Liverpool. Reproduced with permission of Aintree University Hospital.

Perioperative Practice at a Glance, First Edition. Paul Wicker. © 2015 John Wiley & Sons, Ltd. Published 2015 by John Wiley & Sons, Ltd.

This second chapter on postoperative patient care covers monitoring of the patient's temperature and their general care (Figure 32.1).

Temperature status

Body temperature is a critical issue in postoperative care and can result in either hypothermia or hyperthermia. Perioperative hypothermia occurs more often than hyperthermia and is defined as a core temperature of less than 36 °C (ASPN 2001, NICE 2008). Children, elderly patients and patients who have been in theatre for a long time are at risk of hypothermia. Reasons for this include open abdominal or chest wounds, cold IV fluids, medications given before and during surgery, and exposure of the body to a cold theatre environment. The patient's temperature needs to be monitored closely and action taken to return it to within the normal level of 37 °C, plus or minus 0.5 °C (NICE 2008). Forced-air blankets such as Bair Huggers® (3M) or other blankets can help to warm the patient if their temperature is too low; alternatively antipyretics, fanning or tepid sponging can be used if their temperature is too high.

Hypothermia can be identified in a patient who is shivering, has peripheral vasoconstriction and has 'goose pimples' or piloerection of the hair on their body. Patients undergoing general anaesthesia have no control over body heat as they are unconscious and anaesthetic drugs affect their physiology. The result of hypothermia can include skin and tissue breakdown, increased risk of infection, and low blood supply to non-vital organs, the intestinal tract and the skin (ASPN 2001). Cardiac workload can also increase as the arterioles constrict, leading to greater pressure on the heart to pump blood around the body (Stanhope 2006). Increased metabolic activity in cold patients can lead to physiological problems such as a higher risk of shivering, increased carbon dioxide production, respiratory acidosis, increased cardiac output, increased oxygen consumption, decreased platelet function, increased blood loss during surgery, altered drug metabolism and increased risk of cardiac events (Kiekkas et al. 2005).

Core temperature measurement relates to the thoracic, cranium and abdominal cavities. The shell temperature relates to the temperature of the skin or periphery of the body (Stanhope 2006). The core temperature is indicative of the internal temperature of the body, which usually remains fairly stable unless there are extremes of hypothermia. Pulmonary artery catheters, which mirror the temperature of the heart, can measure core temperature, as can oesophageal and nasopharyngeal probes. Oesophageal probes mirror the temperature proximal to the heart, and nasopharyngeal probes mirror the temperature of the hypothalamus. These three methods are invasive and so cannot be used on all patients, but depend on their postoperative status (NICE 2008).

Common peripheral temperature measurement methods and sites include the bladder, skin, dot matrix and liquid crystal thermometers, rectal, oral, axillary and tympanic sites. Bladder temperature measurements are rarely used and require a thermistor in an indwelling Foley catheter within the bladder. Skin temperature sensors, liquid crystal thermometers (attached to the forehead) and dot matrix thermometers (a plastic strip with temperature-sensitive dots that change colour) are rarely used in postoperative recovery, as they tend not to be accurate and may give false or unreliable readings. Rectal temperature measurement is not often carried out, as the rectal temperature is not consistent with the core temperature because of the low blood flow in the rectum (Kiekkas et al. 2009). Axillary temperature monitoring is common and matches core temperature well, unless the patient is hypothermic, and then the skin temperature does not match the core temperature. Finally, tympanic measurements match core temperature very closely, even when the body temperature is changing rapidly. Tympanic temperatures closely match the temperature of the hypothalamus and the blood supply in the internal carotids, which are both close to the tympanic membrane (NICE 2008).

General patient care

The main aims of recovery practitioners when looking after patients in the recovery room are to keep them comfortable and safe (Alfaro 2013). The roles of the recovery practitioner therefore cover many areas other than those discussed here and in Chapter 31, and include the following:

- Observing and recording the functioning of tubes, drains and intravenous fluids, including preventing kinking or blocking of catheters and drainage tubes (Hatfield & Tronson 2009).
- Monitoring areas such as IVs, blood products, urine, emesis and nasogastric tube drainage, and recording their intake and output of fluids.
- Implementing safety measures to protect unconscious or disorientated patients. For example, keeping the patient warm and comfortable, showing the patient how to use the call bell, keeping side rails in the high position, and maintaining a good position for the patient to help breathing, comfort and relaxation (Alfaro 2013).
- Preventing the spread of infection by washing your hands before and after working with each patient, and maintaining aseptic technique when caring for wounds.
- Observing and recording recovery from general, regional, epidural and spinal anaesthesia.
- Engaging the patient in a conversation, whenever possible, to assess the level of orientation and to let the patient know the actions the practitioner is taking and the help that can be offered.
- Relaying information to the patient from the surgeon and anaesthetist about the procedures that have taken place (Alfaro 2013).

Family members may be allowed to sit near the patient in the recovery room. If this is the case, then a recovery practitioner should always be close by the patient in case of sudden changes in condition or emergency situations. This is to support the family and prevent them from being too worried. Most of the recovery practitioner's time is spent at the bedside giving direct patient care, since the observation, recording or care of a patient cannot usually be conducted from any other location.

33 Monitoring in recovery

Figure 33.1 Checking the patient's temperature postoperatively to check for any problems related to hypothermia or hyperthermia

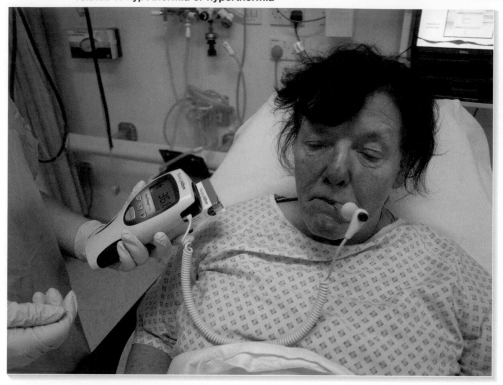

Source: Liverpool Women's Hospital.

Figure 33.2 Complex selection of monitoring devices used to care for patients safely.

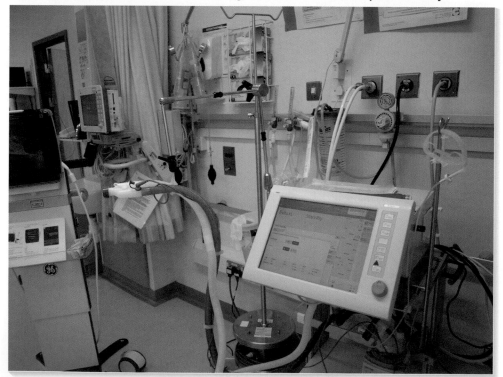

Source: Aintree University Hospital, Liverpool.

Perioperative Practice at a Glance, First Edition. Paul Wicker. © 2015 John Wiley & Sons, Ltd. Published 2015 by John Wiley & Sons, Ltd.

This chapter provides overall guidelines on the need for monitoring of patients in recovery, with the goal of optimising patient safety. However, monitoring of individual patients depends on the needs of each patient, which the recovery practitioner assesses. Postanaesthetic care of the patient may include the regular assessment and monitoring of respiratory and cardiovascular function, neuromuscular function, mental status, temperature, pain, nausea and vomiting, drainage and bleeding, and urine output.

Respiratory monitoring

Assessment and monitoring of respiratory function during recovery, using pulse oximetry, helps in the early detection of hypoxaemia. The practitioner may also detect respirator problems by checking breathing, chest movement and signs of cyanosis in the patient (Hatfield & Tronson 2009). Therefore, regular assessment and monitoring of airway patency, respiratory rate and SpO$_2$ are important during early recovery from anaesthesia. In some recovery units practitioners can extubate patients, but if this is the case they must have been trained formally to undertake this task.

Cardiovascular monitoring

Cardiovascular assessment and monitoring help to identify perioperative complications caused by anaesthetic drugs and surgery. Routine pulse, blood pressure and electrocardiographic monitoring detect any cardiovascular complications and reduce the possibility of adverse reactions, and should always be carried out during the recovery phase.

Neuromuscular monitoring

Most patients undergoing general anaesthesia and intermediate or major surgery receive neuromuscular blocking agents. These drugs paralyse muscles, allowing anaesthesia and surgery to progress. The recovery practitioner can assess neuromuscular function by physical examination, although during anaesthesia it is also common practice to use a neuromuscular blockade monitor that is effective in detecting neuromuscular dysfunction (Jones et al. 1992). Assessment of neuromuscular function helps to identify potential complications, such as difficulty in breathing or moving of limbs. This reduces adverse outcomes, especially in patients who received long-acting non-depolarising neuromuscular blocking agents or who have medical conditions associated with neuromuscular dysfunction.

Psychological monitoring

The effect of anaesthetic drugs, such as propofol or ketamine, and the physiological effects of surgery can influence the patient's mental and psychological condition, causing anxiety, distress, anger and disruption (RCPRCP 2003). Assessment of the patient's mental status and behaviour reduces postoperative complications, such as wound damage, blocking of tubes or removal of catheters by the patient, and reduces the possibility of harm to the patient. Several types of scoring systems are available for such assessment, including those described by the Joanna Briggs Institute (JBI 2011).

Temperature monitoring

The patient's temperature can change radically because of the physiological effects of anaesthesia and surgery, and in recovery due to, for example, the delivery of cold IV fluids or the lack of warming blankets. Routine assessment of patient temperature (Figure 33.1) can help reduce postoperative complications such as hypothermia or hyperthermia (see Chapter 32), detect complications and reduce adverse outcomes during recovery.

Pain monitoring

Analgesics are given during surgery, but may wear off during the recovery phase, leading to postoperative pain. Pain can be assessed by simply asking the patient about their pain, or by asking them to complete a numerical assessment form (Rawlinson et al. 2012). For example, if a patient says that the pain score is 10, then they are seriously in need of analgesia. A score of 1 or 2 may not require analgesics. Routine and regular assessment and monitoring of pain will assist in detecting complications and will help the patient to be pain free and comfortable during their recovery.

Monitoring nausea and vomiting

Postoperative nausea and vomiting (PONV) occur in around 30% of postoperative patients (Smith et al. 2012). This results in conditions such as distress, aspiration into the lungs, poor analgesia, dehydration and damage to surgical wounds. Regular assessment and monitoring of nausea and vomiting will therefore detect complications and improve patient outcomes. Assessing the patient can involve watching their physiological state and asking them how they are feeling. Risk assessment of PONV can also be carried out before surgery (Rawlinson et al. 2012). If a patient does vomit, then anti-emetic drugs such as Ondansetron can be given. Unconscious patients should be placed on their side to lessen the chance of inhaling vomit.

Fluid monitoring

Fluid balance refers to the input and output of fluids in the body to assist metabolic processes. Regular postoperative assessment of the patient's hydration status and fluid management reduces problems and improves patient comfort and satisfaction. Fluid balance can be assessed using blood pressure, pulse, observation of the patient's hydration status, a review of the fluid charts and, if necessary, a review of blood chemistry (Shepherd 2011). Surgical procedures that involve a significant loss of blood or fluids may need extra fluid management.

Urine output and voiding

Assessment of urine output detects complications and can reduce adverse outcomes such as dehydration. Assessment of urine output during recovery is not carried out on all patients, but should be done for selected patients, for example those undergoing urological surgery, or patients who are susceptible to fluid imbalances (Hatfield & Tronson 2009).

Drainage and bleeding

Assessment and monitoring of drainage and bleeding detect complications, reduce adverse outcomes, and should be a routine part of recovery care. Drainage can originate from chest drains or wound drains; excessive blood loss in either case needs to be referred to the surgeon or anaesthetist so that action can be taken if required. Fluid or blood loss should be recorded in the patient's notes and regularly monitored.

34 Maintaining the airway

Figure 34.1   Oral airway and face mask

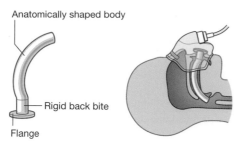

Anatomically shaped body

Rigid back bite

Flange

Figure 34.2   Tracheostomy

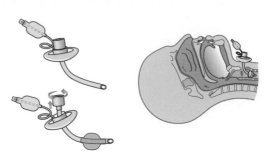

Figure 34.3   Nasopharyngeal airway

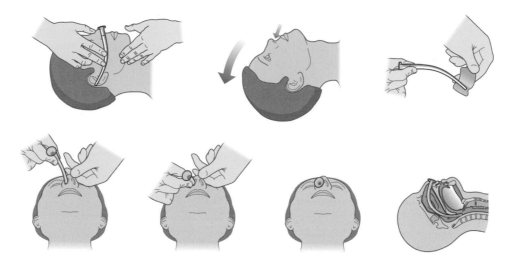

Figure 34.4   Endotracheal tube

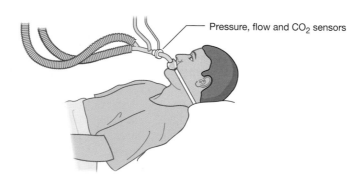

Pressure, flow and CO_2 sensors

Perioperative Practice at a Glance, First Edition. Paul Wicker. © 2015 John Wiley & Sons, Ltd. Published 2015 by John Wiley & Sons, Ltd.

Postoperative patients in the recovery room or PACU will always need airway management and close monitoring to prevent any serious postoperative complications (Scott 2012). If practitioners ignore airway management, then the patient may become hypoxic, resulting in organ failure and eventually death. Therefore, a thorough understanding of the airway management of patients during recovery is essential for practitioners so that they can provide the best care for patients emerging from anaesthetic (AAGBI 2013a). Staffing levels need to be appropriate (AAGBI 2013a) to support patients. A minimum of two staff should be present in the recovery room and a minimum of one member of staff should be allocated to each individual patient until they can maintain their own airway, breathing and circulation. Anaesthetists are responsible for the safe extubation of patients in recovery, but they can delegate this task to appropriately trained practitioners.

Equipment and facilities must also be suitable for the care of unconscious patients. Recovery units are close to operating rooms and must fulfil the requirements of the AAGBI and Department of Health (AAGBI 2013a). Patients need easy access to emergency call systems in the case of sudden emergencies. Oxygen and suction, delivered via pipelines and devices attached to the wall, must be available in each recovery bay (Dolenska et al. 2004). Other equipment needed to monitor breathing and circulation includes pulse oximetry, non-invasive blood pressure monitoring, an electrocardiograph and, if the patient is intubated, a capnographic monitor is needed to monitor CO_2. Patients requiring resuscitation will also need specific drugs, fluids and resuscitation equipment (including a defibrillator), which should be available in every recovery room (AAGBI 2013b).

Physiology of the airway

Airway obstruction can occur because of several reasons, including sedation from drugs such as opioids, the tongue falling back against the posterior pharyngeal wall, foreign bodies in the mouth, false teeth, damaged crowns and throat packs (Dolenska et al. 2004). Partial airway obstruction may result in inspiratory stridor, expiratory wheeze or a crowing noise, whereas complete obstruction results in no chest movement and lack of airflow (AAGBI 2013b). Physiological obstructions can be prevented by placing the unconscious patient in the lateral position with their head tilted backwards and jaw moved forwards (jaw thrust). Instruments such as Yankeur suckers or McGill forceps can be used to remove obstructions.

Breathing results in gas exchange between the lungs and the blood, which supplies oxygen to the tissues and eliminates CO_2. Failure to breathe effectively, caused by pain, drugs, obstruction or laryngospasm, can result in an increase of partial pressure of carbon dioxide ($PaCO_2$), leading to respiratory acidosis (West 2008). Respiratory acidosis can cause tachycardia, vasodilation, coma and cardiac arrest (Aitkenhead et al. 2007). The anaesthetist should be informed as soon as any breathing problems are identified and if necessary the patient may be reintubated.

Circulation

The respiratory and circulatory systems are linked to each other: one provides oxygen and the other supplies that to the tissues. As the circulatory system provides cells with oxygenated blood, an inefficient circulatory system will increase the demands on the patient's respiratory system. Hypovolaemia can result in hypotension, leading to inadequate tissue perfusion and cellular hypoxia as well as a reduction in pulmonary blood flow. This results in an imbalance in the ratio of ventilation and perfusion of oxygen in the body tissues (Scott 2012). Monitoring the circulatory system, blood pressure, pulse and perfusion is therefore important for airway management.

Monitoring of the airway

Regular checking of respiratory status supports the delivery of treatment in case of problems (AAGBI 2013b). Clinical observations provide prompt feedback on the patient's status, whereas monitoring of patients can sometimes be overlooked or provide false readings (Scott 2012). Monitoring is essential for physiological variables such as respiratory acidosis or blood gas analysis. Clinical observation involves checking and assessing the patient's respiratory status. Airway assessments include listening to breathing to identify any obstructions, observing bilateral chest movement, observing for tracheal tug (caused by accessory muscles around the neck), which indicates airway blockage, and irregular breathing patterns indicating partial or complete obstruction (Scott 2012). Observing cyanosis and decreased peripheral perfusion will suggest problems with the airway, breathing and circulatory systems. Pulse oximetry to detect SpO_2 and blood pressure measurements will detect early signs of hypoxaemia and circulatory problems.

Postoperative airway complications

Practitioners often use Yankeur suckers under direct vision to clear the airway of fluids, vomit or sputum. Alternatively, a flexible suction catheter can be passed through an endotracheal tube to remove secretions below the cuff of intubated patients. Care needs to be taken when suctioning, as excessive use may lead to trauma and oedema. Irritation of the vocal chords caused by fluids or foreign bodies may lead to laryngospasm. Laryngospasm is a serious airway complication that occurs as the vocal chords contract, obstructing the airway (Scott 2012). Treatment can involve using the jaw thrust to expose the airway, followed by suctioning and administration of 100% oxygen. If laryngospasm continues, then reintubation may be needed.

Medications such as opioids, muscle relaxants and inhalation agents given during anaesthesia can have ongoing effects postoperatively. The action of these drugs may be reversed, or alternatively the patient may need to be reintubated until the effects wear off.

Discharge criteria

Most recovery rooms have set criteria for the discharge of patients. As a minimum, this should include patients being conscious, able to breathe and maintain their own airway, having reduced pain, being normothermic and free of cardiovascular problems. A handover must also be given to the ward nurse explaining anaesthesia and surgery, any perioperative complications and the anaesthetist and surgeon's postoperative care instructions.

35 Common postoperative problems

Table 35.1   Postoperative complications

The prevalence of postoperative complications in a research study into postoperative patients who had undergone cardiac surgery (Lobo *et al.* 2008), which showed that the patient population had an overall major complication rate of 38.3% and 90-day mortality rate of 20.3%

Complications	Definitions	Frequency
Sepis/severe sepis/septic shock	ACCP/SCCM[1]	135 (22.9)
Extubation failure	Failure to extubate in the first 24 hours after the operation or the need for reintubation within 72 hours after extubation	59 (10.0)
Gastrointestinal dysfunction	Intolerance to feeding after 5 days of the operation or the need for parenteral nutrition	47 (8.0)
Cardiac adverse event	Unexpected cardiac arrest and/or acute myocardial infarction	34 (5.6)
Severe bleeding	Transfusion of more than 2 units of RBC or reoperation was necessary	32 (5.5)
Heart failure	Classical signs and symptoms or worsening in relation to preoperative status	32 (5.5)
Pulmonary oedema	Radiological signs of vascular hypertension and clinical signs of congestion	27 (4.6)
Fistula or anastomosis leak	Abnormal communication between two epithelised surfaces or anastomosis breakdown requiring reintervention	30 (5.1)
Surgical site infection	CDC definitions[2]	30 (5.1)
Shock	Refractory hypotension despite fluid resuscitation and need for vasoacti	24 (4.0)
Nosocomial pneumonia	CDC definitions[2]	10 (1.7)
Urinary tract infection	CDC definitions[2]	10 (1.7)
Venous thromboembolism or pulmonary embolism	Confirmed by spiral CT or perfusion scintilography or autopsy	7 (1.2)
Bloodstream infection	CDC definitions[2]	6 (1.0)
Cerebral vascular accident	Confirmed by CT	6 (1.0)

ACCP/SCCM – American College of Chest Physicians/Society of Critical Care Medicine;
RBC – red blood cells; CDC – Centers for Disease Control; CT – computed tomography.
Results are expressed in N(%)

1. ACCP/SCCMCC (1992)
2. Garner *et al.* (1988)

Source: Lobo *et al.*, 2008. Reproduced under the Creative Commons Attribution License.

Most postoperative problems include issues such as respiratory and cardiovascular status, PONV, pain and bleeding (Hood *et al.* 2011). However, other problems can arise that are more unusual and may not be immediately identified by the practitioner. Practitioners must be aware of issues that can arise when they are not expecting them to occur, so that they can be dealt with quickly (Table 35.1).

Allergy

Allergies happen when the body reacts against foreign substances. These include medicines (such as morphine, codeine or muscle relaxants), blood and blood products, plasma expanders, fluids, foods or latex. Allergies commonly result in rashes, oedema, airway obstruction and hypotension (Hatfield & Tronson 2009). An allergic response that occurs within one hour is called an immediate allergic response. This is considered to be a medical emergency, as the patient may develop anaphylactic shock that may affect the whole body, leading to airway obstruction and hypotension as the main problems. Avoiding allergies in postoperative patients includes giving intravenous drugs slowly while supervising the patient's blood pressure, skin condition and breathing. The anaesthetist needs to be informed of negative reactions to drugs or fluids given to the patient so that relevant action can be taken urgently (Hatfield & Tronson 2009).

Haemorrhage

Haemorrhage can occur following surgery when the patient is in recovery. When cardiac output and blood pressure return to normal, this can lead to dry wounds starting to bleed. Major postoperative bleeding can be identified by evidence of overt bleeding from the wound itself, or bloodstained fluid from a drain. Other signs include cyanosed or white peripheries, hypovolaemia, tachycardia, hypotension, tachypnoea and low-volume urine output (Hatfield & Tronson 2009). Intra-abdominal bleeding can lead to distension of the abdomen. Bleeding is controlled by identifying the source of bleeding, such as leaking arterioles in wound edges, putting pressure on the wound or reapplying a dressing if it is bleeding, or correction of any coagulopathy. To give patients a blood or fluid transfusion, assessment of blood loss and hypovolaemic status will be needed. In some circumstances, the patient may need to return to the operating room for surgery to control an area of internal bleeding.

Septic shock

Septic shock can occur following surgical procedures carried out when the patient is already infected or septic. Other causes include leakage into the abdomen of gastrointestinal contents from the bowel during anastomosis, spreading of microbes from a surgical area when the body has impaired immunity or leucopenia, or contamination from devices or instruments used during surgery or anaesthesia, for example contaminated intravenous cannulas, suction devices or instruments. Cells in the immune system secrete circulating cytokines, which can cause arteriolar dilatation leading to the peripheries becoming warm. Septic shock can also cause a loss of circulating blood volume because of capillary leakage (Hatfield & Tronson 2009). When septic shock becomes serious, the systolic blood pressure can reduce below 100 mmHg, mirroring hypovolaemia. Usually the clinical features of septic shock include pyrexia, hypotension, tachycardia and a warm periphery. To identify the causes of septic shock, venous blood is sent for culture; following identification of the infection, treatment will be started with a combination of effective antibiotics and intravenous fluids. Identification of the focus of the infection is also important as the cause may be, for example, an intravenous catheter or urinary catheter. Further surgery may be needed if infected devices have been inserted into the body or tissue abscesses develop.

Intravascular catheters

Central venous catheters, arterial catheters or peripheral intravenous catheters may cause infection, bleeding or thrombus formation (Hatfield & Tronson 2009). In one research study, complications related to initial catheter placement occurred in 5.7% of cases, sepsis in 6.5% of cases, and mechanical difficulties (such as major venous thrombosis or patient care mishaps) in 9% of cases (Henry & Thomson 2012). Adherence to careful techniques, monitoring of the patient and the use of heparin-coated catheters can help to prevent these incidents. Complications caused by faulty placement of central venous catheters include haemorrhage or pneumothorax, in which case the catheter needs to be removed urgently and the patient may be given surgical treatment and parenteral antibiotic therapy.

Urinary complications

Placement of a urinary catheter can lead to several complications, such as infection, damage to the urethra, internal bleeding, urinary tract infection (Wicker & Cox 2010) and sometimes even death. Aseptic techniques are therefore critical for the care of patients. The distal urethra is colonised with bacteria in 1% of patients. Following surgery, the average infection rate is 10%; however, up to 75% of urological and medical infections are related to a urinary tract infection. One of the most common pathogens is *Escherichia coli* (*E. coli*), and other pathogens can include staphylococci, streptococci and enterococci (Henry & Thomson 2012). If the patient is infected, practitioners should remove the catheter immediately and give antibiotics and fluid therapy to encourage high-volume urine output.

Wound dehiscence

Wounds can burst open during recovery because of coughing leading to a rise of intra-abdominal pressure, or due to poor surgical technique. Often the dehiscence can be deep and concealed, with separation of all layers of the abdominal wall except for the skin. If this is not recognised immediately, and given that the skin remains united, an incisional hernia may develop. Alternatively, an abdominal wound can burst open following surgery, leading to protrusion of a loop of bowel or a portion of the omentum through the wound (Henry & Thomson 2012). However, the chance of this happening is low, as closure of the abdominal wall is performed using suitable suture materials that are slowly absorbed or non-absorbable, and are also strong and resilient. Management of dehiscence depends on the impact on the wound site, but the result can be a return to the operating room for resuturing of the wound (Wicker & Cox 2010).

Other issues

Many other complications can happen postoperatively, such as pressure sores, upper gastrointestinal bleeding, respiratory complications and myocardial infarction. Recovery practitioners therefore need a thorough understanding of all possible complications so that they can keep the patient safe from harm.

Managing postoperative pain

Figure 36.1   A pain rating scale

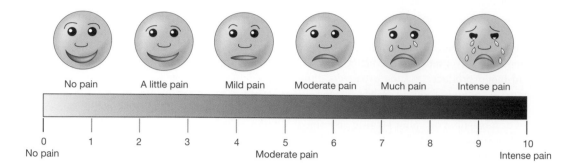

No pain   A little pain   Mild pain   Moderate pain   Much pain   Intense pain

| 0 | 1 | 2 | 3 | 4 | 5 | 6 | 7 | 8 | 9 | 10 |

No pain   Moderate pain   Intense pain

**Figure 36.2   A PCAM® syringe pump which monitors the patients use of pain killers.
The patient administers the pain killer by pressing the button attached to the black cable**

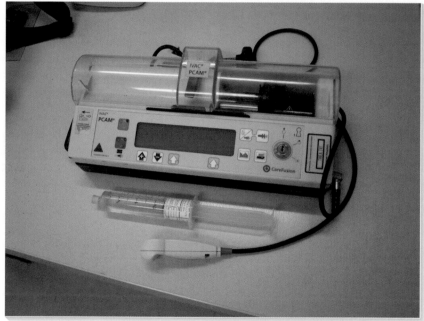

Source: Aintree University Hospital, Liverpool.

Reducing postoperative pain requires practitioners to monitor, assess and treat pain effectively (Wicker & Cox 2010). Inadequate pain control may result in increased morbidity or mortality, leading to further postoperative complications. Data suggests that local anaesthetics are the most effective analgesics, followed by opioids and non-steroidal anti-inflammatory agents (Kehlet 1998). Managing postoperative pain improves patient comfort and satisfaction and encourages earlier mobilisation. Pain relief also reduces pulmonary and cardiac complications and improves recovery time (Kehlet 1998). There are several reasons why patients are not always given pain relief, for example lack of knowledge or understanding, complications associated with opioids, poor pain assessment, and inadequate staffing in the recovery room.

Concept of pain

Pain is a subjective experience, therefore assessing pain depends mostly on the person experiencing it (Wicker & Cox 2010). A practitioner cannot assess pain in a patient unless the patient describes or shows signs of suffering pain. One patient may suffer pain but be able to control their perception of it, while another patient may feel less pain but suffer more as a result. Pain is therefore what the patient says hurts, and their emotional response to it (Hatfield & Tronson 2009).

Effects of pain

Pain has systemic effects on the body, caused by physiological and emotional reactions to the source of the pain. Pain contributes to postoperative nausea and vomiting because of raised anxiety levels and effects on the vomiting centre in the brain. There is also a risk of increased blood pressure, leading to problems such as cardiac ischaemia, headache, increased bleeding from wounds or damaged tissues (Hatfield & Tronson 2009). Other effects of pain include an increased metabolic rate, decreased hepatic and renal blood supplies, abnormal bowel function and breathing difficulties.

Pain physiology

Pain physiology is complex, so it will only be covered superficially here. Nociceptors, which are pain receptors found in tissues throughout the body, send impulses to sensory nerves, which then carry the sensation of pain to the spinal cord and from there to the brain (Hatfield & Tronson 2009). Once it is in the brain, the pain is analysed and acted on by other parts of the brain. For example, if a man was burned by a hot item, he would scream and let go. Then he would cool down the burnt area with cold water and consider treatment needed to protect the area from further damage. At the same time, areas of the central nervous system would increase blood pressure and pulse, sweating and anxiety levels (Wicker & Cox 2010). The area of pain is also likely to become inflamed and oedematous due to the release of chemicals from the cells. White cells and macrophages then flood the area with chemicals in an effort to clean away dead cells and start the repair process, which leads to further pain by stimulating the nociceptors.

Managing pain

The **first stage** in managing pain is to find out its cause. Postoperative pain is caused by surgery, especially if the surgery was major. Pain can originate from muscles that have been divided, from skin grafts, from organs in the body, such as a bowel that has been divided, and any other areas where tissues have been cut or damaged during surgery. Psychological factors also play a part in pain perception. However, patients will feel less pain if they received support from practitioners to alleviate the pain through medicines or by being moved into a more comfortable position (Wicker & Cox 2010).

The **second stage** is to assess the pain. The primary way to assess pain is to ask patients – if they say they are in terrible pain, then they will need urgent help to reduce the level of pain. Several different types of pain scales have also been introduced over the years and these can help further in assessing the pain that the patient feels (Figure 36.1).

The **final stage** is to help reduce pain by using drugs, and to reduce their side effects to a minimum. Opioids remain the best painkillers to give to patients, although they do have serious side effects, including respiratory depression, bradycardia, pruritus, sedation, nausea and vomiting, hypotension and reduction in bowel function (Wicker & Cox 2010). Treating nausea and pruritus with antihistamines may cause additional effects on sedation and respiratory depression.

Systemic opioids

Drugs can be administered via oral, rectal, sublingual, transdermal, subcutaneous, intramuscular, intrathecal, epidural, inhalational or intravenous routes. Patient-controlled analgesia is often used for intravenous infusion using a syringe pump (Figure 36.2) and is the best option, as it provides consistent levels of pain relief for the patient (Etches 1994). Drugs that are frequently used include morphine, meperidine and Fentanyl.

Nonsteroidal anti-inflammatory drugs (NSAIDS)

NSAIDS are commonly used to treat inflammation and pain, and do not have the same side effects as opioids. NSAIDS inhibit the COX-2 enzyme, which reduces the production of prostaglandins (Ramsay 2000). This helps to reduce pain, fever and vasodilatation. However, by blocking prostaglandins, they also increase tissue inflammatory responses and affect pain perception. These analgesics may be safer than opioids and will help in the management of acute postoperative pain.

Regional techniques

Epidural and spinal opioids can provide good levels of analgesia, although side effects can still occur. Local anaesthetics do reduce or eliminate pain, but they may cause hypotension and muscle weakness that may slow down postoperative mobilisation of the patient.

Non-pharmacologic techniques

These can include electrical stimulation of peripheral nerves, which may affect pain-inhibitory pathways, acupuncture or massage.

There are many research projects looking at further advances in postoperative pain control, which hopefully will result in less postoperative pain for patients.

37 Managing postoperative nausea and vomiting

Figure 37.1 Physiology of vomiting

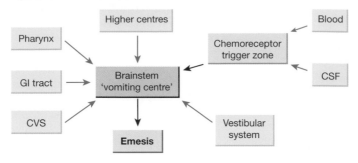

Figure 37.2 Act of vomiting

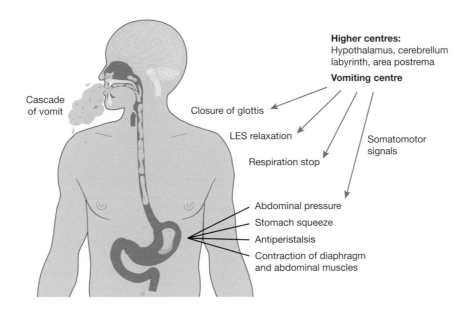

Postoperative nausea and vomiting (PONV) is a common complication following surgery and anaesthesia, leading to other problems that can cause the patient discomfort and pain, and prolong their stay in recovery. Around 10% of patients develop PONV immediately after surgery, and around 30% of patients develop PONV within 24 hours (Wilhelm *et al.* 2007; Chetterjee *et al.* 2011).

Physiology of vomiting

Vomiting is managed via the brain and the central nervous system (Figure 37.1). Chemicals or drugs in blood and CSF trigger the chemoreceptor trigger zone, called the area postrema. This is located at the base of the fourth ventricle, outside the blood–brain barrier (Chetterjee *et al.* 2011). The chemoreceptor trigger zone, and other areas such as afferent neurons from the pharynx and higher cortical centres (e.g. the visual centre), send signals to the brain stem vomiting centre, which sends signals to the diaphragm, stomach and chest muscles, causing them to forcibly contract. This results in vomiting or emesis (Figure 37.2; Chetterjee *et al.* 2011).

There are three stages of vomiting. First, nausea presents the person with the urge to vomit; at the same time they feel sensations in the head and stomach and usually the back of the throat. Secondly, retching is the contraction of chest and abdominal muscles, without the person actually vomiting. Stomach contents move backwards and forwards as the proximal and distal ends of the stomach relax and contract. Thirdly, vomiting occurs when stomach contents are expelled from the mouth as the stomach, duodenum and chest muscles all contract forcibly. Vomiting stops once the respiratory and abdominal muscles relax (Tinsley & Barone 2012).

Risk factors

There are many risk factors related to PONV, such as being a child over the age of 3 or an adult under the age of 50; having a preexisting condition such as a history of motion sickness or anxiety; being female – women are more prone to PONV than men because of the presence of female hormones (Mathias 2008); being obese, due to gastric volume and retention of anaesthetic drugs in adipose tissues (Chetterjee *et al.* 2011); type and length of surgery; and the use of morphine and diamorphine. Non-smokers are also more susceptible to PONV than smokers, because chemicals in tobacco smoke increase the metabolism of some drugs used in anaesthesia, reducing the risk of PONV (Miaskowski 2009). Postoperative complications following PONV include dehydration, electrolyte imbalances, ocular disturbances, pulmonary complications, wound dehiscence, haematoma development, patient discomfort and delayed discharge from the recovery room (Tinsley & Barone 2012).

Prevention of vomiting

Patient satisfaction is reduced if they suffer PONV. Furthermore, there may be problems such as wound damage due to extreme vomiting, and patients may inhale vomit and suffer respiratory problems as a result. Steps to consider during anaesthesia include using regional techniques or total intravenous anaesthesia (TIVA) rather than volatile anaesthetic agents. Managing pain using NSAIDs or regional/local anaesthesia rather than opioids is also useful if appropriate for the patient. In recovery, patients need fluid therapy using crystalloids or colloids, oxygen therapy during the early stages of recovery, and if possible the use of acupuncture, which is known to reduce the risk of PONV (Wilhelm *et al.* 2007). Suction using a Yankaur or flexible sucker may be required, and if the patient is still semi-conscious the anaesthetist needs to be informed urgently so the patient can be reintubated.

Anti-emetic therapy

The two main groups of anti-emetics are antagonists and agonists. Antagonists include dopaminergic, cholinergic, histaminergic, 5-HT3 and NK-1 drugs (Smith *et al.* 2012). Antagonists are chemicals that reduce the physiological activity of chemical substances (such as opiates); they act by blocking receptors within the nervous system. Agonists are medications that combine with a receptor on a cell and initiate a reaction or activity that prevents neurotransmitter release to the chemoreceptor trigger zone or vomiting centre in the brain. Agonists include dexamethasone and cannabinoids.

Metoclopromide is a D_2 receptor antagonist in the stomach, gut and chemoreceptor trigger zone. It is often prescribed and is most effective in young children (Chetterjee *et al.* 2011). Dosage is usually 0.1 mg/kg in children, and higher for adults.

Droperidol is a D_2 receptor antagonist and an α-adrenergic agonist. Dosages up to 2.5 mg can be given. This drug also causes sedation and side effects include long QT syndrome, which increases the risk of irregular heartbeats.

Hyoscine (Scopolamine) is anticholinergic and is effective for PONV associated with vestibular inputs (sense of movement in the inner ear). This drug can also produce muscarinic side effects including blurred vision, confusion, diarrhoea and shortness of breath (Chetterjee *et al.* 2011).

Cyclizine is an H_1 receptor antagonist that also produces anticholinergic responses. The effective dose is around 50 mg. It can produce side effects such as mild sedation, dry mouth and blurred vision.

Ondansetron is a $5-HT_3$ receptor antagonist. The $5-IIT_3$ receptor is a serotonin receptor found in terminals of the vagus nerve and in certain areas of the brain (Smith *et al.* 2012). Ondansetron is one of the most effective anti-emetics and can be given in doses of 4 mg up to 8 mg. It is, however, one of the most expensive antiemetic drugs and can cost up to £5.99 for a 2 ml ampoule.

Dexamethasone is an effective anti-emetic at a dose of 8 mg. It is a member of the glucocorticoid class of steroid drugs that has anti-inflammatory and immunosuppressant properties. Its anti-emetic properties activate the glucocorticoid receptors in the medulla.

Conclusion

In many circumstances it is most effective to use a combination of drugs that have different mechanisms of action to increase their anti-emetic properties. Practitioners can improve patient satisfaction and reduce the direct costs of PONV by monitoring and taking action for patients at risk of nausea and vomiting.

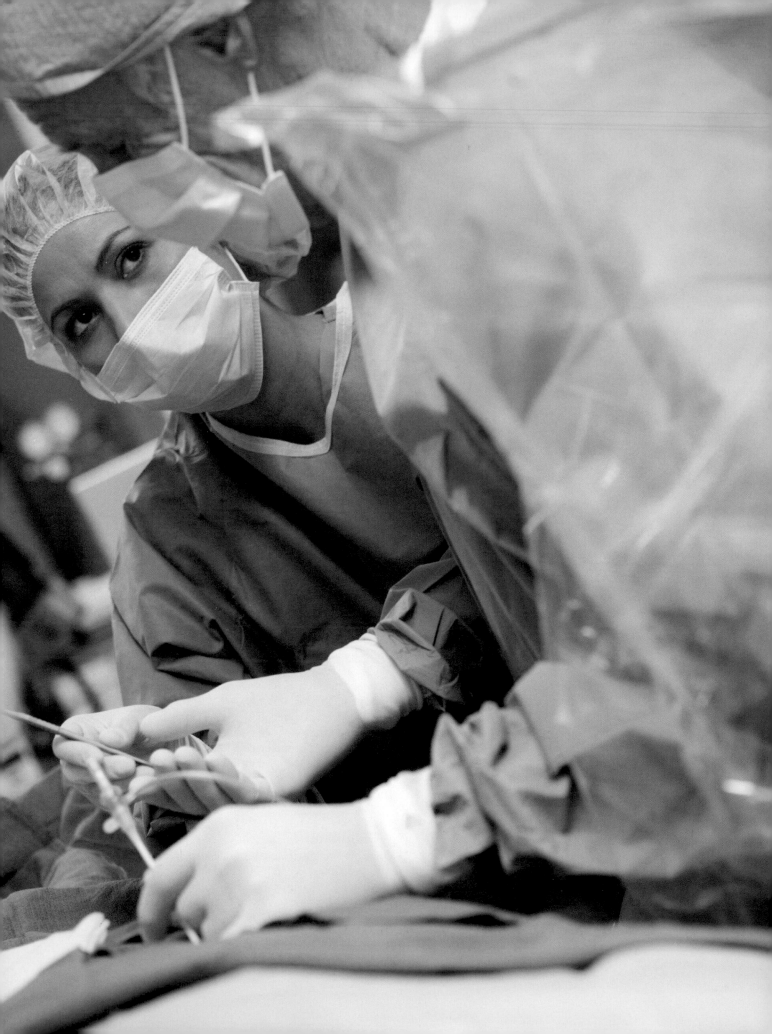

Perioperative emergencies

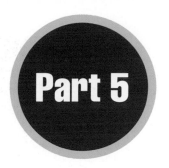

Part 5

Chapters

38 Caring for the critically ill 84
39 Airway problems 86
40 Rapid sequence induction 88
41 Bleeding problems 90
42 Malignant hyperthermia 92
43 Cardiovascular problems 94
44 Electrosurgical burns 96
45 Venous thromboembolism 98
46 Latex allergy 100

38 Caring for the critically ill

Box 38.1 Principal recommendations for caring for the critically ill

- There is a need to introduce a UK-wide system that allows rapid and easy identification of patients who are at high risk of postoperative mortality and morbidity. (Departments of Health in England, Wales and Northern Ireland)
- All elective high-risk patients should be seen and fully investigated in preassessment clinics. Arrangements should be in place to ensure that more urgent surgical patients have the same robust work-up. (Clinical directors and consultants)
- An assessment of mortality risk should be made explicit to the patient and recorded clearly on the consent form and in the medical record. (Consultants)
- The postoperative care of the high-risk surgical patient needs to be improved. Each Trust must make provision for sufficient critical care beds or pathways of care to provide appropriate support in the postoperative period. (Medical directors)
- To aid planning for the provision of facilities for high-risk patients, each Trust should analyse the volume of work considered to be high risk and quantify the critical care requirements of this cohort. This assessment and plan should be reported to the Trust Board on an annual basis. (Medical directors)

Source: Findlay *et al*. (2011).

Figure 38.1   A recovery practitioner caring for a high-risk patient following major surgery

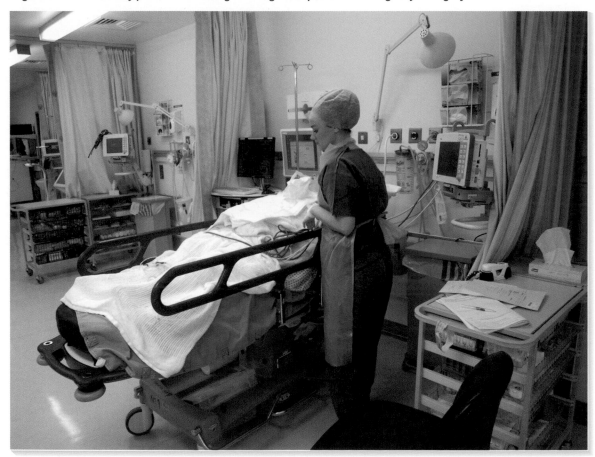

Source: Aintree University Hospital, Liverpool.

As the population in the UK ages, the risk of harm during surgery and anaesthesia is rising. Although the preassessment of high-risk patients happens before surgery, there are often unresolved issues following surgery. For example, a lack of beds in intensive care units (ICU) or high-dependency units (HDU) can compromise postoperative care. However, the surgery is likely to go ahead, as surgeons and anaesthetists are under pressure to continue because of targets imposed on them by the government, and because of the need to avoid surgical cancellations. As the number of high-risk patients increases over the coming years, it is important to improve patient care and reduce morbidity and mortality (Pearse *et al.* 2006).

Critical risk areas

The National Confidential Enquiry into Patient Outcome and Death (NCEPOD) published a report in December 2011 entitled 'Knowing the risk: A review of the perioperative care of surgical patients' (Findlay *et al.* 2011). This enquiry investigated the care of patients undergoing elective and emergency surgery, and their state of health up to 30 days later. The report highlighted a high mortality rate in 'high-risk' surgical patients. The caseload of high-risk surgical patients is likely to rise in the coming years and that will have an increased impact on physical resources (such as recovery rooms, ICU and HDU). There will also be increased pressure on practitioners, as the UK government does not currently recognise a need for an increased number of perioperative practitioners in operating departments and critical care areas.

Bhattacharyya *et al.* (2002) undertook a study in orthopaedic surgery that identified five critical risks during surgery: chronic renal failure, congestive heart failure, chronic obstructive pulmonary disease, hip fracture and an age greater than 70 years. The NCEPOD report also identified that between 5% and 10% of patients should be considered as high risk (Findlay *et al.* 2011). Its other key findings included the following:

- Only 48% of high-risk patients received good-quality care.
- 57% of high-risk patients were overweight.
- 20.5% of patients who died within 30 days postoperatively had inadequate preoperative fluid management.
- Patients who suffered intraoperative complications had a 30-day mortality of 13.2% compared to 5.7% in those without complications.
- Inadequate intraoperative monitoring was associated with a threefold increase in mortality.
- 8.3% of high-risk patients who should have gone to an area with a higher level of care postoperatively did not do so.
- Postoperative complications had affected outcome in 56/213 (26%) of cases.

There are of course many other issues that need to be considered. For example, up to 39% of surgical patients have anaemia, which is also linked to increased morbidity or mortality (Wu *et al.* 2007). Older patients also have a greater risk of impaired nutritional status, which can lead to more profound wound complications (Greene *et al.* 1991) and poor healing. Older patients have a lower physiological reserve, which can be affected by anaesthetic drugs, resulting in dementia or confusion postoperatively. However, this can be improved by using magnesium (Vizcaychipi 2013). Surgical site infections can also be initiated because of nasal colonisation with *Staphylococcus aureus* or MRSA, especially in orthopaedic patients (Schwarzkopf *et al.* 2010).

Improvements in patient care

Normally, high-risk elective patients are assessed and problems are identified before surgery. Postoperative management can be compromised because of a lack of resources, such as insufficient beds in ICU or HDU, and because of pressures on surgeons and anaesthetists to meet targets set by the hospital or the government. The NCEPOD report identified four particular areas in which to improve patient care:

- Identification of 'high-risk' patients
- Improved preoperative assessment, triage and preparation
- Improved intraoperative care
- Improved use of postoperative resources (Findlay *et al.* 2011)

Identifying high-risk patients can be difficult because a high surgical caseload leads to fewer opportunities for identifying problems. According to the NCEPOD report (Findlay *et al.* 2011), around 20% of high-risk patients were not assessed preoperatively and therefore did not have their high risks identified. This in turn could lead to morbidity and mortality issues.

High-risk patients in recovery

High-risk surgery represents around 12.5% of surgical procedures, but can result in 83.3% of deaths (Pearse *et al.* 2006). The recovery room provides postoperative high-dependency care, or intensive care, in order to address the need for improved care for these patients (Figure 38.1). Recovery rooms are usually open 24 hours a day and if they preserve the same staffing levels at night as during the day, this reduces the risk of poorer 'out-of-hours' care. Evidence-based protocols should be established to ensure that each high-risk patient receives standardised care in order to reduce the risk of complications. Standardised processes that can help in the care of high-risk patients include ventilation, haemodynamic management, monitoring and pain management. Setting up and running a recovery room in this way will have cost implications, but the results will be lower postoperative morbidity and a reduced stay, which should help to lower costs. An efficient and effective recovery room can therefore improve surgical outcomes, reduce postoperative morbidity and mortality and lead to cost savings (Simpson & Moonesinghe 2013).

Conclusion

The NCEPOD report (Findlay *et al.* 2011) highlights several recommendations for improving the care of high-risk patients (Box 38.1). A standardised system of rapid and easy identification of patients who are at high risk of postoperative mortality and morbidity needs to be introduced nationally. Furthermore, all elective high-risk patients should be seen and investigated in preassessment clinics. If the patient is at risk of death, then this should be recorded on the consent form and made explicit to the patient. Trusts need to provide sufficient critical care beds or pathways of care to provide high-risk patients with the appropriate level of support in the postoperative period. In conclusion, the number of high-risk patients is high and is likely to significantly increase in the coming years as the population becomes older. Reducing morbidity and mortality in these patients is therefore a priority.

39 Airway problems

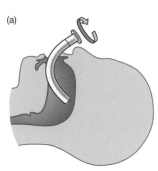

Figure 39.1 Insertion of oral airway
The airway is first inserted upside down, and then reversed to insert into the trachea

(a)

(b)

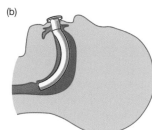

Figure 39.2 Ventilation using a mask and bag
Two practitioners make ventilation more effective and easier to control

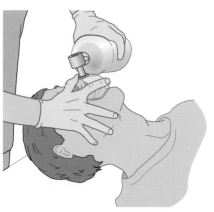

1 Person: difficult, less effective

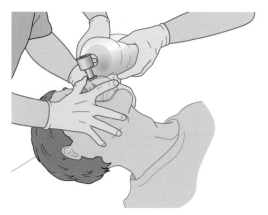

2 Person: easier, more effective

Perioperative Practice at a Glance, First Edition. Paul Wicker. © 2015 John Wiley & Sons, Ltd. Published 2015 by John Wiley & Sons, Ltd.

Critically ill patients can suffer from respiratory failure for several reasons. Inability to breathe properly can be caused by trauma to the chest muscles and ribs, sputum retention, pneumonia, respiratory depression caused by anaesthetic drugs, and frailty or malnutrition in the elderly. Cardiovascular problems can also affect the pulmonary arteries and veins, leading to issues such as heart failure, fluid overload and pulmonary hypertension or embolism. Airflow obstruction can also happen because of chronic obstructive pulmonary disease or asthma. Some of the factors that increase the risk of respiratory problems include smoking, thoracic surgery, obesity, upper abdominal surgery and preexisting pulmonary diseases. Elderly patients are also at high risk of respiratory problems (Jevon & Ewens 2002).

The main risks in airway management include failure to assess and plan for potential airway complications; failure to achieve airway control; complications following surgery, for example airway injuries or injury to the larynx; and practitioners' own issues, such as anxiety, performance problems and avoidance of responsibility (Ball 2011).

The early recognition of airway problems and early treatment may prevent even further deterioration of the patient and will provide a good basis for effective resuscitation (Loftus 2010). Effective airway management enables gas exchange between the blood and the alveoli, delivering oxygen and removing carbon dioxide. It will also protect the lungs from injury due to aspiration of fluids such as gastric contents or blood secretions. Inhalation of fluids interferes with gas exchange either by physical obstruction or by instigating bronchospasm or inflammation (Ball 2011). Gastric contents are acidic and highly toxic, leading to serious damage to the lungs and airways if inhaled, and they may also contain lumps of food that can block the airway (Loftus 2010).

Assessing the airway

When assessing a critically ill patient, the first step should be to assess the airway. If the patient responds verbally to any questions then there is usually no airway issue. However, if the patient does not respond verbally then there are likely to be respiratory problems that will need urgent attention (Jevon & Ewens 2002). If the patient loses consciousness, then this can result in loss of airway control, loss of gag and coughing reflexes, and increased risk of aspiration of gastric contents into the lungs. An airway problem can be detected by observing:

- Inability to speak coherently
- Peripheral or central cyanosis
- Dyspnoea, tachypnoea or apnoea
- Perspiration and tachycardia
- Reduction in consciousness, increased agitation or thrashing around (Jevon & Ewens 2002)

Airway control

A patient who is breathing but is hypoxic needs urgent application of a Hudson oxygen mask, ideally with a reservoir bag attached and with high-flow oxygen from the wall outlet (Loftus 2010;

Figure 39.2). The high-flow oxygen may cause the patient to reduce their breathing rate, but this is not an issue as it is unlikely to result in hypoxia because of the high oxygen flow rate. Using a pulse oximeter will assess oxygen saturation and establish whether the delivery of oxygen is improving the patient's saturation (Jevon & Ewens 2002). On recovery from hypoxia, the oxygen rate can be reduced to 5 litres per minute or lower. Close observation of the patient will ensure that the saturation level does not fall again (Ball 2011).

If breathing does not improve with use of an oxygen mask, then other measures will have to be taken, such as lifting the chin and providing a jaw thrust, using suction devices to remove foreign bodies or inserting a Guedel airway (Figure 39.1) or nasopharyngeal airway (Loftus 2010). At this point the anaesthetist needs to be aware of the issue and will have to be called urgently if the patient is in recovery. Complete blockage of the airway will require reintubation using either a laryngeal mask (LMA) or an endotracheal tube (ETT), or if required a tracheostomy.

In the absence of an anaesthetist, if the patient stops breathing or becomes severely hypoxic or cyanosed, then use of a bag, valve and mask system will be required until the anaesthetist arrives (Loftus 2010).

Tracheostomy

In a situation in which the patient cannot be intubated and the airway is blocked, then a tracheostomy may need to be undertaken. Indications for tracheostomy in critically ill patients include weaning off long-term mechanical ventilation, excessive secretions and inability to cough well, protection of the airway if it is damaged or obstructed, and maintaining the airway when there is an upper airway obstruction.

There are various types of tracheostomy tubes, made of either plastic or metal. The tube can be cuffed or uncuffed. Mechanically ventilated patients use a cuffed tube, so that oxygen does not escape around the edges of the tube, but they will not enable the patient to speak. An uncuffed tube is used when patients can breathe by themselves. The tubes can also be single lumen or they can have an inner cannula. The inner cannula can be removed and cleaned, leaving the outer tube in place (Loftus 2010). The tube can also be fenestrated or non-fenestrated. The fenestrations allow patients to talk with a tracheostomy in place, but they cannot be used in ventilated patients. Finally, the tube can either be flanged or unflanged; in some cases the flange is adjustable.

Tube sizes of around 10 mm are used for female patients and around 11 mm for males (Loftus 2010). The tube must not be too large or it may cause damage to the trachea, resulting in necrosis. Problems arising following insertion of the tracheostomy include accidental displacement of the tube, blockage by sputum or phlegm and haemorrhage caused by damage to the surrounding tissues (Ball 2011). Removal of the tracheostomy tube can be undertaken once the airway is patent. However, risks following removal of the tube include obstruction due to aspiration, sputum retention, damage to the trachea and difficulty with oral reintubation if it is required.

40 Rapid sequence induction

Box 40.1   Sedation

Barbiturates/hypnotics
- Thiopental (Pentothal), Methohexital (Brevital): Short onset (10–20) seconds, duration 5–10 minutes; may reduce intracranial pressure (ICP), cerebro protective; side effects histamine release, hypotension, bronchospasm.

Non-barbiturates
- Etomidate (Amidate): A non-barbiturate hypnotic; decreases ICP/intraocular pressure (IOP); rapid onset, short duration; minimal haemo-dynamic effects; no histamine release; increases seizure threshold; no malignant hyperthermia reported. Watch for myoclonus, vomiting, may decrease cortisol synthesis (adrenal insufficiency). Dose 0.3 mg/kg IV.
- Propofol: A sedative hypnotic, extremely rapid onset (10 seconds), duration of 10–15 minutes, decreases ICP, can cause profound hypotension. Dose 1–3 mg/kg IV for induction, dose 100–200 mcg/kg/min for maintenance.
- Ketamine: A dissociative anaesthetic; rapid onset, short duration; potent bronchodilator, useful in asthmatics; increases ICP, IOP, intragastric pressure (IGP); contraindicated in head injuries; increases bronchial secretions. 'Emergence' phenomenon can occur, though rarely in children less than 10 years old; emergence reactions occur in up to 50% of adults. Dose 1–2 mg/kg.

Opiates
- Fentanyl: A broad dose–response relationship; can be reversed with naloxone; rapid acting (<1 minute), duration of 30 min; does not release histamine; may decrease tachycardia and hypertension associated with intubation; seizures and chest wall rigidity have been reported. Dose 2–10 mcg/kg IV.
- Morphine sulphate: A longer-onset (3–5 minutes) and duration (4–6 hours); may not blunt the rise in ICP, hypertension and tachycardia as well as Fentanyl, can cause histamine release. Dose 0.1–0.2 mg/kg IV.

Benzodiazepines
- Midazolam, Diazepam and Lorazepam provide excellent amnesia and sedation; broad dose–response relationship; reversed with Flumazenil (Romazicon). Doses required are higher for rapid sequence induction than for general sedation.
  Midazolam: A slower-onset (3–5 minutes) than barbiturate/hypnotic agents; considered short acting (30–60 minutes); does not increase ICP; causes respiratory and cardiovascular depression. Dose 0.1–0.4 mg/kg IV.
  Diazepam and Lorazepam: Moderate/long-acting agents; longer onset time than Midazolam; may be more beneficial postintubation for sedation.

Box 40.2   Neuromuscular blocking (NMB) agents

Depolarising agents
- Succinylcholine: Stimulates nicotinic/muscarinic cholinergic receptors; gold standard drug for 50 years; onset 45 seconds, duration 8–10 minutes. Dose adults 1.5 mg/kg IV; children 2.0 mg/kg IV. Inactivated by pseudocholinesterase; prolonged paralysis seen with pregnancy, liver disease, malignancies, cytotoxic drugs, certain antibiotics, cholinesterase inhibitors, organophosphate poisoning. Adverse reactions: muscle fasciculations, hyperkalaemia, bradycardia, prolonged neuromuscular blockade, trismus (Masseter spasm) usually in children and treated with a nondepolarising NMB; malignant hyperthermia; increases ICP/IOP/IGP, causes muscle pain that can be minimised by a 'priming' dose of NMB; bradycardia in children under 10 years due to higher vagal tone; malignant hyperthermia from excessive calcium influx through open channels treated with IV Dantrolene.

Non-depolarising agents
- Pancuronium: Long-acting agent (45–90 minutes); slow onset (1–5 minutes); renal excretion; vagolytic tachyarrythmias common. Dose 0.10–0.15 mg/kg IV.
- Vecuronium: Duration of 30–60 minutes; onset of 1–4 minutes; hypotension may occur from loss of venous return and sympathetic blockade; mostly biliary excretion. Dose 0.1 mg/kg; 'priming dose' 0.01 mg/kg.
- Rocuronium: Has the shortest onset of the non-depolarising agents (1–3 minutes); duration 30–45 minutes; tachycardia can occur. Dose 0.6–1.2 mg/kg.

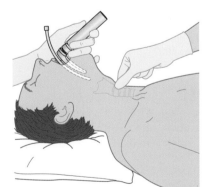

Figure 40.1   Patient undergoing rapid sequence induction
The anaesthetist is inserting the endotracheal tube while the practitioner is applying cricoid pressure to prevent gastric reflux from the stomach into the lungs

Perioperative Practice at a Glance, First Edition. Paul Wicker. © 2015 John Wiley & Sons, Ltd. Published 2015 by John Wiley & Sons, Ltd.

Rapid sequence induction (RSI) is the simultaneous administration of a potent sedative agent and a neuromuscular blocking agent to induce unconsciousness and muscular paralysis to enable endotracheal intubation. RSI also minimises the risk of gastric aspiration (AAGBI 2009). Important reasons for using RSI may include urgent surgery, urgent oxygenation and a full stomach. Normally the patient will be preoxygenated, will have no ventilation during intubation and will have cricoid pressure applied until the endotracheal tube is inserted.

The classic approach to RSI has four stages: preoxygenating with eight vital breaths; injecting IV thiopentone and succinylcholine; applying cricoid pressure; and finally intubating.

The RSI approach is used in many situations such as ruptured aortic aneurysms, ectopic pregnancies and trauma cases, and its main purpose is to anaesthetise the patient as quickly as possible while trying to avoid aspiration of stomach contents. In the UK, the classic approach to RSI with associated cricoid pressure is still advocated by the Royal College of Anaesthetists. However, across the world, including in the UK, modifications are increasingly being made to the classic approach that can improve patient outcomes by reducing side effects and complications (DAS 2014). The modified approach to RSI has often been described as the 7Ps: Preparation, Preoxygenation, Pretreatment, Paralysis with induction, Positioning, Placement and Postintubation management.

Preparation (T(time) – 10 minutes)

Preparation of the patient occurs 10 minutes before intubation (DAS 2014). The patient is evaluated using the LEMON approach: Look at the patient and observe for problems; Evaluate using the 3-3-2 rule: three of the patient's fingers should be able to fit into their mouth when open, three fingers should comfortably fit between the chin and the throat, and two fingers in the thyromental distance (distance from thyroid cartilage to chin); Mallampati assessment to predict the ease of intubation, assessing the visibility of the base of the uvula, faucial pillars (the arches in front of and behind the tonsils) and soft palate – Class 1 means full visibility, progressing to Class 4, which means that only the hard palate is visible; Obstruction, checking for obstruction of the airway; Neck mobility, ensuring neck is mobile to allow for the chin tilt and jaw thrust (DAS 2014).

Preoxygenation (T – 5 minutes)

Patients are preoxygenated with 100% oxygen for 5 minutes to allow a limit of around 3–5 minutes of apnoea before desaturation of less than 90% occurs (DAS 2014). However, a danger with preoxygenation is that it can sometimes mask oesophageal intubation, as the patient will not show immediate signs of hypoxia.

Pretreatment (T – 3 minutes)

Pre-treatment lowers the patient's physiological responses to intubation (AAGBI 2009). This minimises bradycardia, hypoxaemia, the cough/gag reflex and increases in intracranial, intraocular and intragastric pressures (DAS 2014). Medications used include lignocaine, which helps to blunt the rise in intracranial pressure associated with airway manipulation; opioids, which offer sedation and pain relief; atropine, which can minimise vagal effects, bradycardia and secretions, given in doses of 0.02 mg/kg, minimum 0.1 mg IV, max 1 mg, 3 minutes prior to intubation; and defasciculating medication, which decreases muscle fasciculations caused by the depolarising agents (succinylcholine). Usually the agents used are the non-depolarising blocking agents (vecuronium, pancuronium etc.) at 1/10 of the standard dose.

Paralysis with induction (zero)

Cricoid pressure is applied as the induction agent and neuromuscular blocking agent are injected (Hernandez et al. 2004). Applying cricoid pressure (Sellick's manoeuvre) during endotracheal intubation prevents aspiration of gastric contents and helps with visualisation of the glottis. Using the thumb and index finger, 20–30 Newtons of pressure are applied on the cricoid cartilage (just below the thyroid prominence) to occlude the oesophagus (Hein & Owen 2005). Sedatives are administered to produce unconsciousness with little or no cardiovascular effects (DAS 2014; Box 40.1). Sedatives include barbiturates/hypnotics, non-barbiturates, neuroleptics, opiates and benzodiazepines. The drugs most often used are propofol and thiopental (AAGBI 2009). Propofol is most common these days because it has a rapid onset of around 10–40 seconds and lasts for up to 10–15 minutes. It has few side effects but can sometimes cause profound hypotension. Thiopental is still used and is effective with a short onset of 5–10 seconds and duration for 5–10 minutes, although it does have various side effects including histamine release, hypotension and bronchospasm. Other rarely used sedatives include etomidate and ketamine. Opiates, such as Fentanyl and morphine, and benzodiazepines, such as Midazolam, Diazepam or Lorazepam, may also be given to provide analgesia, amnesia and sedation. More often benzodiazepines are given following intubation to induce longer-term sedation (AAGBI 2009).

Neuromuscular blocking agents (NMB) induce paralysis of skeletal muscles (Box 40.2). Depolarising agents exert their effect by binding with acetylcholine receptors at the neuromuscular junction, causing sustained depolarisation of the muscle cells (fasciculations). Non-depolarising agents bind to acetylcholine receptors in a competitive, non-stimulatory manner, with no receptor depolarisation and no fasciculations. The drugs most often used are succinylcholine and rocuronium (Perry et al. 2008). Succinylcholine, a depolarising agent, has an onset of 45 seconds and duration of 8–10 minutes. Rocuronium, a non-depolarising agent, is commonly used and has an onset of 1–3 minutes and duration of 30–45 minutes.

Placement of endotracheal tube (T + 30 seconds)

The process for intubating the patient (Figure 40.1) involves allowing the sedative to work; applying cricoid pressure (assistant); ensuring complete neuromuscular blockade of the patient; intubation using appropriate equipment; ventilation with bag-valve mask; additional doses of sedatives/NMB if necessary; confirming correct ETT placement; maintaining cricoid pressure until the cuff is inflated; and establishing ventilator parameters (DAS 2014).

Postintubation management

Following intubation, steps taken include securing the tube, monitoring pulse oximetry, assessing vital signs frequently and, if required, obtaining a chest X ray and arterial blood gases, restraining the patient to prevent them falling off the table, and considering long-term sedation.

41 Bleeding problems

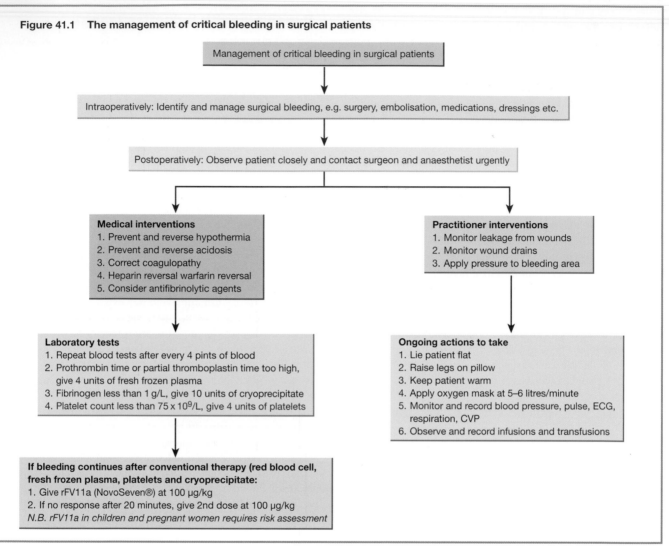

Figure 41.1 The management of critical bleeding in surgical patients

Management of critical bleeding in surgical patients

Intraoperatively: Identify and manage surgical bleeding, e.g. surgery, embolisation, medications, dressings etc.

Postoperatively: Observe patient closely and contact surgeon and anaesthetist urgently

Medical interventions
1. Prevent and reverse hypothermia
2. Prevent and reverse acidosis
3. Correct coagulopathy
4. Heparin reversal warfarin reversal
5. Consider antifibrinolytic agents

Practitioner interventions
1. Monitor leakage from wounds
2. Monitor wound drains
3. Apply pressure to bleeding area

Laboratory tests
1. Repeat blood tests after every 4 pints of blood
2. Prothrombin time or partial thromboplastin time too high, give 4 units of fresh frozen plasma
3. Fibrinogen less than 1 g/L, give 10 units of cryoprecipitate
4. Platelet count less than 75×10^9/L, give 4 units of platelets

Ongoing actions to take
1. Lie patient flat
2. Raise legs on pillow
3. Keep patient warm
4. Apply oxygen mask at 5–6 litres/minute
5. Monitor and record blood pressure, pulse, ECG, respiration, CVP
6. Observe and record infusions and transfusions

If bleeding continues after conventional therapy (red blood cell, fresh frozen plasma, platelets and cryoprecipitate:
1. Give rFV11a (NovoSeven®) at 100 µg/kg
2. If no response after 20 minutes, give 2nd dose at 100 µg/kg
N.B. rFV11a in children and pregnant women requires risk assessment

Perioperative Practice at a Glance, First Edition. Paul Wicker. © 2015 John Wiley & Sons, Ltd. Published 2015 by John Wiley & Sons, Ltd.

Intraoperative or postoperative bleeding can be a risk depending on the patient's condition and the particular surgery (Figure 41.1). Conditions that can affect bleeding include haemophilia A; haemophilia B; Von Willebrand's disease (a deficiency or abnormality of a plasma coagulation factor creating a tendency to bleed; Kozek-Langenecker et al. 2013); deficiency of blood factors VII, VIII, IX, X and XI; factor-specific inhibitors (for example antithrombin III, protein S and protein C; when activated, these proteins inactivate specific clotting factors); platelet dysfunction; and hypofibrinogenaemia (deficiency of fibrinogen in the blood leading to an acute haemorrhagic state brought about by inability of the blood to clot) or dysfribrinoginaemia (abnormal fibrinogen in the blood leading to abnormalities including bleeding and thrombosis; Kozek-Langenecker et al. 2013). The past history of patients offers guidance on the need for laboratory investigations (Chee et al. 2008). Examples include previous surgical bleeding requiring transfusion; return to theatre or readmission for haematoma/bleeding; a history of significant spontaneous bleeding; recurrent epistaxis; recurrent GIT bleeding; haemarthrosis (bleeding in joint spaces); retroperitoneal bleeding (bleeding in the space behind the peritoneum); muscle bleeds; menorrhagia; iron deficiency; hysterectomy for menorrhagia; petechiae (a small red spot on the body caused by broken capillary blood vessels); and easy bruising (Chee et al. 2008; Mansour et al. 2012). Drugs can also increase bleeding, for example antiplatelet agents and anticoagulants, drugs associated with thrombocytopaenia and herbal medications such as garlic, ginseng and Ginkgo biloba (Kozek-Langenecker et al. 2013).

Massive blood loss is defined as the replacement of total blood volume or transfusion of more than 10 units of blood within 24 hours. For example, a 70 kg adult needs an estimated replacement of 4–5 litres of blood lost, or the transfusion of 16–20 units of packed red blood cells (RBC). Massive blood loss can also be defined as replacing 50% of circulating blood volume in less than 3 hours, or bleeding of more than 150 ml/minute (Rossaint et al. 2010).

Giving colloids to patients can also cause bleeding problems because of haemodilution of clotting factors. Dextran has a significant impact on bleeding, especially low molecular weight dextrans, which increase microvascular flow, reduce clot strength and impair platelet function (Rossaint et al. 2010). Gelatins such as Haemaccel and Gelofusin have a lesser impact on haemostasis (Mansour et al. 2012). Thrombocytopaenia is the most common haemostatic abnormality during and after a massive transfusion. This can cause microvascular bleeding, for example oozing from mucosa, wounds and puncture sites. A platelet count of 50×10^9/litre during active bleeding should be sufficient for normal haemostasis provided that platelet function is intact. However, there may be variation in platelet counts depending on the type of transfusion being carried out. Drugs can be given to patients to reduce bleeding, including antifibrinolytic agents, aprotinin, tranexamic acid, EACA (epsilon-aminocaproic acid), Desmospressin (DDAVP), fibrin sealants and rVIIa (NovoSeven). NovoSeven is highly effective and is a recombinant human coagulation Factor VIIa (rFVIIa), intended for promoting haemostasis by activating the extrinsic pathway of the coagulation cascade (Kozek-Langenecker et al. 2013). It is a vitamin K-dependent glycoprotein consisting of 406 amino acid residues and is structurally similar to human plasma-derived Factor VIIa (Martinowitz et al. 2001). The primary side effect is an allergic response, as NovoSeven is made from animal proteins. It is given in doses of 100 µg/kg and can cost £6000 or more for a 70 kg adult (Martinowitz et al. 2001).

Managing rapid blood loss in surgery

Once the source of bleeding is identified, the surgeon should apply pressure using gauze or packing and then, if possible, repair the affected area of tissues or blood vessels. Various haemostatic tools and processes include haemostatic agents, fibrin glues, hypogastric artery ligation and specialised pelvic packing techniques (Gallop 2005). Stopping bleeding in the abdominal cavity requires the urgent application of pressure with a finger or sponge stick, followed by securing blood vessels with clamps, sutures or clips. If injury occurs to vessels such as the aorta, vena cava or common iliac vessels due to the removal of nodes, or needle or trocar injuries during laparoscopy, then the first step in managing great vessel injuries is applying pressure (Gallop 2005). The vessel should then be compressed proximally and distally using vascular clamps. The vessel tear can be closed using nylon or monofilament polypropylene sutures. If intraoperative bleeding persists despite artery ligation, a pelvic pack may be left in place for two to three days. The patient will then need to be transferred to intensive care, to correct problems such as acidosis, coagulopathy and hypothermia. After 48 to 72 hours, the packs are gently removed with saline drip assistance. If haemostasis still has not been achieved, repacking or further surgery may be needed (Gallop 2005).

Managing rapid blood loss in recovery

The surgeon and anaesthetist need to be informed as soon as ongoing and massive blood loss is observed in a patient, so that they can take immediate action. Massive blood loss leads to hypovolaemia, therefore urgent blood transfusion is required to reduce further problems (Hatfield & Tronson 2009). Blood loss after surgery can happen because of problems with the wound internally or externally, and problems with sutures, ties or damaged blood vessels. Bleeding may also start when the patient's blood pressure rises as they regain consciousness. Monitoring of wounds and wound drains is important and if more than 100 ml of blood is collected within 30 minutes, then the surgeon needs to be informed (Hatfield & Tronson 2009).

Actions to reduce blood loss can include laying the patient flat; giving the patient high levels of oxygen; raising their legs (to improve central circulation); monitoring blood pressure, pulse, ECG and respiration; and observing infusions and transfusions (Hatfield & Tronson 2009). If bleeding persists, it is likely that the patient will need to return to theatre for further surgery.

Malignant hyperthermia

Box 42.1 EMHG guidelines: Recognising an MH crisis

Anaesthetic trigger agents are:
- all volatile (inhalation) anaesthetic agents;
- succinylcholine

Clinical signs

Early signs
- Metabolic: Inappropriately elevated CO_2 production (raised end-tidal CO_2 on capnography, tachypnoea if breathing spontaneously); increased O2 consumption; mixed metabolic and respiratory acidosis; profuse sweating; mottling of skin.
- Cardiovascular: Inappropriate tachycardia; cardiac arrhythmias (especially ectopic ventricular beats and ventricular bigemini); unstable arterial pressure.
- Muscle: Masseter spasm if succinylcholine has been used. Generalised muscle rigidity.

Later signs
- Hyperkalaemia; rapid increase in core body temperature; grossly elevated blood creatine phosphokinase levels; grossly elevated blood myoglobin levels; dark-coloured urine due to myoglobinuria; severe cardiac arrhythmias and cardiac arrest; disseminated intravascular coagulation.

Differential diagnosis
- Insufficient anaesthesia, analgesia or both; infection or septicaemia; insufficient ventilation or fresh gas flow; anaesthetic machine malfunction; anaphylactic reaction; phaeochromocytoma; thyroid crisis; cerebral ischaemia; neuromuscular disorders; elevated end-tidal CO_2 due to laparoscopic surgery; ecstasy or other dangerous recreational drugs; malignant neuroleptic syndrome.

Box 42.2 EMHG guidelines: Managing an MH crisis

Start treatment as soon as an MH crisis is suspected
- Immediately: Stop all trigger agents; hyperventilate with 100% O_2 at high flow; declare an emergency and call for help; change to non-trigger anaesthesia (TIVA); inform the surgeon and ask for termination or postponement of surgery; disconnect the vaporiser.
- Dantrolene: Give Dantrolene 2 mg kg^{-1} IV (ampoules of 20 mg are mixed with 60 ml sterile water); Dantrolene infusions should be repeated until the cardiac and respiratory systems stabilise; the maximum dose (10 mg kg^{-1}) may need to be exceeded.
- Monitoring: Continue routine anaesthetic monitoring; measure core temperature; consider inserting arterial, central venous line, urinary catheter; obtain blood samples for testing K^+, CK, arterial blood gases, myoglobin and glucose; check renal and hepatic function and coagulation; check for signs of compartment syndrome; monitor the patient for a minimum of 24 hours (ICU, HDU or in a recovery unit).

Symptomatic treatment
- Treat hyperthermia: 2000–3000 ml of chilled (4 °C) 0.9% saline IV; surface cooling using wet, cold sheets, fans and ice packs placed in the axillae and groin; other cooling devices if available; stop cooling once temperature <38.5 °C.
- Treat hyperkalaemia: dextrose 50%, 50 ml with 50 IU insulin (adult dose); $CaCl_2$ 0.1 mmol kg^{-1} IV (e.g. 7 mmol=10 ml for a 70 kg adult); dialysis may be required.
- Treat acidosis: hyperventilate to normo-capnoea; give sodium bicarbonate IV if pH <7.2.
- Treat arrhythmias: amiodarone 300 mg for an adult (3 mg kg^{-1} IV). β-blockers (e.g. propranolol/ metoprolol/esmolol) if tachycardia persists.
- Maintain urinary output >2 ml kg^{-1} h^{-1}: frusemide 0.5–1 mg kg^{-1}; mannitol 1 g kg^{-1}; fluids: crystalloids (e.g. lactated Ringer's solution or 0.9% saline) IV.

Consult your local Malignant Hyperthermia Investigation Unit about the case.

Source: Glahn *et al.*, 2010.
Reproduced with permission of Oxford University Press and the European Malignant Hyperthermia Group.

Malignant hyperthermia (MH) is a condition that is inherited by families and often develops into a severe reaction following a dose of anaesthetic agents. It causes a rapid rise in body temperature and produces severe muscle contractions. MH is not the same as hyperthermia, which is due to medical emergencies such as heat stroke or infection. MH is very dangerous, requiring early recognition and prompt treatment, and may lead to severe illness or death. Therefore it is important that the patient tells the surgeon and anaesthetist before having any surgery or anaesthesia if a member of their family has had problems with general anaesthesia or there is a known family history of MH (Heller 2011).

As MH is inherited, only one parent has to carry the disease for a child to inherit the condition. MH may also occur with muscle diseases such as multi-minicore myopathy and central core disease. Multi-minicore disease (MmD) is a recessively inherited neuromuscular disorder characterised by multiple cores on muscle biopsy and clinical features of a congenital myopathy (Jungbluth 2007). Central core disease is a disorder that affects muscles used for movement (skeletal muscles). This condition causes muscle weakness that ranges from being almost unnoticeable to severe (GHR 2007). In people with muscle abnormalities, muscle cells have an abnormal protein on their surfaces. The protein does not affect muscle function significantly until the muscles are exposed to an anaesthetic drug that can trigger a reaction. When a person with this condition is exposed to these drugs, muscle cells release calcium and the muscles contract and stiffen at the same time, followed by a dramatic and dangerous increase in temperature (Jungbluth 2007).

MH usually occurs during or after surgery following the use of anaesthetic drugs. This also includes areas such as accident and emergency departments, dental surgeries, surgeon's clinics and intensive care units. MH is rare, especially with the increasing use of total IV anaesthesia (TIVA), which can lead to a potential for reduced awareness of the condition (Glahn *et al.* 2010).

Diagnosis

Diagnosis of people with MH usually happens after they have a serious reaction following general anaesthesia. Surgeons or anaesthetists will suspect that MH is developing if the patient demonstrates typical symptoms of high fever and rigid muscles. Blood tests showing changes in body chemistry can indicate the presence of MH. These include high levels of the muscle enzyme CPK (creatine phosphokinase) and electrolyte changes (Glahn *et al.* 2010). Blood tests that show signs of kidney failure can also show indications of MH. However, if MH is not recognised and treated quickly, the patient may suffer from cardiovascular disorders or even cardiac arrest during surgery.

Symptoms

Early symptoms of MH (Box 42.1) include a quick rise in body temperature to 40 °C or higher (Heller 2011). There are also rigid or painful muscles, especially in the jaw. The skin often becomes flushed and excessive sweating develops. The patient will also exhibit an abnormally rapid or irregular heartbeat and rapid or uncomfortable breathing, leading to confusion or disorientation. Other symptoms of MH include bleeding, dark brown urine, muscle aching, muscle rigidity and stiffness, and low blood pressure

(Glahn *et al.* 2010). There is also usually muscle weakness or swelling after MH has subsided. Tests may include Chem-20 (UCSF 2013). This group of tests is performed on the blood serum and includes testing for total cholesterol, total protein and various electrolytes. Electrolytes in the body include sodium, potassium, chlorine and many others. The remainder of the tests measure chemicals that reflect liver and kidney function. Chem-20 helps provide information about the body's metabolism (UCSF 2013). It gives the anaesthetist information about how the kidneys and liver are working, and can be used to evaluate values such as blood sugar, cholesterol and calcium levels. Other tests include genetic testing to look for defects in the RYR1 gene (involving moving calcium ions within muscle cells), muscle biopsy and urine myoglobin (muscle protein) determination (UCSF 2013).

Prevention

If the patient has MH it is important for them to tell their doctor before having surgery with general anaesthesia. Using certain medications can prevent the complications of MH during surgery. For example, TIVA is less likely to cause MH than is general anaesthesia. Patients with MH must avoid stimulant drugs such as cocaine, amphetamine (speed) and ecstasy, as these drugs may cause more problems (Heller 2011). Genetic counselling is recommended for anyone with a family history of myopathy, muscular dystrophy or malignant hyperthermia.

Expected duration

With prompt treatment, symptoms of MH should resolve within 12–24 hours. However, if a severe reaction occurs before starting treatment, complications may develop. These can include respiratory or kidney failure. These complications may not improve for days or weeks and some physical or physiological damage may be protracted, for example myoglobinuria, elevated potassium levels and coagulation status. In ICU, treating and monitoring patients undergoing MH lasts for a minimum of 36 hours (MHAU 2013).

Treatment (Box 42.2)

During an episode of MH, wrapping the patient in a cooling blanket can help reduce fever and the risk of serious complications. Drugs such as Dantrolene, lidocaine or β-blockers can help with heart rhythm problems (Glahn *et al.* 2010). Various medications will be used to control the heart beat and stabilise the blood pressure. Giving intravenous and oral fluids as well as medication will help to preserve kidney function (Glahn *et al.* 2010). Oxygen will also need to be administered because of the difficulty in breathing and the high metabolic rate, leading to hypoxia (Heller 2011). Ongoing monitoring of vital signs is essential in case of sudden changes in the patient's condition.

Repeated or untreated episodes of MH can lead to kidney failure. Possible complications also include amputation of limbs, breakdown of muscle tissue (rhabdomyolysis), compartment syndrome (swelling of the hands and feet and problems with blood flow and nerve function), disseminating intravascular coagulation (abnormal blood clotting and bleeding), heart rhythm problems, kidney failure, metabolic acidosis, respiratory dysfunction (fluid build-up in the lungs), weak muscles (myopathy) or muscular dystrophy (deformity), and death (Heller 2011).

43 Cardiovascular problems

Figure 43.1a Cardiovascular system

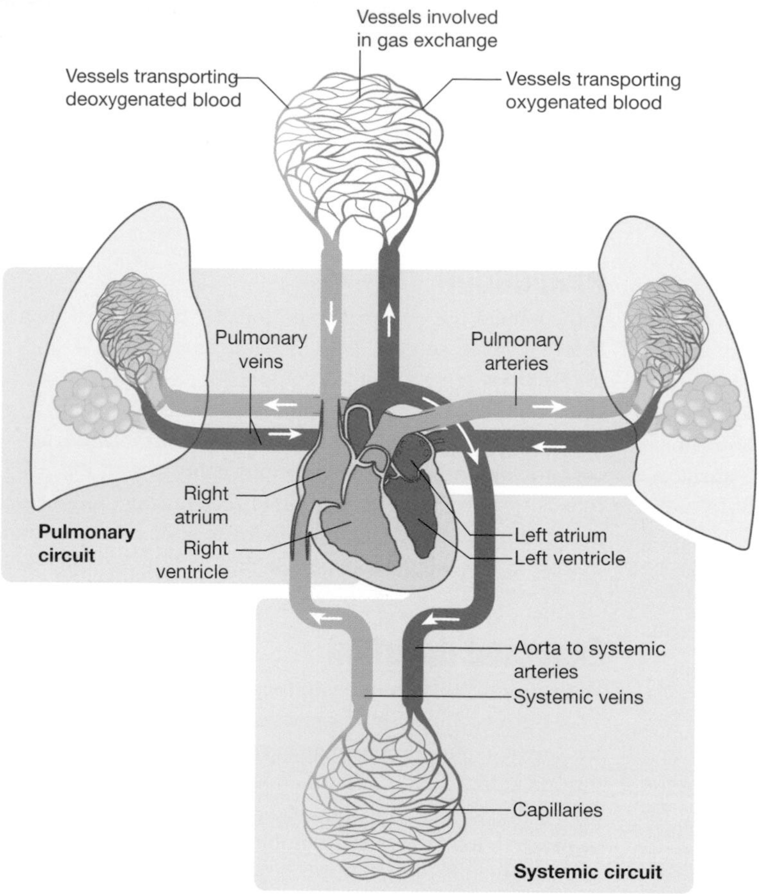

Vessels involved in gas exchange

Vessels transporting deoxygenated blood

Vessels transporting oxygenated blood

Pulmonary veins

Pulmonary arteries

Pulmonary circuit

Right atrium

Right ventricle

Left atrium

Left ventricle

Aorta to systemic arteries

Systemic veins

Capillaries

Systemic circuit

Figure 43.1b Ischaemic heart attack

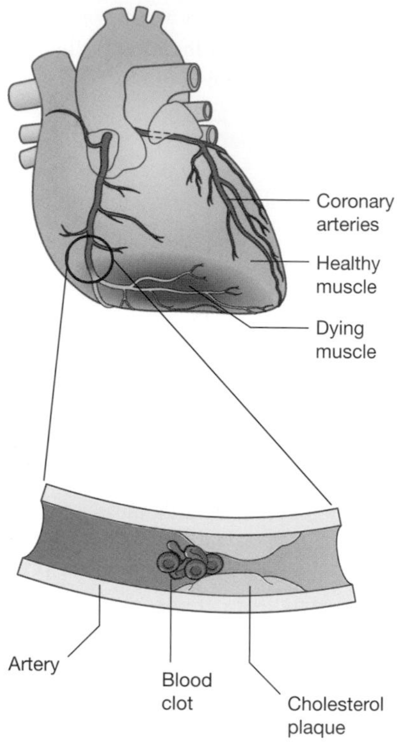

Coronary arteries

Healthy muscle

Dying muscle

Artery

Blood clot

Cholesterol plaque

Figure 43.2   Replacement of blocked coronary arteries using blood vessels from arms or legs

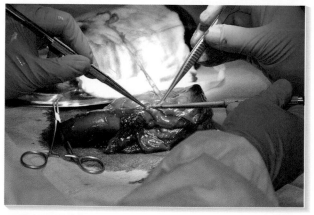
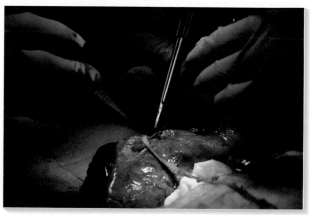

Source: Medical Illustration, University Hospital of South Manchester. Copyright: UHSM Academy.

Patients undergoing non-cardiac surgery may need cardiovascular management where heart disease is a potential source of complications during surgery. Cardiac and respiratory systems are very much intertwined and rely on each other to maintain health and safety in the patient (Figure 43.1a). Cardiac problems may arise in patients with asymptomatic ischaemic heart disease (IHD; Figure 43.1b), left ventricular (LV) dysfunction and valvular heart disease (VHD) who are undergoing procedures that cause prolonged haemodynamic and cardiac stress (ESC 2009). The increasing acceleration in the ageing of the population will have a major impact on perioperative patient management (Sear & Higham 2002). Elderly people require surgery four times more often than the rest of the population (ESC 2009). Age, however, is responsible for only a small increase in the risk of complications; greater risks are associated with significant cardiac, pulmonary and renal diseases (Sear & Higham 2002). The number of affected individuals is likely to be higher in countries with high CVD mortality, particularly in Central and Eastern Europe. These conditions should, therefore, have a greater impact on evaluating patient risk than age alone (ESC 2009).

Preoperative evaluation

Surgical factors that influence cardiac risk are related to the urgency, magnitude, type and duration of the procedure, as well as the change in core body temperature, blood loss and fluid shifts (Aresti et al. 2014). Every operation elicits a stress response. This response is initiated by tissue injury and mediated by neuroendocrine factors, and may induce tachycardia and hypertension. Fluid shifts in the perioperative period add to the surgical stress, increasing myocardial oxygen demand (Aresti et al. 2014). The extent of such changes is proportionate to the extent and duration of the surgery. All these factors may cause myocardial ischaemia and heart failure.

To assess the risk of cardiac problems during surgery, a detailed physical and physiological history, an assessment of exercise tolerance and a resting ECG are used for an initial estimate of perioperative cardiac risk (Qazizada & Higgins 2013). Physical examination includes assessments such as measuring blood pressure, assessment of blood flow in the carotid and jugular vessels, testing of the lungs and examination of the extremities for oedema and vascular integrity (Qazizada & Higgins 2013). Other assessments include stress testing, obesity, age and echocardiography.

Hypertension

Hypertension is a common problem during surgery and is present in almost a quarter of the population (Aresti et al. 2014). Hypertension can increase cardiovascular problems, because of the irregular rise and fall in blood pressure. During induction of anaesthesia blood pressure can fall, while postoperatively blood pressure might rise because of pain or anxiety. These changes can lead to myocardial ischaemia, heart failure and stroke. Patients may be taking antihypertensives regularly, but the use of these needs to be assessed and may be stopped before surgery. For example, ACE inhibitors (including captopril, enalapril and ramipril, which cause vasodilation and are used to treat high blood pressure

and heart failure) and angiotensin 11 receptor agonists can lead to hypotension during surgery (Fleisher et al. 2007). Hypertensive patients are those with systolic blood pressure higher than 160 mmHg and diastolic blood pressure higher than 100 mmHg. Carrying out blood pressure monitoring during surgery and postoperatively can support stabilisation of blood pressure (Fleisher et al. 2007).

Arrhythmias

Arrhythmias are another complication in patients undergoing non-cardiac surgery, and this has been a common problem for many years (Goldman et al. 1977). The presence of arrhythmias can signal issues such as cardiac abnormalities, drug toxicity or metabolic issues (Aresti et al. 2014). Management of arrhythmias is therefore important to prevent further complications arising. Atrial fibrillation is common in elderly patients and can produce myocardial ischaemia, increased myocardial activity leading to higher oxygen demand, intracardiac emboli and cerebrovascular accidents, including strokes (Fleisher et al. 2007). Cardiac surgery may also be needed to replace coronary arteries that have become blocked by emboli (Figure 43.2). Ventricular arrhythmias are less serious, but can lead to further arrhythmias following surgery. ECG monitors will detect arrhythmias and will indicate signs of altered pulse rates and blood pressure changes. The patient may then suffer from poor perfusion of blood throughout their body, which may result in cardiac arrest (Fleisher et al. 2007).

Aortic stenosis

Aortic stenosis, the abnormal narrowing of the aortic valve by calcification, can arise when patients develop arrhythmias and heart failure. As the valve narrows, the left ventricle has to pump harder to maintain blood circulation (Aresti et al. 2014). As the left ventricle increases in size due to the extra effort, it becomes stiffer leading to lower aortic pressure and a reduction in oxygen demand for the myocardium. As the disease progresses, cardiac output falls, leading to angina, ischaemia and other cardiovascular abnormalities. Patients with severe aortic stenosis should have this treated prior to undertaking any other general surgery.

Congestive heart failure

Congestive heart failure is a weakness of the heart that leads to a build-up of fluid in the lungs and surrounding body tissues. Blood pools in the veins because the heart does not pump efficiently enough to allow it to return. Symptoms may vary from the most minimal symptoms to sudden pulmonary oedema or lethal shock. Symptoms worsen as the body tries to compensate for the condition, creating a vicious circle (Aresti et al. 2014). The patient has trouble breathing, at first during exertion and later even at rest. Treatment is directed towards increasing the strength of the heart's muscle contraction, reduction of fluid accumulation and elimination of the underlying cause of the failure. Diuretics, β-blockers and ACE inhibitors are the most commonly used drugs for treating this condition (Aresti et al. 2014). ACE inhibitors can cause hypotension following anaesthesia and may not be used before surgery.

44 Electrosurgical burns

Figure 44.1 Diathermy burns
Forearm and hand – 50 days after the surgery

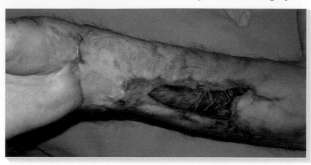

Source: Demircin et al. (2013). Reproduced with permission of the Romanian Society of Legal Medicine.

Figure 44.3 An electrosurgical burn

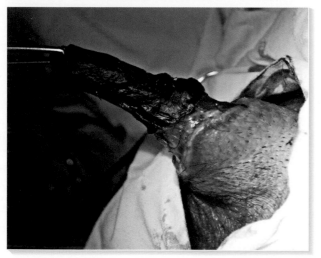

Figure 44.2 Diathermy burns
Atrophy and contracture of the forearm and hand

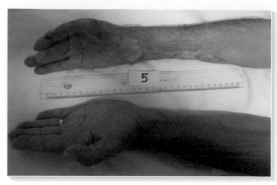

Source: Demircin et al. (2013). Reproduced with permission of the Romanian Society of Legal Medicine.

This 38-year-old patient underwent a circumcision. Instead of using bipolar electrosurgery, the surgeon used monopolar electrosurgery. As the current returned up the penis towards the return electrode, the vessels in the penis became coagulated, leading to necrosis. After two weeks the penis was amputated. This event occurred about 9 years ago. Bipolar electrosurgery would have prevented this from occurring, as the current would only have passed through the tissues held between the tines of the bipolar forceps

Source: Jiang et al. (2004). Reproduced with permission of Shanghai Materia Medica, Shanghai Jiao Tong University.

Most surgical procedures use electrosurgery (diathermy) to cut or coagulate tissue by using high-frequency current. The current is at radio frequency, meaning that it can escape from the wire or even the tip of the active electrode if it is not touching the patient's tissues, and can travel through the air (Wicker 1991). Adjusting the voltage and current produces the desired clinical effects of desiccation (coagulation), fulguration (spray) or cutting. Staff should focus on using electrosurgery safely, maintaining the electrosurgical unit (ESU) and its proper range of settings, ensuring correct pad placement, ensuring that the patient is safe and observing other electrical devices within the range of the electrosurgical unit (Wicker 1991). Safe use of electrosurgical units will reduce the potential for patient harm before, during and after surgical procedures.

However, if electrosurgery is applied without knowledge of the harm it can cause, it can lead to two main contributors to patient injury: thermal burns and burns caused by explosions or fire (Wicker 1991).

Thermal burns

Thermal burns can lead to serious burns and tissue damage (Figure 44.1). Isolated electrosurgical units have reduced the number of surgical burns, because electrosurgical current is not connected to earth or ground. Thermal burns received by the patient during an electrosurgical procedure can be attributed to misuse of the ESU and can happen at the active electrode or return electrode site, or at an alternate site where the patient is touching a metal object such as the edge of the operating table or the Mayo stand. Serious burns can also occur when the ESU settings are too high and the current is applied for a long time. Three other problems attributed to stray energy burns are insulation failure, capacitive coupling and direct coupling (O'Riley 2010). Insulation failure involves breakdown of the insulation covering the wire and active electrodes used during minimally invasive procedures, leading to burning of tissues.

Capacitance is the passing of currents between two conductors that are separated by an insulator. This can happen in minimally invasive procedures, where capacitive coupling occurs between an insulated electrode and a surrounding metal trocar with plastic screw threads (O'Riley 2010), leading to tissue burns. Direct coupling is contact between the active electrode and tissue. Unintended direct coupling may occur due to faulty insulation on an active electrode.

Methods of reducing electrical burns include inspecting all active electrodes for insulation damage before use, avoiding contact with metal instruments when using an active electrode and using bipolar forceps when possible. A return electrode (also called a grounding pad or patient plate) must be used for monopolar electrosurgery to activate the generator and to reduce the risk of injury. Actions taken when attaching the return electrode include inspecting and recording the skin area underneath the return electrode; observing for skin-to-skin contact and for contact pathways from metal or jewellery or stray radio frequency currents; avoiding the pad being placed over bony prominences, on top of burned,

scarred or hairy tissue or distal to the tourniquet; and placing the pad close to the operative site (O'Riley 2010).

Avoiding burns to hands may involve changing gloves regularly during prolonged electrosurgery and ensuring that the surgeon and assistant are not touching the patient's tissues when electrosurgery is applied. Electrosurgical current operates at radio frequency, allowing the current to pass through insulated wire, even more so if it is secured to the drapes with a metal towel clip or clamp. If the cable is coiled, the insulation can also become damaged and expose the metal wire inside. Under these circumstances, the current can leave the electrode and divert to other places. Similarly, broken insulation can lead to sparks jumping from the cable to patient tissues or a surgeon or assistant's hand, leading to burns. Thermoelectric burns can also be caused by the concentration of monopolar electrosurgical current through a narrow tissue area, such as the penis, fingers or periphery of the body. Minimally invasive surgery also increases the risk of burns due to faulty insulation, direct coupling and capacitive coupling (Prasad et al. 2006; O'Riley 2010; Valleylab 2013).

Explosion and fire

The National Reporting and Learning System (NRLS) identified 33 incidents of fire during 2011 that involved either skin preparation and/or electrosurgery. Four incidents caused death or severe harm to the patient (NRLS 2012).

Explosion and fire may occur when electrosurgical sparks ignite flammable gases or solutions. Flash fires can occur following the release of oxygen into the air when the concentration is high. Releasing less oxygen, while ensuring that the patient receives the right amount, can help minimise the risk of oxygen-related fires.

The 'fire triangle' is a combination of fuel, an ignition source and oxygen. Fuels such as alcoholic skin-prepping agents, drapes and gowns and the patient's hair can start fires during surgery. Alcohol-based prepping solutions can cause the most harm, since they release vapours as the prep solution evaporates. Therefore, ensure that surgical sites are dry before commencing surgery, and prevent pooling around the site of surgery (AFPP 2011).

The ignition source is the active electrode, which can ignite fuels in an oxygen-rich environment or in the presence of alcoholic vapours. Alcohol solutions must be allowed to dry around the surgical site, and the active electrode should not be used away from the surgical site.

Explosion sometimes happens when abdominal gases are present during colonoscopy, or are released during colon resections in laparotomies. Sparks generated by electrosurgery can lead to serious explosions and harm to both the patient and the surgeon (Dhebri & Afify 2002; Prasad et al. 2006)

The most effective safety system in electrosurgery is when ODPs, nurses, surgeons and anaesthetists understand the safe and correct way to use electrosurgery devices and units. A basic understanding of electrosurgery and adherence to the necessary precautions by all staff will help to provide a safe environment for both patients and staff.

45 Venous thromboembolism

Figure 45.1   Action of intermittent pneumatic compression (IPC) on blood vessels

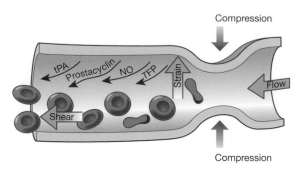

Figure 45.2   Action of IPC on blood and lymphatic supplies

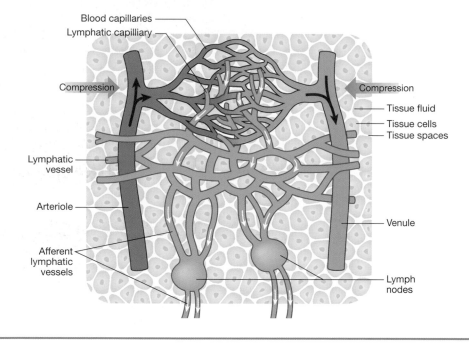

Patients undergoing surgery, especially those with previous cardiovascular problems and those undergoing long procedures, are at high risk of developing venous thromboembolism (VTE), comprising deep vein thrombosis (DVT) and pulmonary embolism (NICE 2011). Over 25 000 patients each year in the UK die because of VTE and around 20% of patients undergoing major surgery suffer from DVT. Orthopaedic surgery can lead to even higher rates (40%) of DVT if thromboprophylaxis, which is any measure taken to prevent coronary thrombosis, is not put in place (Narani 2010; NICE 2011).

Physiology of DVT

DVT occurs because of thrombi forming in the deep veins of calf muscles or the proximal veins of the leg (Narani 2010). Inactivity leads to thrombi developing, therefore patients undergoing long operations can develop VTE (DH 2010). In most circumstances thrombi are formed in the calf, and their presence is unknown until the patient wakes up and feels pain or discomfort. However, DVT in the calf can lead to a pulmonary embolus developing (DH 2010; NICE 2011). Development of a pulmonary embolus can lead to respiratory and cardiovascular problems, which are, of course, high risks for all patients. The coagulation cascade and fibrinolysis, which helps restore blood vessel patency by reducing occlusive thrombus formation, determine the end result of thrombus formation (Narani 2010).

Treatment options

NICE guidance (2011) recommends that any patients undergoing major orthopaedic surgery should receive thromboprophylaxis using either medication or mechanical means. Patients at risk of DVT or pulmonary embolism may be given medication such as low molecular weight heparin, warfarin or aspirin. Chemoprophylaxis for all patients involves the use of anticoagulant pharmacological treatment to reduce coagulation (Narani 2010). Some drugs, such as aspirin, can also produce major side effects including an increased risk of bleeding, which could become a problem for patients undergoing surgery (Augistinos & Ouriel 2004). Intermittent pneumatic compression (IPC) devices (Figures 45.1 and 45.2), which are usually compression stockings or intermittent compression devices, are normally used with medication. Patients undergoing orthopaedic surgery are at high risk of developing VTE and are often given chemoprophylaxis before and after surgery to help prevent these problems (Desciak & Martin 2011).

Mechanical prophylaxis

Mechanical prophylaxis includes events such as early mobilisation, leg exercises, use of graduated compression stockings (GCS) and use of IPC devices. Unlike chemoprophylaxis there is little associated risk of bleeding, assuming that GCS and IPC devices are not applied over open wounds (Wienert *et al*. 2005). GCS are specialised stockings that can be either knee or thigh length. Once GCS are fitted correctly and IPC are switched on, they exert circumferential or sequential pressure, mechanically preventing venous distension and reduce pooling of blood in the deep veins. However, in some cases they are not used, especially in patients with peripheral vascular disease or diabetic neuropathy (Agnelli 2004).

Intermittent compression devices (ICD)

ICD apply mechanical pressure on limbs to help blood circulation. Indications for their use include acute and sub-acute injuries to reduce oedema and pain due to swelling; postsurgical oedema; preventing DVT formation; reducing postsurgical oedema such as venous oedema, lymphoedema and lipoedema; foot or ankle ulcers; peripheral arterial disease; and hemiplegia, which is total paralysis of the arm, leg and trunk on the same side of the body (Wienert *et al*. 2005; DH 2010).

The presence of peripheral vascular disease is the main indication for not using IPC devices or GCS (Augistinos & Ouriel 2004). Other contraindications include fractured limbs, open wounds, compartment syndrome, congestive heart failure, gangrene, dermatitis, DVT and thrombophlebitis (Wienert *et al*. 2005).

The ICD is wrapped around a limb and connected with hoses to a unit. Air or cold water flows through the appliance, either sequentially or circumferentially, and on a constant or intermittent basis. Sequential pressure (SP) is when the appliance is divided into various compartments and the compartments are filled from distal to proximal areas. Circumferential pressure (CP) is when the appliance is filled simultaneously and equal amounts of pressure are applied to all parts of the extremity. Pressure rises with the ON cycle and drops with the OFF cycle. CP can be used to prevent the formation of oedema. Movement of fluids is caused by various pressure gradients. Two pressure gradients are being utilised. External compression causes the gradient between the tissue hydrostatic pressure and the capillary filtration pressure, and reduces the pressure, encouraging reabsorption of interstitial fluids (DH 2010). A gradient is also formed between the distal portion of the extremity (high pressure) and proximal portion (low pressure) because the tissues are being compressed, which forces fluids to move from high-pressure to low-pressure areas (Wienert *et al*. 2005). If the extremity is elevated, both gradient pressures are enhanced by gravity, encouraging a speedier venous drainage. Low pressure (35–55 mmHg) has been shown to increase venous velocity substantially. Because debris is removed from the area, fresh blood flow is increased significantly to the area following treatment. During ON time the blood flow to the area is decreased because of the external pressure. During OFF time the blood flow is restored, allowing venous and lymph vessels to absorb fluids.

Precautions

The ICD needs to be applied carefully, following the manufacturer's and the hospital's clinical guidelines and policies. Precautions when using this device include checking the distal extremity to ensure that blood circulation is present, and these checks need to be carried out throughout the treatment period. Practitioners should check that objects are not lodged within the appliance and that the fabric is not folded, as this may cause further damage (Wienert *et al*. 2005). Potential complications when using ICD include nerve palsy, neurovascular compression, ischaemia, compartment syndrome, pulmonary embolism and genital lymphoedema (Wienart *et al*. 2005).

Latex allergy

Figure 46.1 **Some of the tissues affected following an allergic reaction**

The early phase of the allergic reaction typically occurs within minutes, or even seconds, following allergen exposure and is also commonly referred to as the immediate allergic reaction or Type I allergic reaction. The reaction is caused by the release of histamine and mast cell granule proteins by a process called degranulation, as well as the production of leukotrienes, prostaglandins and cytokines, by mast cells following the cross-linking of allergen-specific IgE molecules bound to mast cell FcεRI receptors. These mediators affect nerve cells, causing itching, smooth muscle cells causing contraction (leading to the airway narrowing seen in allergic asthma), goblet cells causing mucus production, and endothelial cells causing vasodilatation and oedema

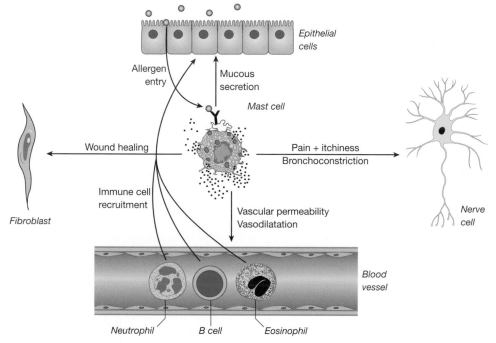

Source: Adapted from Wikipedia © Sabban, Sari (2011)

Development of an *in vitro* model system for studying the interaction of Equus caballus IgE with its high-affinity FcεRI receptor (PhD thesis), The University of Sheffield. Reproduced under the Creative Commons Attribution License.

Latex is extracted from rubber trees and is composed of natural proteins. The latex is processed by adding chemicals that result in strength, elasticity and stability. Sensitivity to latex and the development of allergies have increased because of the higher number of latex products in the operating department, the most common use being surgical gloves (Mercurio 2011). Latex allergies occur in both patients and staff who are exposed to latex, and some individuals are at higher risk because of conditions they have. Many staff develop latex allergies through the the regular and frequent use of latex gloves or other devices in the operating department that contain latex. Individuals who suffer from different allergies, for example asthma, hay fever, allergic dermatitis or food allergies, such as to avocado, strawberry, banana and chestnuts, can develop latex allergies quickly (Katz 2005). Females develop allergies to latex more often than males. Although the reasons for this are unknown, it may be caused by exposure to latex during gynaecological and obstetric procedures (Katz 2005).

Reducing problems with latex

Managers should support the reduction of latex use wherever possible, as long as it does not interfere with safe patient care. Informing and training staff in the safe use of latex products, together with risk assessments, should address the dangers and risks to health (Mercurio 2011). **Team leaders** need to encourage staff to follow hospital policies (Brown 1999). This can include following Control of Substances Hazardous to Health (COSHH) guidelines and ensuring that these are applied and used by staff and contractors. Staff should be trained and records kept of the instruction and training that has been given. Incidents relating to latex should be reported and recorded (Sussman & Gold 2014). **Perioperative practitioners** also need to know the dangers of latex allergy and how to address them by following hospital policies and guidelines (Brown 1999). For example, personal protective equipment should be worn correctly and appropriately and removed before eating food or drinking; personal hygiene should be practised at a high standard; any problems, risks, issues, defects or events related to latex or the development of allergies need to be reported to managers (Mercurio 2011). When anybody develops a latex allergy, this should be reported to the manager as soon as possible. A member of staff will also need to go to the occupational health service for support and treatment options.

Dangers of latex

Latex irritates the skin and mucous membranes and is known to be a sensitiser, a substance that has the ability to cause allergy (Brown 1999). Allergy can affect people in different ways (Figure 46.1), but the three reactions to latex are irritation, delayed hypersensitivity and immediate hypersensitivity. **Irritation** is a non-allergic reaction leading to a characteristic dry and itchy rash. Normally this reaction disappears after contact with the latex stops (Katz 2005). **Delayed hypersensitivity** is also known as allergic contact dermatitis. Normally this is caused by the chemicals used in the manufacturing process, which lead to an allergic reaction. The patient affected by these chemicals can develop red rashes, blisters and papules, and the skin may become hard and leathery (Sussman & Gold 2014). **Immediate hypersensitivity** is activated by Immunoglobulin E (IgE), which is an antibody, and is a reaction to the natural protein residue found in natural rubber latex. Once the person touches latex symptoms appear quickly, although they usually reduce rapidly when contact with the latex has ceased. Body reactions to immediate hypersensitivity include urticaria (hives), oedema, rhinitis, conjunctivitis and asthma. More serious problems include anxiety, shortness of breath, anaphylaxis, tachycardia, hypotension and cardiovascular collapse, potentially leading to serious complications or death (Katz 2005).

Treatment for severe allergic reaction

Drugs are used to treat severe allergic reactions. Epinephrine can relax muscles in the airways and contract blood vessels, reducing the effects of the allergy (Sussman & Gold 2014). Diphenhydramine is very effective at reducing allergic responses. It is an antihistamine and provides anticholinergic (inhibits acetylcholine), antitussive (reduces coughing), anti-emetic and sedative effects. Salbutamol can also be given as a bronchodilator, which reduces constriction of the airways (Sussman & Gold 2014). The patient should be placed in a head-down position (Trendelenberg) and administered oxygen by nasal cannula if they have cardiovascular or respiratory symptoms. The patient needs to be monitored carefully and should never be left alone (Sussman & Gold 2014).

Managing the perioperative environment

Patients allergic to latex should be first on the operating list in order to reduce exposure to latex allergens in the environment (Katz 2005). During anaesthesia, bacterial and viral filters can be attached to the airway tubes to prevent the inhalation of latex particles. Since the main risks to the anaesthetised patient are from actual contact with latex, removing latex from the operating room and the use of latex-free products are essential in the management of high-risk patients (Mercurio 2011). Anaesthetic drugs are sometimes presented in glass vials with latex rubber bungs. These bungs can contaminate the solutions, and can also be injected into patients via the needle that was used to mix the drug with water. Operating tables must be latex free or covered with sheets to prevent contact with the patient (Katz 2005).

Postoperative management

Allergic reactions can occur up to 60 minutes after the patient receives the anaesthetic. If the case is short, then patients should stay in recovery for at least an hour so that they can be monitored in case allergic reactions start. All staff in recovery should understand the signs and symptoms of latex allergy, such as rash, bronchospasm and discomfort. Drugs including anti-emetics and analgesics need to be latex free. Any equipment used should also be latex free, especially oxygen masks, tubing and tape. Following an allergic reaction to latex, discharge of the patient back to the ward will be at the discretion of the anaesthetist.

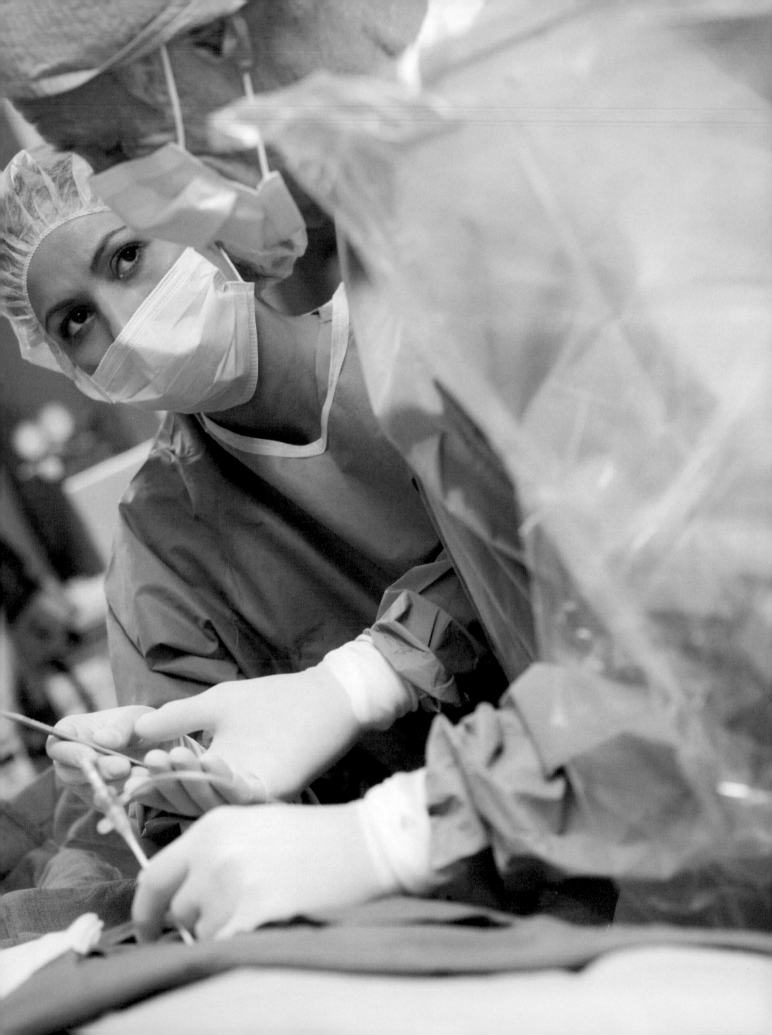

Advanced surgical practice

Part 6

Chapters

47 Assisting the surgeon   104

48 Shaving, marking, prepping and draping   106

49 Retraction of tissues   108

50 Suture techniques and materials   110

51 Haemostatic techniques   112

52 Laparoscopic surgery   114

53 Orthopaedic surgery   116

54 Cardiac surgery   118

55 Things to do after surgery   120

47 Assisting the surgeon

Figure 47.1 **A patient undergoing wound closure following a fasciotomy due to trauma damage to his leg**
The surgical care practitioner is assisting the surgeon by attaching loops to the skin to help close the wound. The wound will not close completely because of the expanded leg muscles

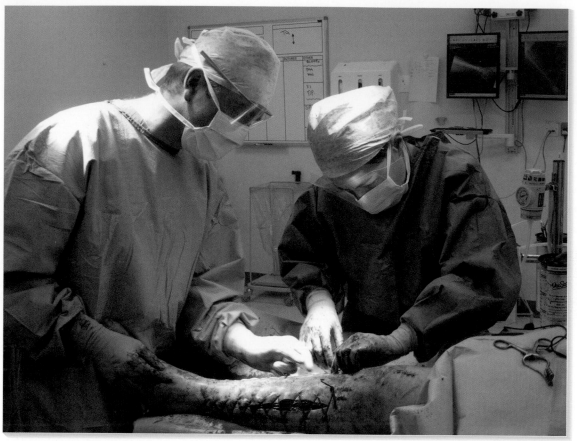

Source: Aintree University Hospital, Liverpool.

This chapter is about the roles of the Surgical First Assistant (SFA) and Surgical Care Practitioner (SCP), who assist surgeons. There has been confusion in the past because of the range of different titles, training courses and expectations from trusts and private hospitals. Over the past few years, the Royal College of Surgeons and the Perioperative Care Collaborative have helped to clarify the roles of the surgeon's assistant. The idea of a perioperative practitioner assisting surgeons started as early as 1993, and the first cardiac surgeon's assistant was Suzanne Holmes, who introduced the role of the SCP (Holmes 1994). Since then there have been several concerns about the role of the non-medical surgeon's assistant and the details of the role have been updated to ensure patient and staff safety (Jones *et al.* 2011).

Surgical First Assistant

To act as an SFA, registered practitioners must have undertaken an SFA module that has been benchmarked against the national competencies, and also undertake additional training in specific surgical techniques. The SFA also has to have their role risk assessed within their job description, which is supported by the hospital or organisation (PCC 2012). The SFA must be accompanied by a scrub practitioner, because the dual role of SFA and scrub practitioner cannot normally be maintained due to the difference in the roles. The dual role must be risk assessed and supported by a hospital policy that both the SFA and the scrub practitioner are allowed by their employer to carry out this role in specific circumstances. The knowledge and skills of the SFA role (excluding pre- and postoperative visits) have now been provided in the preregistration curriculum document for the BSc (Hons) in Operating Department Practice, which was written by the College of Operating Department Practitioners (2011). The role of the SFA has been supported by the Royal College of Surgeons in a statement made in 2011. This statement identified the need for clarification of the role and highlighted the need for quality-assured competencies and accreditation to help develop multidisciplinary surgical teams (RCS 2011).

Roles and responsibilities

The SFA may undertake various roles, but is limited in some areas. Preoperatively, the SFA may undertake preoperative visits to improve communication between surgical wards and operating theatres. The SFA also supports the Surgical Safety Checklist, ensuring that it is carried out before the start of surgery and participating in the five steps of the process (PCC 2012). During surgery the SFA undertakes tasks such as catheterisation, assisting in patient positioning, skin preparation, draping, tissue retraction, cutting of sutures, assisting with haemostasis, applying indirect electrosurgery, applying suction, holding instruments and cameras during minimally invasive surgery, and assisting with wound closure and application of dressings (Whalan 2006; PCC 2012). Practitioners who have undertaken the postregistration SFA modules can be supported by their hospital to undertake these tasks. ODPs who have completed the module as part of the preregistration BSc (Hons) in ODP will need to demonstrate competencies as defined nationally, and will also need preceptorship to develop their skills further. Registered practitioners can only undertake the role of SFA if their hospital has a policy in place and the role is part of their job description and contract of employment (PCC 2012).

Surgical Care Practitioner

Between 2004 and 2006 the Department of Health, the Royal College of Surgeons and other organisations assessed the role of the SCP to ensure that SCP were trained to the same level as junior surgeons (DH 2006; Jones *et al.* 2011). An SCP curriculum was developed (DH 2006) and the SCP role was defined as 'A non-medical practitioner, working in clinical practice as a member of the extended surgical team, who performs surgical intervention, preoperative and post-operative care under the direction and supervision of a consultant surgeon' (RCS 2011). The role of the SCP continued to be under scrutiny until 2012, when the Royal College of Surgeons in association with Edge Hill University and other parties rewrote the SCP curriculum and endorsed the validation of every programme for SCP training to ensure that the core competencies of the SCP were nationally recognised and that the role of the SCP remained safe and effective.

Roles and responsibilities

Once qualified, the SCP may still be in a position of needing to learn particular surgical skills. For example, if general surgery was the main speciality during training as an SCP, a move into orthopaedics would need different skills and knowledge. In the first month of the SCP's role in the job, the SCP would take part in core skills such as patient preparation, patient positioning, tissue exposure, application of suction, indirect application of electrosurgery, camera holding, superficial suturing of skin and so on (Whalan 2006). The SCP would also learn how to carry out pre- and postoperative visiting of the patient, and also read and understand local policies and protocols. As the SCP develops skills, the skills will be enhanced. For example, skin closure can be carried out under the direct supervision of the surgeon using either skin clips or sutures. Other skills that can be learned over time include tying surgical knots, insertion and suture of wound drains, assistance with haemostasis and retraction of skin, tissues, and organs (Figure 47.1; Whalan 2006). The SCP will also be expected to join in ward rounds, attend meetings and observe patients in outpatient clinics. Other skills that need to be learned outside of the operating room include, for example, X-ray evaluation, wound care evaluation, postoperative assessment of the patient's condition, personal organisation and critical thinking skills. Eventually the SCP will develop enough skills, knowledge and understanding to be able to support the surgeons fully in their specific field of surgery.

48 Shaving, marking, prepping and draping

Figure 48.1 Shaving the patient prior to surgery

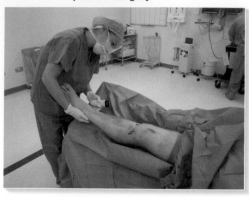

Figure 48.2 Disposal of swabs and instruments following prepping of skin

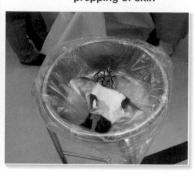

Figure 48.3 Common draping for major abdominal cases

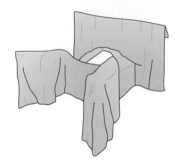

Figure 48.4 Draping the patient's leg using a drape with a central hole for the leg to go through

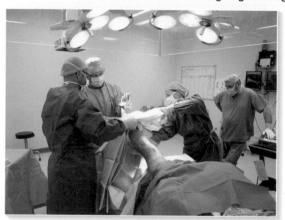

Figure 48.5 Draping the patient by covering their top, bottom and side – here the leg is being wrapped by a drape

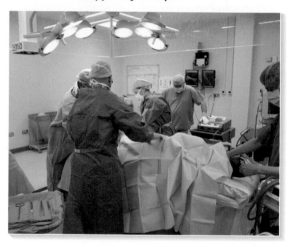

Figure 48.6 Marking the patient

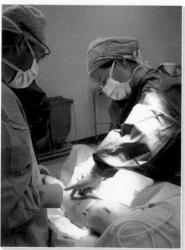

Source: All photos from Aintree University Hospital, Liverpool.

everal actions need to be taken before starting surgery, including (but not limited to) anaesthetic preparation of the patient (Part 2), positioning of the patient (Part 3), applying antithrombotic devices (Part 5), shaving, marking the operative sites, prepping the skin and draping.

Shaving

Shaving of an area (Figure 48.1) depends on the planned surgery. Removing hair is important, because it harbours bacteria that can contaminate wound areas. Electric clippers are preferable to razor blades because they minimise the risk of cutting the skin (Whalan 2006). Shaving normally happens immediately before surgery in the anaesthetic room or operating room. Sometimes, for example during trauma emergencies or emergency aortic aneurysms, shaving may not happen as the patient needs surgery urgently to survive. With the help of patients, electrodes should be placed on an area of skin free from hair, although if necessary a hairy patient may need the area to be shaved.

Skin marking

Skin marking using an indelible surgical skin-marking pen is normally an important procedure and the surgeon or an SCP will carry it out before surgery. Sometimes there may be extra marking once the surgery has started (Figure 48.6). Carefully marking the skin preoperatively will help to identify the surgical site, indicate the final appearance of the wound and help to establish the method of closure of the wound (PPSA 2008). Marking arrows or symbols on the skin is essential to pinpoint the surgical area and to avoid surgery on the wrong site.

Skin preparation

Skin prepping is painting clean skin with an antiseptic solution to reduce the chance of contamination of the wound area (Hemani & Lepor 2009). The SCP or SFA may carry out this task. The antiseptic solutions usually used are Betadine (povidone-iodine, brown solution) or chlorhexidine (pink solution). Both can either be alcohol or water based. The surgical assistant will prep the skin, or assist the surgeon if required (Hemani & Lepor 2009). The surgical assistant will be given a swab on a Rampley sponge holder and a small container of the skin prep solution.

Painting the skin should be done in a systematic way, not randomly (AST 2008). The first area to paint is over the site of the incision. Next, start painting from the incision site outwards as far as necessary. For example, the whole abdomen may be painted for a laparotomy, and the whole upper leg and surrounding areas may be painted for a hip replacement or insertion of femoral nail. Any dirty or contaminated areas, such as the umbilicus or groin, should be painted last to prevent the spread of contamination (AST 2008).

Often Betadine is used first, then the area is cleaned again using chlorhexidine to prevent the skin staining postoperatively. Sensitive areas, such as the eyes and mouth, need to be protected if the antiseptic agent is used close to them (Whalan 2006). Swabs and solutions are disposed of after prepping is complete (Figure 48.2).

Draping

Draping (Figures 48.3, 48.4 and 48.5) is carried out by two people to ensure sterility and correct placement of the drapes according to the skin markings, and following drying of alcoholic prep solutions. Surgeons often carry out draping with the help of the SCP or SFA. SCPs can also drape patients with the help of the scrub practitioner. Draping involves setting up a sterile area around the site of the surgery, normally covering the patient's entire body and leaving the site of surgery exposed. Drapes are normally sealed around the site of surgery using either adhesives on the drapes, or sterile self-adhesive sheets of soft, clear plastic material (for example Opsite or Ioban®) to prevent blood or fluids flowing under the drapes. This also helps to fix drapes into place so that they do not move (Davidson *et al.* 2003). Self-adhesive plastic sheets are attached to the patient in the following way: the sheet is opened, the surgeon and assistant hold its corners, the scrub practitioner removes the paper sheet underneath to expose the adhesive surface, and then the sheet is lowered into position and smoothed out, removing air bubbles, by using a gauze pack (Whalan 2006).

Usually the surgical field is draped in tandem with the surgeon. Therefore, the SCP would stand on the opposite side of the table to the surgeon and follow the surgeon's actions. In most circumstances (such as abdominal surgery), four small drapes are placed around the surgical field, then two large drapes are placed on the top end and lower end of the patient. If a limb is being draped, then a large drape with a hole in it can be used, along with a drape wrapped around the limb and secured with a crepe bandage. During insertion of a dynamic hip screw (DHS) and plate into the broken neck of the femur, a vertical isolation drape can be used. This is secured to an overhanging pole and then attached to the patient's leg by an adhesive. Drapes can also be secured by blunt towel clips (Whalan 2006), although these are rarely used now because drapes are usually disposable and have adhesive linings.

Drapes should be handled carefully and not allowed to touch the floor or be contaminated by either the patient or other members of staff. Any drapes hanging below waist level are considered to be unsterile (Whalan 2006). A barrier is formed between the surgeon and the anaesthetist to prevent contamination of the anaesthetist or patient by blood and fluids that may splash from the wound site, and to prevent contamination of the surgical field from the unsterile anaesthetic area (Davidson *et al.* 2003).

Shaving, marking, prepping and draping should therefore all be carried out according to local hospital policies and regulations, and in accordance with best practice.

49 Retraction of tissues

Figure 49.1 (a) Deavers retractors, (b) Langenbecks retractors, (c) rake retractor, (d) Balfour self-retaining retractor and (e) Travers self-retaining retractor

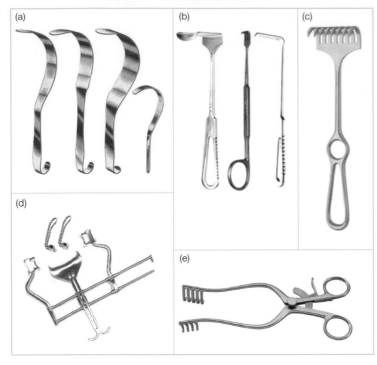

(a)

(b)

(c)

(d)

(e)

Figure 49.2 (a) Transanal surgical retractor, for hip surgery, (b) table-mounted Omni-flex® retractor for hip surgery

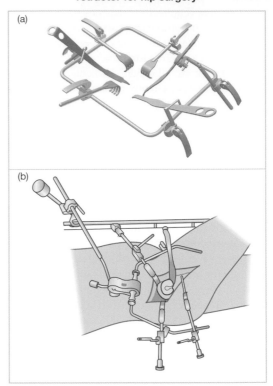

(a)

(b)

Figure 49.3 Retraction of tissues using a self-retaining retractor and a Hohmann's retractor

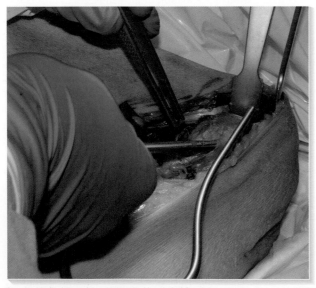

Source: Medical Illustration, University Hospital of South Manchester. Copyright: UHSM Academy.

Figure 49.4 Curved Travers retractor

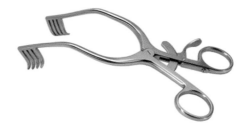

Figure 49.5 Gelpi self-retaining retractor

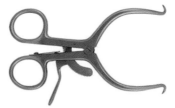

Perioperative Practice at a Glance, First Edition. Paul Wicker. © 2015 John Wiley & Sons, Ltd. Published 2015 by John Wiley & Sons, Ltd.

Surgical assistants are often needed to retract tissues, to expose the area of tissue being operated on. This role can be taken on by either an SCP or SFA, or by a scrub practitioners (during minor surgery), depending on hospital policies and regulations. Retractors can be either hand held or self-retaining. The potential dangers of retraction include damage to nerves, structures and organs.

Holding retractors

The surgeon will show the surgical assistant how to place and hold the hand-held retractor and to pull on the tissues to expose the surgical site. In some circumstances, retraction can be high risk because it requires flexion of your neck, arm and back muscles, as well as long periods of standing (Spera & Lloyd 2011). This can lead to aches and pains as well as possible musculoskeletal injuries, especially if the retraction is at an odd angle and the tissues are heavy or tight, requiring excessive pulling. Therefore, you should be careful to pull the retractor only as much as is needed to expose the surgical site (Whalan 2006). If you hold the manual retractor close to your body, rather than reaching out or pulling a retractor away from or lateral to the body, it will help you to maintain a good posture. When you are holding a manual or hand-held retractor, position yourself at the optimal working height and posture by either lowering or raising the operating table, using a stool to sit on, or using a platform to raise your height. The best posture to adopt is standing upright and facing towards the site of the operation (Whalan 2006). As an alternative, using self-retaining retractors reduces the chances of pain, fatigue and injury, and allows you to carry out other actions (Spera & Lloyd 2011).

The surgical procedure, as well as the patient's physical characteristics, determines the type of retractor required. Manual retraction is sometimes employed by holding gauze pads, stay sutures, sloops or swabs to retract the bowel while undertaking a laparotomy (Goodman & Spry 2014). Normally, manual retraction is needed only for short periods of time. Once in place, self-retaining retractors, such as Travers or Balfour retractors, provide a good view of the surgical site and usually need no handling. Hand-held retractors, for example Langenbecks and rake retractors, can be placed quickly and carefully and are easily repositioned and also removed if required (Spera *et al.* 2011).

The use of minimally invasive procedures has increased over the years and has resulted in the development of different types of laparoscopic retractors that are capable of many different uses in many different ways. However, changing the instrument during a laparoscopy can be time consuming and also risky, because the instruments may not be within the view of the surgeon or the assistant. Nevertheless, the use of minimally invasive retractors reduces the need for assistants to hold retractors for a long period of time (Whalan 2006).

Managing retractors

Hand-held retractors include Langenbeck, Kocher, Lahey, Deaver and Hohmann retractors (Figures 49.1 and 49.3). Examples of self-retaining retractors include Norfolk-Norwich, Travers and Balfour.

There are also table-mounted retractors that are used for major cases, and may be employed alongside hand-held retractors to give extra retraction along tissue edges (Figure 49.2). Examples of table-mounted retractors include Universal Ring, Omnitract and Iron Intern® retractors.

Hand-held retractors

Hand-held retractors come in all shapes and sizes. Some of them are fitted with handles; others only have flat edges, which can be uncomfortable to the surgical assistant and painful in the long term (Kirkup 1996). Some hand-held retractors also have sharp points, for example cat's paws and skin hooks. These retractors should be handled carefully to prevent holes in gloves, damage to tissues and damage to surgeons and assistant's hands or fingers.

Normally there is little need to pull hard on a retractor, as this can cause tissue damage. If the retractor has no handle, hold it lightly and close to the proximal end. Ensure that your hand does not move down the shaft of the instrument or you will end up holding it close to the distal end, which may lead to your hand being in the wound as well, obstructing the surgeon's view and possibly resulting in a sharps injury (Whalan 2006). Also, make sure that you maintain the angle and tension that the surgeon asks of you. If holding the retractor becomes painful, let the surgeon know and suggest another type of retractor. The surgeon will place the lip of the retractor in the wound and it needs to be kept in place throughout the surgery.

Self-retaining retractors

Surgeons usually place self-retaining retractors (Figures 49.4 and 49.5) in the best position without relying on the assistant to do this. This helps the surgeon to view the anatomy better and exposes the surgical site. Self-retaining retractors are placed in the tissue area and then opened as wide as required (Kirkup 1996). Once in place, these retractors usually stay there, although hand-held retractors may also be needed to assist with retracting wound edges.

Table-mounted retractors

Table-mounted retractors are usually fixed in place by the surgeon, with the help of the assistant. Various table-mounted retractors exist and it is best to learn how to position the retractor by observing the surgeon or asking a practitioner who has used such retractors before. The retractors are presented by the scrub practitioner to the surgeon in pieces, and the surgeon and assistant then assemble the retractor and organise it to be clamped to the operating table in the correct position. Once it is in position, retractor blades are added to the retractor as required for the surgery (Whalan 2006).

The best way to find out more about retractors is to read the manufacturers' written guides, or to ask either surgeons or scrub practitioners about them before the start of surgery.

50 Suture techniques and materials

Figure 50.1 Methods for releasing clips attached to suture materials

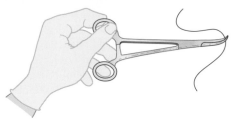

Left-handed grip, to release clip

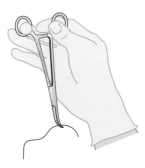

Reverse right-handed grip, to release clip

Figure 50.3 Suturing a damaged blood vessel and ligating other blood vessels in close proximity

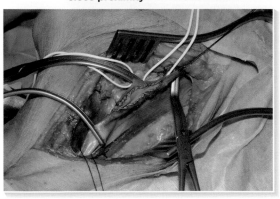

Figure 50.2 Examples of suture techniques

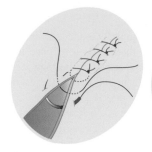
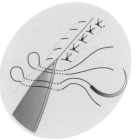

Interrupted suture · Interrupted mattress sutures

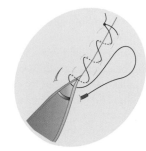
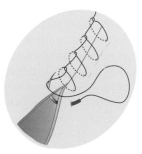

Continuous sutures · Continuous interlocking suture

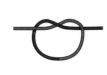
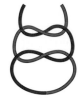
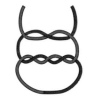

Half-hitch knot · Reef knot · Surgical knot (reef knot is doubled)

Source: Medical Illustration, University Hospital of South Manchester. Copyright: UHSM Academy.

Perioperative Practice at a Glance, First Edition. Paul Wicker. © 2015 John Wiley & Sons, Ltd. Published 2015 by John Wiley & Sons, Ltd.

The role of the surgeon's assistant during suturing is to assist the surgeon by either cutting the sutures or holding the suture material to keep it out of the surgeon's way, or maintaining tension so that the suture does not become slack. A suture includes a needle attached to suture material; a 'tie' is a piece of surgical suture material with no needle attached that is used to tie blood vessels or areas of tissue.

Assisting the surgeon

When holding and following suture material, you must remember to release it when the surgeon completes the suture and pulls the suture material through the tissue. If you release too early, the suture will become slack and the tissues may not join together; if you release too late, then the suture might snap (Whalan 2006). Long suture material can also become entangled with retractors or instruments, so you need to be aware of this to make sure that it does not happen (Semer 2001).

Another action that surgical assistants may undertake is releasing artery forceps clipped to bleeding points that have been tied. As artery clips close with a ratchet, to open the clip you need to hold it with your thumb and forefinger, using the right hand if possible, and with your middle and ring finger put pressure on the clip to open the ratchets (Figure 50.1; Whalan 2006). The act of removing a clip takes three steps. First, the artery forcep is lifted to enable the surgeon to pass a ligature around the tissue just below the tip of the artery forcep. Next, lower the artery forcep so that the surgeon can start tying a knot around the tissue or vessel to prevent bleeding (Whalan 2006). Once the surgeon is satisfied that the tissue has been tied properly, they will ask you to take the clip off using the technique already mentioned. The scrub practitioner will then give you scissors to cut the tie. When a blood vessel needs to be ligated (tied with a surgical tie) and is in a difficult place to access, then ties may be loaded onto long artery forceps, or on Lahey forceps, which have a 45° angle at the tip. The tie attaches to the clip like a 'bowstring' and can be passed under the blood vessel (Whalan 2006). The surgeon then takes a long pair of artery forceps, grasps the tie near to the tip of the forceps, then releases the tie and pulls it around the vessel and ties it using a surgical knot. This is repeated a little further down the blood vessel and then the vessel is cut through the middle portion between the two ties.

Suture techniques

Suturing is carried out either as single sutures (interrupted) or continuous sutures (Figures 50.2 and 50.3). Interrupted sutures include the 'over and over' suture, where the needle is inserted into the wound edges, passed underneath the skin and tissues and out the other side, then knotted (Semer 2001). The 'mattress' suture involves passing the suture through the skin, under the tissues and out the other side, and then passing it back to the point of origin in the same way, but down a pathway approximately 1 or 2 mm from the original pathway. In other words, this forms a loop, which is tied on one side of the wound. A continuous suture can be threaded under and over the tissue in a continuous fashion. Alternatively, it can be a 'continuous interlocking suture', which is twisted around the previous suture in order to make it more firm (Semer 2001). Knot tying is another important skill to learn. The securest knots are created when a loop is placed over another loop, as in a granny knot or half hitch. Another type is the reef knot, which is composed of two half hitches placed beside each other. When pulled together they tighten securely and are less likely to unravel. It is important for the SCP to undertake clinical workshops using simulation to practise suturing and learn more about suturing techniques.

Suture materials

The ideal suture material is easy to handle, does not cause tissue reactions, allows knots to be tied securely and is sterile and non-allergenic. The choice of suture material depends on various elements, including its properties, absorption rate, ability to knot, the type of tissue being sutured and the type of needle that is attached to it (Semer 2001; McDermott 2014; STO 2014).

Needle points come in a variety of shapes and sizes. Conventional cutting needles are triangular, with a flat surface on the external curve of the needle. Reverse cutting needles are the same but reversed. Round-bodied needles are sharp but have a round body, similar to a bent pin. Taper-cut needles have a triangular shape, allowing for cutting of tissues on all sides. Blunt-point needles are used to penetrate muscle and fascia and to reduce needlestick injuries to both the patient and the surgical staff (Semer 2001).

Natural suture materials include silk, linen and stainless-steel wire, which are all non-absorbable. Stainless-steel wire is used mainly for thick and heavy tissues, especially bone. An example is the use of stainless-steel wire to bond together the sternum (breast bone) following cardiac surgery (STO 2014).

Synthetic materials are either absorbable or non-absorbable. Absorbable suture material includes Dexon®, Vicryl® and PDS®. Dexon is either braided or monofilament and provides a strong material to assist in wound healing of soft tissues or ophthalmic procedures (Asali 2014). Vicryl is braided and therefore flexible, and is used for skin, subcutaneous tissues and muscles. PDS is monofilament, very strong and is often used for major wounds. It drops to around 80% of its tensile strength after 14 days. Non-absorbable sutures include nylon, Dacron® (polyester) and Prolene®. These materials remain strong, durable and long lasting and are used in various operations, such as skin closure, hernias, laparotomies and orthopaedic surgery (Asali 2014).

51 Haemostatic techniques

Figure 51.1 Coagulation of blood

The coagulation of blood is dependent on the actions of enzymes and activity by blood cells. The end result, following the activation of coagulation by thrombin, is the formation of a blood clot that acts as a plug to stop further bleeding. During the healing phase, as the vessel repairs itself, the clot starts dissolving in a phase known as fibrinolysis. During this phase the clots dissolve, releasing fibrin fragments.

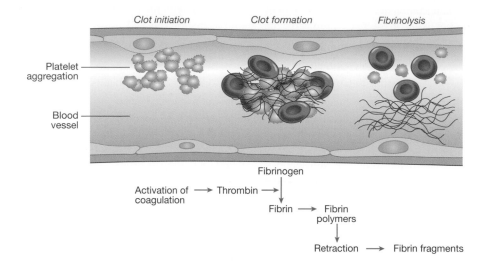

Figure 51.2 Use of diathermy to stop bleeding

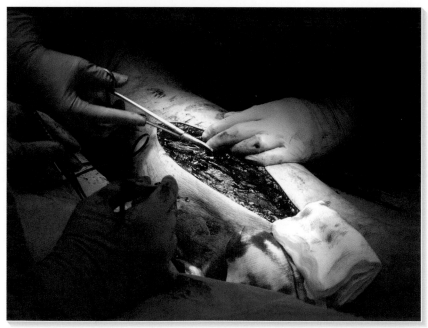

Source: Aintree University Hospital, Liverpool.

Perioperative Practice at a Glance, First Edition. Paul Wicker. © 2015 John Wiley & Sons, Ltd. Published 2015 by John Wiley & Sons, Ltd.

The word 'haemostasis' comes from Greek, *haem* meaning 'blood' and *stasis* meaning 'stop'. It is used for intraoperative bleeding, which always occurs, caused by the cutting of blood vessels. Normally, the surgeon will immediately apply pressure to the bleeding site and then employ some form of haemostatic technique to prevent further bleeding (Hakim & Canelo 2007). At this point, the surgical assistant would be responsible for using a Yankauer sucker to remove the remaining blood from the area.

The most common methods of stopping bleeding include the use of electrosurgery, clipping and tying vessels, and suturing or ligating vessels. Other techniques include compressing the area with a finger; adding topical haemostatic material such as cellulose gauze; using argon gas with electrosurgery to create superficial necrosis; or using ultrasonic instruments to cause coagulation of tissues (Niles 1999).

Assisting with haemostasis
Minor bleeding

Minor bleeding may require no action at all (Figure 51.1), as it often stops because of coagulation of the blood. Pressing on the wound site or patting the area with a gauze swab can also stop minor bleeding. Pressing on the area and then removing the swab can help the surgeon to identify the bleeding spot and electrosurgery can then be applied if necessary. Items used to pat the bleeding area include gauze swabs, packs (if there is a great deal of bleeding), peanuts (a small piece of gauze shaped like a peanut) attached to artery clips, or a swab attached to the end of a large Mayo artery forceps or Rampley's forceps, which are often called a 'swab on a stick'.

Major bleeding

Major bleeding will require more sustained action. Artery clips can be used to clamp blood vessels that have started bleeding. Once they stop bleeding, if they are not essential for the area they are supplying, they may be sutured or ligated to prevent further bleeding. Sutures can also seal blood vessels or bleeding points using either a figure-of-eight type suture, or passing the needle through the blood vessel and then tying the vessel off with the suture material. Using a suture in this way increases the likelihood of the suture material staying in place. You may need to assist the surgeon by dabbing the area to expose the bleeding point, and cutting the suture or tie.

Electrosurgery is also used frequently to stop bleeding (Niles 1999). The surgeon may conduct the electrosurgery by applying the active electrode directly to the bleeding point. Alternatively, they may grasp the bleeding point with a pair of forceps or artery forceps and then tell you to apply electrosurgery to the distal end of the instrument. The electrosurgical current travels down the instrument, through the patient and back towards the electrosurgical generator via the return electrode. Occasionally the surgeon may incur minor burns if the blade slips and touches their hand, or if they have a hole in their glove.

Wound drains are also applied to wounds if there is bleeding to drain fluid or blood to ensure that it does not accumulate within the wound. Surgeons normally introduce the drain into the wound themselves, as they are fully aware of where to place it and how to avoid any damage, and may then attach it to the patient using a suture. The assistant will be responsible for cutting off the spike on the end of the drain using a pair of heavy scissors, such as Mayo scissors, and connecting the drain to a drainage bottle or bag.

Haemostatic agents

Bleeding from areas such as bony surfaces, organ tissues, friable and damaged vessels, and multiple capillaries can usually not be managed through mechanical means such as clips or electrosurgery. The surgeon will choose the chemical to use, which can help to prevent bleeding (Hakim & Canelo 2007).

Pharmacological agents can be given preoperatively to improve or enhance clot formation. Epinephrine causes vasoconstriction and can reduce bleeding. Vitamin K plays an important part in the coagulation process, so this can be given preoperatively to help prevent bleeding (Samudralla 2008). Protamine reverses the action of heparin; however, it can cause anaphylaxis, acute pulmonary vasoconstriction and right ventricular failure. Other chemicals that can be used include desmopressin, which improves coagulation, and lysine, which helps to reduce bleeding (Moss 2013).

Topical haemostatic products are often used during surgery (Samudralla 2008). Passive devices include substances such as cellulose or porcine gelatins, contained within an absorbable sponge or foam pad with a topical haemostatic agent, such as collagen, which is then applied to the bleeding site (Hakim & Canelo 2007). These devices slow down bleeding and can absorb several times their own weight in fluids. More active haemostatic agents, such as topical thrombins, support the coagulation cascade in blood by stimulating fibrinogen resulting in the formation of a fibrin clot, normally within 10 minutes (Samudralla 2008). Thrombin is an enzyme that supports haemostasis, inflammation and cell signalling, and helps to produce a fibrin clot by helping to convert fibrinogen to fibrin (Moss 2013). Despite being more expensive, active haemostatic agents control local bleeding more effectively than passive haemostats, and they can be applied to large wound areas using pumps or spray kits (Moss 2013). Surgeons can also use a saturated gelatin sponge to apply them directly to the bleeding site (Moss 2013).

There are many other haemostatic agents in use, including flowable haemostatic agents that can block the flow of blood, and sealants, for example made from fibrin and albumin, which also form a barrier to block the flow of blood (Moss 2013). Control of surgical bleeding is a primary concern for the surgeon and their assistant and therefore knowledge and understanding of haemostatic agents are important.

52 Laparoscopic surgery

Figure 52.1 Laparoscopic surgery – placement of equipment for optimum viewing

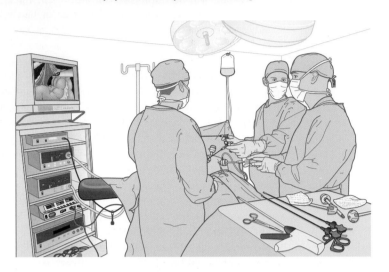

Figure 52.2 Laparoscopic surgery in gynaecology

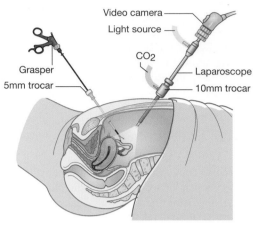

Video camera
Light source
CO_2
Grasper
Laparoscope
5mm trocar
10mm trocar

Figure 52.3 Laparoscopic cholecystectomy

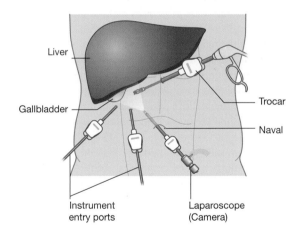

Liver
Gallbladder
Trocar
Naval
Instrument entry ports
Laparoscope (Camera)

Figure 52.4 Laparoscopic colorectal surgery

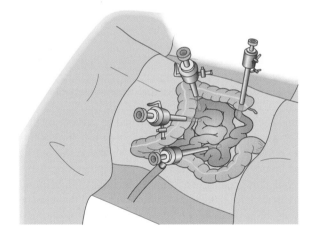

Perioperative Practice at a Glance, First Edition. Paul Wicker. © 2015 John Wiley & Sons, Ltd. Published 2015 by John Wiley & Sons, Ltd.

The role of the SFA and SCP is to aid and facilitate the surgeon to ensure that they are focusing on performing safe and effective surgery. This chapter focuses on the SCP, who will perform higher-level duties during laparoscopies.

To undertake these roles it is essential that the team as a whole uses a safe approach, employing the WHO surgical safety checklist as well as hospital policies and procedures. You will also need a fundamental or basic knowledge of laparoscopic techniques and equipment, and be familiar with the particular procedure being carried out (Rothrock 1999). As you gain more experience, it is likely that you will learn more about laparoscopic surgery, and you will gain enough experience to understand the key elements of laparoscopies.

Your knowledge and understanding are based on the surgeon's teaching, which includes improving the safety and efficacy of laparoscopic procedures. For example, intracorporeal knot tying is different to the normal knot tying in non-laparoscopic surgery (Ferzli 2011). A good way to learn laparoscopic techniques is in simulation labs. Things to learn in the simulation lab include handling of the camera, focusing on the surgical field and retraction using various instruments. Other items of importance to learn from the surgeon include comorbidities, which are other illnesses that may be associated with the main need for surgery, and issues with patient anatomy such as hernias, scars and obesity, which can affect laparoscopic surgery. For example, a morbidly obese male patient may need longer trocars and different instruments than the average 70 kg male (Rothrock 1999).

Before surgery

Before laparoscopic surgery, the surgeon may ask you to help prepare the operating room (Figure 52.1; Chiu et al. 2008). Issues of which you need to be aware include the appropriate positioning of the surgeon and the patient. Monitors, foot pedals and equipment need to be placed according to the surgery. For example, if the surgeon is going to be on the right side of the table, then the electrosurgical foot pedal should also be on the right side of the patient, and the video monitor should be easily viewed by the surgeon and their assistants. Cables need to be strategically placed to ensure that they do not contaminate the surgeon or risk being damaged or disconnected. It is also worthwhile discussing the need for instruments and equipment with the scrub practitioner before the start of surgery, to ensure that everything required is available either on the instrument trolley or ready for use within the operating room (Chiu 2008).

During surgery

Intraoperatively, the experienced surgical assistant should be familiar with the relevant surgical techniques (Figures 52.2, 52.3 and 52.4; Kaar 1999). Essential areas can include, for example, being familiar with the different techniques involved in achieving inflation of the peritoneum (pneumoperitoneum). You must also be aware of the need to monitor and observe safe parameters, including the flow rate of gas and the intra-abdominal pressure during insufflation and throughout the surgery. For instance, incomplete abdominal wall penetration can result in air collecting outside the peritoneum, or between different levels of tissues, rather than being within the abdomen itself. Other issues could include adhesions that can interfere with the surgery, visceral injuries that can cause problems such as infection or bleeding (Ferzli 2011), or fire caused by the light lead.

At the start of surgery, correct trocar placement is essential; while it is normally the surgeon in charge of the surgery who places these trocars, the SCP may be asked to do so (Rothrock 1999). Consider the size of incision required, which depends on the size of the trocar. Insert the trocar under supervision in a careful and controlled manner, following the manufacturer's guidelines, and ensure that it is placed in the correct position. The best position will ensure perfect access to the site of surgery, easy holding and manipulating of instruments inserted, minimum chance of instruments from different trocars interfering with each other, and the best visualisation of the surgical area (Rothrock 1999).

Being able to hold and manipulate the camera effectively is important for the success of all laparoscopic procedures (Bradley 2014). This role can be undertaken by either an SCP or an SFA, depending on hospital policies and regulations, as well as the expertise of the camera holder. Problems can arise with cameras, including camera fogging caused by moisture within the abdomen, displacement of the trocar, or simply wrong settings on the video equipment (Bradley 2014). Occasionally, electrosurgery can interfere with the view on the video screen because of the electrosurgical current causing the screen to flicker (Chiu et al. 2008). Whether or not these issues can be resolved depends on the skills and expertise of the assistant. For example, you need to ensure that you are holding the camera at the optimal angle and horizon for the surgeon to see the operative site, which can be especially important when instruments are inserted or withdrawn during surgery.

Training and development

The surgical assistant therefore needs to have a detailed knowledge of the instruments used during laparoscopy, including retractors, cutters, tissue forceps, suction and irrigation, and suturing instruments (Ferzli 2011). All these instruments come in different sizes and shapes, but most will also be supplied along with a detailed explanation by the manufacturer of how to use them. To train effectively for the role of laparoscopic surgeon's assistant, various methods of learning can be adopted; for example, simulation workshops and teaching videos are common in most hospitals or universities. Learning from the surgeon can also improve your ability.

Depending on the situation and if hospital policies and regulations allow this to happen, SCPs can transition from assistant to surgeon, as long as they are being monitored and supervised by an experienced consultant surgeon.

53 Orthopaedic surgery

Figure 53.1   Arthroscopy

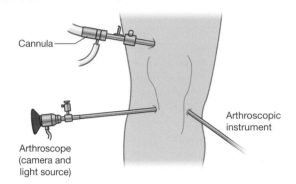

Cannula

Arthroscope
(camera and
light source)

Arthroscopic
instrument

Figure 53.2   Hip replacement

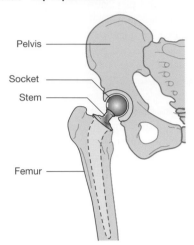

Pelvis

Socket

Stem

Femur

Figure 53.3   Knee-replacement surgery

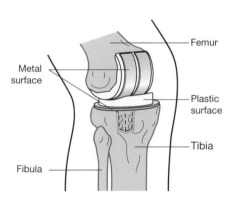

Femur

Metal
surface

Plastic
surface

Tibia

Fibula

Figure 53.4   Tibial surgery requiring insertion of nail

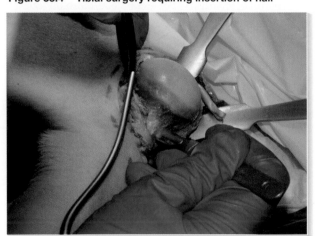

Source: Medical Illustration, University Hospital of South Manchester.
Copyright: UHSM Academy.

Orthopaedic surgery is divided into elective and trauma. Elective surgery includes surgery such as arthroscopies, joint replacement, spine repair and repair of bones that are malformed. Trauma orthopaedics deals mostly with broken bones and joints, and also involves tissue repair and vascular surgery in extreme cases, mostly caused by accidents. This chapter looks at the help needed by the surgical assistant during orthopaedic surgery (Jones *et al.* 2012); for details about the steps taken during orthopaedic surgery, check the reference list.

Specific factors in orthopaedic surgery

Serious bone infection can result in the patient receiving an amputation. Therefore, in most operating rooms, orthopaedic surgeons expect anybody in the operating room to cover their hair totally using an orthopaedic hood, rather than a surgeon's cap. This reduces the chance of hair falling into the wound and leading to bone infection. Wearing 'space-suits' or 'togas' that cover the individual from head to foot reduces the chance of blood splashing into the eyes, mouth or face. This also reduces the chance of infection for the patient and the member of staff (AAOS 2011).

As a surgical assistant, it is important that you have a knowledge and understanding of orthopaedic anatomy, given the potential issues with arteries, veins, nerves and the structure of bones and joints (Palan *et al.* 2009). It is also your responsibility to point out any areas of danger (such as cutting through an artery while using a power saw) to the surgeon, as they will focus mainly on the bone that they are repairing (Palan *et al.* 2009).

Arthroscopic knee surgery

To prepare a patient for knee arthroscopy (Figure 53.1), after anaesthesia a tourniquet will be applied proximally to the limb being operated on, and inflated once the surgeon is ready. One side of the distal end of the table may be removed so that the leg flexes at 90°. As the assistant, you may need to move the leg at the surgeon's request or flex it to open the joint more. A fluid, normally saline or 5% glycine, is first injected inside the joint via a cannula to expand it so that the scope can view inside the joint. Small joints such as wrists or ankles do not usually require fluid, although at times they may need a little.

Normally the scrub practitioner will hand over instruments to the surgeon. However, as a surgical assistant you can hold instruments ready for the surgeon, especially if the surgeon is using different instruments one after the other, at the same time. The surgeon will normally hold the camera and the instrument in each hand so they can easily see what they are doing. This will need little help from you while they are looking at the patella-femoral and medial compartments; however, after they move into the lateral compartment you will be requested to cross the leg over the opposite knee and hold it carefully in place. The leg may need to be repositioned at the request of the surgeon. Following completion of the surgery, the fluid is evacuated from the wound and the wound is sutured, dressed and bandaged. The tourniquet is then deflated and removed (Whalan 2006).

Elective joint replacement

Information about joint replacements is usually supplied in detail in manuals by the company providing the implants. A major complication of joint surgery is infection, therefore meticulous attention must be given to sterility to ensure that infection does not occur (Rothrock 1999). One way to support asepsis is to change gloves after prepping and draping, as contamination can occur without you realising it. After draping, the next step is to assist the surgeon in setting up for surgery. This can be complex, as it includes setting up suction, electrosurgery, irrigation, drills, saws and so on. Tubes and cables should be attached to the drapes to prevent them from slipping off the table.

Total hip replacements are normally carried out using a lateral approach (Figure 53.2). The patient will be in a lateral position and the upper leg will need to be lifted to complete the prepping and draping. The femoral head is dislocated from the hip joint and when this happens the leg's position needs to be controlled by you or the surgeon. Total knee replacements (Figure 53.3) are also complex and start with a midline incision, eversion of the patella and then gently flexing the knee to a 90° angle (AAOS 2012). You will be asked to retract tissues to expose the joint and also to protect structures such as collateral ligaments, the patellar tendon and the popliteal artery (Whalan 2006). When the bone has been shaped to fit the implants, bone cement is mixed and the implants are inserted and positioned properly. The knee is then placed flat and the wound is sutured and dressings applied.

Trauma orthopaedics

In most trauma cases an image intensifier (portable, live-view X-ray machine) is needed and must be set up before the surgery starts. The patient's broken limbs will need to be lifted for the skin to enable prepping and draping. When lifting the leg, it is important that some traction is applied to ensure that the broken bones do not grind together or cause damage to local tissues (Whalan 2006). You may need to maintain alignment of the bone ends while the surgery takes place, to prevent further damage and to ensure that the fracture is reduced. Internal fixation relates to plates, screws or nails (Figure 53.4); external fixation involves using an external fixator. During the procedure taking live X rays regularly checks that the bone ends are aligned.

Postoperatively, in elective or trauma surgery, the damaged limb's distal blood supply should be checked, and all X rays and case notes need to be taken with the patient to the recovery room.

54 Cardiac surgery

Figure 54.1   Aortic valve replacement

(a)

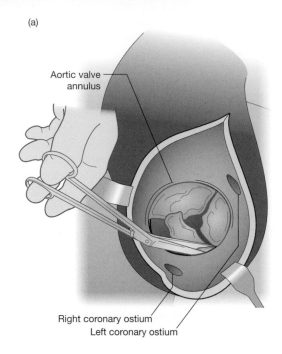

Aortic valve
annulus

Right coronary ostium
Left coronary ostium

(b)

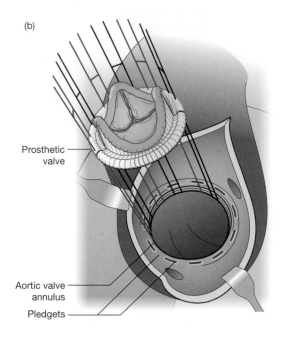

Prosthetic
valve

Aortic valve
annulus

Pledgets

Sutures are passed through the aortic valve annulus,
reinforced with pledgets, then passed through the sewing
ring of the prosthetic valve

Figure 54.2   Mechanical bicuspid aortic valve

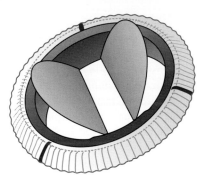

**Figure 54.3   Aortic valve from a pig
(porcine bioprosthesis**

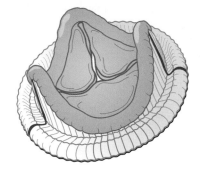

Cardiac surgery is complex and can include surgical events such as resection of ventricular aneurysm, repair of diseased or damaged valves, pulmonary embolectomy, pericardiectomy and revascularising of the ischaemic myocardium (Rothrock 1999).

Cardiac surgical procedures are too detailed to explain in full in this chapter, but as an example, aortic valve replacement involves the excision and replacement of a non-functioning valve (Figure 54.1; Goldman 2008). Aortic valve replacement may involve open or minimally invasive surgery, depending on the health of the patient and the skills of the surgeon. Using open surgery, the sternum is split using an electric saw, the chest opened and the heart exposed. Cardiopulmonary bypass (CPB) is started and clamps are attached to the aorta. The beating of the heart is then stopped by using hypothermia and/or cardioplegic drugs (Goldman 2008). The heart is opened and the damaged aortic valve is excised. Valves are replaced using autografts (the patient's own pulmonary valve), allografts (from a human cadaver), mechanical valves (Figure 54.2) or xenografts from pigs (Figure 54.3; Goldman 2008). The heart is then repaired and once the surgery is complete, the beating of the heart is started again and the chest is closed using heavy wire sutures (Phillips 2007).

Approaches to cardiac surgery can include open surgery using a standard sternotomy, and minimally invasive endoscopy. For example, an aortic valve replacement can be undertaken using either a standard or a mini-sternotomy, and a saphenous vein can be removed from the leg and used to replace blocked coronary arteries endoscopically (Phillips 2007).

Employing a minimally invasive technique, the surgeon can operate through a keyhole incision using a scope. Minimally invasive procedures include repairing heart valves, pulmonary embolectomy, coronary artery bypass grafts and transmyocardial revascularisation (Goldman 2008). Minimally invasive techniques may also include the use of lasers, ultrasound, cryosurgery, radio-frequency ablation and robotic surgery, among others. Cardiac procedures were always performed using CPB, where the patient's blood is diverted from the body, oxygenated and reperfused, bypassing the heart and lungs. Nowadays, due to changes in cardiac surgery techniques, this is not always required (Phillips 2007). Advantages associated with 'off pump' procedures include quicker recovery, decreased need for blood transfusion, and fewer side effects and complications (Goldman 2008).

The patient's haemodynamics and other physiological functions are continuously monitored during cardiac surgery, using ECG, pulse oximeter, blood pressure monitors and so on. Specific cardiac monitors are also used with arterial lines, central venous pressure and Swan-Ganz lines to measure intra-cardiac pressures (Phillips 2007).

Hypothermia is often induced during cardiac surgery to lower the body's metabolic and oxygen requirements. Hypothermia can be induced using iced saline around the heart, by cooling the blood being returned to the patient from the CPB, or by using cooling blankets that blow cold air around the body (Goldman 2008).

Cardioplegic drugs, containing potassium, are injected into the coronary arteries every 15–20 minutes to stop the heart from beating, until cardiac surgery is completed. Body temperature is then restored to normal and the potassium is flushed out, enabling the heart to start beating again. Defibrillation may be needed to restore the effective activity of the heart.

Role of the surgeon's assistant

The main purpose of your role is to maintain the ideal environment for the surgeon to complete the procedure effectively and efficiently (Rothrock 1999). Before surgery, the patient's angiogram results, chest X rays, thoracic CT scans and any other information gained preoperatively must be available for the surgeon to consider.

Prepping and draping are performed no differently to most types of surgery. Skin prep is normally Betadine and/or chlorhexidine. Draping normally involves four square drapes around the wound site, and two large drapes above and below the wound sites, covering the patient. An Opsite adhesive plastic sheet may be used to cover the wound site and to help prevent infection.

The sternotomy is the most common way of opening the chest for heart surgery. An incision is made from the sternal notch to the xiphisternum and you will need to retract the tissue edges so that the surgeon has a clear view of the sternum. The saw is then applied to the bone and the sternum is divided (Whalan 2006). Suction and electrosurgery will also be needed to keep the area clear of blood, as the sternum is vascular. This may be carried out by the surgeon or you, depending on requirements. Once bleeding has stopped, the surgeon will place a self-retaining retractor into the wound to hold it open. After cutting through the fat below the sternum, the surgeon will then start opening the pericardium. To assist with this you can use a pair of Debakey's forceps to grasp the pericardium to provide counter traction while the surgeon is cutting the pericardium and exposing the heart (Whalan 2006). You may also assist the surgeon in applying retraction sutures to lift the heart anteriorly to provide easier access.

Depending on the surgery required, you will need to assist the surgeon by holding instruments, retracting tissues, applying electrosurgery and suction, following suture materials, and assisting with starting cardiopulmonary bypass (Whalan 2006). As an SCP, you may be entitled (depending on your experience and hospital policies) to harvest long saphenous veins or radial arteries for grafting onto the heart. Following sutures can be difficult given that most sutures are either 5/0 or 6/0 when suturing valves or grafting small blood vessels, so in these circumstances you have to hold the suture material carefully and gently. Once the operation is complete, you will be asked to help the surgeon suture the sternum using wire sutures. This involves holding each wire vertically as the surgeon twists the wires. The surgeon will then cut all the wires, close the wound and apply dressings with your help.

55 Things to do after surgery

Figure 55.1 Surgeon and assistant shaking hands after successfully completing surgery

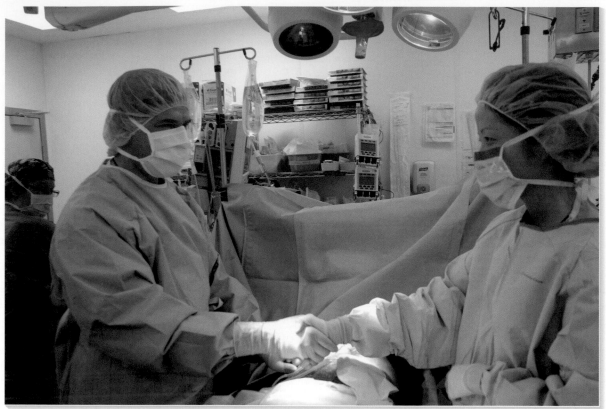

Source: Staff Sergeant David Dobrydney. Reproduced with permission of http://www.dvidshub.net/

Perioperative Practice at a Glance, First Edition. Paul Wicker. © 2015 John Wiley & Sons, Ltd. Published 2015 by John Wiley & Sons, Ltd.

When the SCP or SFA starts assisting the surgeon, it is essential that they understand each other's roles. According to Rothrock and Seifert (2009), the surgeon or anaesthetist cannot produce good-quality patient care by themselves, since teamwork and collaboration are essential in operating rooms to ensure that the patient receives the best possible treatment and care (Rothrock & Seifert 2009; PCC 2012). When doctors, assistants and practitioners all work together, this helps with staff satisfaction and also patient well-being. Poor communication can result in 'never events' happening, and can also increase the risk of harm to patients (Rothrock & Seifert 2009). It is therefore worth keeping in mind that interprofessional working and communication between all members of staff, and all professionals, can lead to a focus on patient-centred care and effective teamwork.

Postoperatively, surgical assistants can take on a huge number of tasks, including inserting or removing monitoring devices, drains or catheters, advising recovery staff on the medication required by the patient, and checking dressings and sutures.

Similarly, perioperative practitioners in operating rooms always work hard. Wearing lead coats can be tiring, as well as scrubbing all day for several operations. It is therefore worthwhile understanding that surgeons need practitioners, or they simply cannot carry out their surgery. With this in mind, it is useful to consider helping practitioners with some of the multiple small jobs they have to carry out before the next patient comes into theatre (Whalan 2006). For example, rather than leaving heavy X-ray gowns on the floor or sitting on stools, consider hanging them up on the rail outside the theatre. Helping practitioners to transfer the patient from the operating table to the bed will give you more respect and also help you engage with the theatre staff, so that in future they will also help you more when you need assistance (Whalan 2006).

An SCP with appropriate qualifications may also be asked to assist the surgeon in prescribing the patient's medications or writing treatment orders specifically for that patient. Medications may need to be continued, withheld or modified, depending on the surgery and anaesthesia that have been undertaken. In cardiac surgery antihypertensives are usually continued, whereas anticoagulants may well be temporarily withheld. Additional medications may include anti-emetics, analgesics, antibiotics and subcutaneous heparin injections (Whalan 2006). Intravenous or other fluids will also usually be used postoperatively. Treatment orders not related to medicines include routine observations, positioning of the patient, fasting status, drain management and anything else required for the patient postoperatively.

Normally the doctor who undertakes the surgery will write the operation record (Rothrock 1999). However, as an SCP it is not unlikely for the surgeon to ask you to do the writing, although this will take a great deal of practice. The most common ways for recording operation notes include writing them on a template provided in the patient's notes, completing a template on a computer in the operating theatre and printing it out later, or dictating the note and leaving it to a secretary to type and print out. Brief notes can be written that summarise the surgery being undertaken. The first point to note is the positioning of the patient, whether it is supine, prone, lithotomy and so on. The incision should then be described, for example transverse across the abdomen, lateral for the hip or lower right side of the abdomen for appendectomy. The next stage is to describe the surgery and what was discovered during it. For example, for a hip replacement you may identify the damage to the head of the femur and the acetabulum, the implant that was used, the type of cement, how tissue structures were protected, some of the instruments used, the incision and its location, sutures used for closing the wound and the type of dressing applied. You would also add any particular problems that may have been discovered and were not known prior to the surgery (Whalan 2006).

Once you have completed the report on the surgery, you may wish to assist the theatre staff with preparing the operating room for the next patient. This is likely to be well received by theatre staff given the reduced number of staff used in operating rooms. If you did start mopping the floor, not only would this be useful to the staff, they would find it surprising and also admire you for your help, which in turn will lead to better support with the next case. As a surgical assistant you will be aware of the relationships between practitioners and surgeons, but at the same time you need to understand that you should be friendly, helpful and confident, rather than arrogant or dominating.

Postoperative complications, for example surgical infections, are fairly common and postoperative antibiotics may need to be given (Rothrock 1999). If the patient is hypothermic that may also lead to other complications such as shivering, pain and poor recovery. If you are present when postoperative complications develop, you may find yourself getting involved in assisting practitioners and alerting surgeons and anaesthetists of the problems as they arise (Rothrock 1999).

If you are currently in training as an SFA or SCP, you probably need to keep a record of the operations in which you assisted, depending on the requirements of the programme. You may be given a log book to record this in or alternatively you can design your own folder or use electronic means for recording the events. It is important to record them as soon as possible after the surgery, because otherwise you may well forget some important points.

Your next task, of course, may be to introduce yourself to the next patient, and prepare for the next case. Your role is always moving on…

References and further reading

1 Preoperative patient preparation

References

Euliano, T. Y. & Gravenstein, J. S. (2004) *Essential Anesthesia: From Science to Practice*. Cambridge University Press, Cambridge.

Goodman, T. & Spry, C. (2014) *Essentials of Perioperative Nursing*. Jones & Bartlett, Burlington, MA.

Hatfield, A. & Tronson, M. (2009) *The Complete Recovery Book* (4th edn). Oxford University Press, Oxford.

O'Neill, J. (2010) Chapter 4: Perioperative Communication. In: P. Wicker & J. O'Neill (2010) *Caring for the Perioperative Patient*, pp. 134–178. Wiley-Blackwell, Chichester.

Wicker, P. (2010) Chapter 7: Preoperative preparation of perioperative patients. In: P. Wicker & J. O'Neill (2010) *Caring for the Perioperative Patient* (pp. 247–270). Wiley-Blackwell, Chichester.

Wicker, P. & O'Neill, J. (2010) *Caring for the Perioperative Patient*. Wiley-Blackwell, Chichester.

Further reading

Association for Perioperative Practice (2011) *Standards and Recommendations for Safe Perioperative Practice* (3rd edn). Association for Perioperative Practice, Harrogate.

Association of Anaesthetists of Great Britain and Ireland (2010) *Preoperative Assessment and Patient Preparation: The Role of the Anaesthetist 2*. AAGBI, London.

National Institute for Clinical Excellence (2003) *Preoperative Tests: The Use of Routine Preoperative Tests for Elective Surgery*. NICE, London.

Phipps, W., Sands, J. & Marek, J. (1999) *Medical Surgical Nursing: Concepts and Clinical Practice*. Mosby, St Louis, MO.

Zambouri, A. (2007) Preoperative evaluation and preparation for anesthesia and surgery. *Hippokratia*, 11 (1), 13–21. http://www.ncbi.nlm.nih.gov/pmc/articles/PMC2464262/ [accessed on 11 June 2013]

Websites

Preoperative care. http://www.surgeryencyclopedia.com/Pa-St/Preoperative-Care.html [accessed on 11 June 2013]

Surgical preparation. http://www.lef.org/protocols/health_concerns/surgical_preparation_01.htm [accessed on 11 June 2013]

Videos

Preoperative assessments: http://www.youtube.com/watch?v=wl7Td5ehgI4 [accessed on 19 September 2014]

Preoperative patient education for hip surgery: http://www.youtube.com/watch?v=FCvCqwai2W4 [accessed on 19 September 2014]

Pre- and postoperative care: http://www.youtube.com/watch?v=XZq1gExGh8k [accessed on 19 September 2014]

Wound care after surgery: http://www.youtube.com/watch?v=uKYjySkG-3Y [accessed on 19 September 2014]

2 Theatre scrubs and personal protective equipment

References

Association of PeriOperative Registered Nurses (2012) *Perioperative Standards and Recommended Practices*. AORN, Denver, CO.

Association for Perioperative Practice (2011) *Standards and Recommendations for Safe Perioperative Practice* (3rd edn). AFPP, Harrogate.

British Standards Institution (2004) *Personal Protective Equipment. Occupational Footwear BS EN ISO 20347*. BSI, London.

British Standards Institution (2006) *Surgical Masks. Requirements and Test Methods BS EN 14683:2005*. BSI, London.

Department of Health (2010) *Uniforms and Workwear: Guidance on Uniform and Workwear Policies for NHS Employers*. http://webarchive.nationalarchives.gov.uk/+/www.dh.gov.uk/en/publicationsandstatistics/publications/publicationspolicyandguidance/DH_114751 [accessed 11 June 2013]

Goodman, T. & Spry, C. (2014) *Essentials of Perioperative Nursing*. Jones and Bartlett Learning, Burlington, MA.

National Institute for Health and Clinical Excellence (2008) *Clinical Guideline 74 – Surgical Site Infection: Prevention and Treatment of Surgical Site Infection*. NICE, London.

Petty, L., Wakeman, J. & Simcock, W. (2005) Surgical gloves in the perioperative setting. *Dissector*, 33 (1), 13–18.

Phillips, N. (2007) *Berry and Kohn's Operating Room Technique* (11th edn). Mosby-Elsevier, St Louis, MO.

Woodhead, K., Taylor, E.W., Bannister, G., Chesworth, T., Hoffman, P. & Humphreys, H. (2002) *Behaviours and rituals in the operating theatre: A Report from the Hospital Infection Society Working Party on Infection Control in Operating Theatres*. Journal of Hospital Infection. 51: 241–255.

Further reading

Conway, N., Ong, P., Bowers, M. & Grimmett, N. (2014) *Clinical Pocket Reference: Operating Department Practice*. Clinical Pocket Reference, Oxford. www.clinicalpocketreference.com.

Wicker, P. & O'Neill, J. (2010) *Caring for the Perioperative Patient*. Wiley Blackwell, Oxford.

Websites

Operating Room Orientation Manual. http://www.utmb.edu/surgery/clerks/Operating_room_orientation.asp [accessed 19 September 2014]

Operating Theatre dress policy (Royal United Hospital Bath). http://www.ruh.nhs.uk/about/policies/documents/clinical_policies/blue_clinical/Blue_741_Operating_Theatre_Dress.pdf [accessed 27 June 2013]

Videos
Operating theatre etiquette for medical students [and practitioners]. http://www.youtube.com/watch?v=E3VX-Ij6ch8 [accessed 19 September 2014]

Surgical attire. http://www.youtube.com/watch?v=wpquzdJaMc4 [accessed 19 September 2014]

Surgical attire and environment. http://www.youtube.com/watch?v=cjWC7JSliqc [accessed 19 September 2014]

3 Preventing the transmission of infection

References
AFPP (2011) *Standards and Recommendations for Safe Perioperative Practice* (3rd edn). Association for Perioperative Practice, Harrogate.

Centre for Disease Control (CDC) (1998) Perspectives in disease prevention and health promotion update: Universal precautions for prevention of transmission of human immunodeficiency virus, hepatitis B virus and other blood borne pathogens in healthcare settings. *Morbidity and Mortality Weekly Report*, 37 (24), 377–388.

Goodman, T. & Spry, C. (2014) *Essentials of Perioperative Nursing* (5th edn). Jones & Bartlett Learning, Burlington, MA.

National Institute for Health and Clinical Excellence (2012) *Infection: Prevention and Control of Healthcare-associated Infections in Primary and Community Care*. NICE, London. http://www.nice.org.uk/nicemedia/live/13684/58656/58656.pdf [accessed 7 November 2013]

NHS Estates (2002) *Infection Control in the Built Environment*. Department of Health, London.

Pratt, R. J., Pellowe, C. M., Wilson, J. A., Loveday, H. P., Harper, P. J., Jones, S. R., McDougall, C. & Wilcox, M. H. (2007) Epic2: National evidence-based guidelines for preventing healthcare associated infections in NHS Hospitals in England. *Journal of Hospital Infection*, 65 (Supplement), S1–S64.

Tanner, J. & Parkinson, H. (2002) Double gloving to reduce surgical cross-infection. *Cochrane Database Systematic Reviews*, 2002 (3), CD003087.

World Health Organization (2006) *Health-care Facility Recommendations for Standard Precautions: Key Elements at a Glance*. WHO, Geneva. http://www.who.int/csr/resources/publications/4EPR_AM2.pdf [accessed 30 June 2013]

Further reading
Association of PeriOperative Registered Nurses (2012) *Perioperative Standards and Recommended Practices*. AORN, Denver, CO.

Rutala, W. & Weber, D. (2010) Guidelines for disinfection and sterilisation of prion-contaminated medical instruments. *Infection Control and Hospital Epidemiology*, 21 (2), 107–117.

World Health Organization (2009) *WHO Guidelines on Hand Hygiene in Health Care*. WHO, Geneva.

Websites
2007 Guidelines for Isolation Precautions. http://www.cdc.gov/hicpac/pdf/isolation/Isolation2007.pdf [accessed 19 September 2014]

Standard Precautions and Infection Control. http://www.ashm.org.au/images/publications/monographs/HIV_viral_hepatitis_and_STIs_a_guide_for_primary_care/hiv_viral_hep_chapter_13.pdf [accessed 19 September 2014]

Videos
Ayliffe hand-washing technique. http://www.youtube.com/watch?v=EwjDShmfFHM [accessed 19 September 2014]

Hand washing technique – WHO approved. http://www.youtube.com/watch?v=vYwypSLiaTU&list=PLC82BD6AD79164052 [accessed 19 September 2014]

Infection prevention in the operating room. http://www.youtube.com/watch?v=TuYEcS_bezU [accessed 19 September 2014]

Standard precautions. http://www.youtube.com/watch?v=nb_zEnB3oCs [accessed 19 September 2014]

4 Preparing and managing equipment

References
Association for Perioperative Practice (2011) *Standards and Recommendations for Safe Perioperative Practice* (3rd edn). AFPP, Harrogate.

Association of Anaesthetists of Great Britain and Ireland (2012) *Checking Anaesthetic Equipment*. AAGBI, London.

Cunnington, J. (2006) Facilitating benefit, minimising risk: Responsibilities of the surgical practitioner during electrosurgery. *Journal of Perioperative Practice*, 6 (4), 195–202.

Department of Health (2013) *Management and Decontamination of Surgical Instruments Used in Acute Care*. DH, London. https://www.gov.uk/government/publications/management-and-decontamination-of-surgical-instruments-used-in-acute-care [accessed 5 July 2013]

Goodman, T. & Spry, C. (2014) *Essentials of Perioperative Nursing* (5th edn). Jones & Bartlett Learning, Burlington, MA.

Health and Safety Executive (1999) *Management of Health and Safety at Work*. HSE, Richmond.

The National Archives (1999) *The Management of Health and Safety at Work Regulations*. TNA, London. http://www.legislation.gov.uk/uksi/1999/3242/contents/made [accessed 5 July 2013]

Wicker, P. & O'Neill, J. (2010) *Caring for the Perioperative Patient*. Wiley-Blackwell, Oxford.

Further reading
British Standards Institute (2003) Medical devices. *Quality Management Systems: Requirements for regulatory purposes BS EN ISO 13485*. BSI, London.

World Health Organization (2003) *WHO Manual for Surveillance of Human Transmissible Spongiform Encephalopathies Including Cariant Creutzfeldt Jakob Disease*. WHO, Geneva. www.who.int/bloodproducts/TSE-manual2003.pdf [accessed 7 July 2013]

Websites
Managing medical devices. http://www.mhra.gov.uk/Publications/Safetyguidance/DeviceBulletins/CON2025142 [accessed 19 September 2014]

Medicines and Healthcare Products Regulatory Agency. http://www.mhra.gov.uk/#page=DynamicListMedicines [accessed 19 September 2014]

Videos
Infection prevention in the operating room – healthcare training. http://www.youtube.com/watch?v=TuYEcS_bezU [accessed 19 September 2014]

Surgical infection control procedures. http://www.youtube.com/watch?v=B4UvmJ5NpA4 [accessed 19 September 2014]

Surgical instrument tracking and management. http://www.youtube.com/watch?v=85ZjZFbBbUs [accessed 19 September 2014]

5 Perioperative patient care

References
Davey, A. (2005) The caring practitioner. In: A. Davey & C. Ince (2005) *Fundamentals of Operating Department Practice* (pp. 29–33). Greenwich Medical Media, London.

De Bleser, L., Depreitere, R., De Waele, K., Vanhaecht, K., Vlayen, J. & Sermeus, W. (2006) Defining pathways. *Journal of Nurse Management*, 14 (7), 553–563.

Lemmens, L. (2008) *Strategies to Improve Patient Care*. Gildeprint Drukkerijen, Enschede.

Macario, A., Horne, M., Goodman, S., Vitez, T., Dexter, F., Heinen, R. & Brown, B. (1998) The effect of a perioperative clinical pathway for knee replacement surgery on hospital costs. *Anaesthesia and Analgesia Journal*, 86 (5), 978–984.

University of Connecticut Health Centre (2013) *Perioperative Plan of Care*. University of Connecticut Health Centre, Farmington, CT.

World Health Organization (2009) *Surgical Safety Checklist*. WHO, Geneva. http://www.nrls.npsa.nhs.uk/resources/?EntryId45=59860 [accessed 15 July 2012]

Further reading

Current Nursing (2012) *Application of Roy's Adaptation Model in Nursing Practice*. http://currentnursing.com/nursing_theory/application_Roy%27s_adaptation_model.html [accessed 12 July 2013]

Gruendemann, B. & Fernsebner, B. (1995) *Comprehensive Perioperative Nursing*. Jones & Bartlett Learning, London.

Rothrock, J. (2007) *Alexander's Care of the Patient in Surgery* (14th edn). Elsevier, St Louis, MO.

Wicker, P. & O'Neill, J. (2010) *Caring for the Perioperative Patient*. Wiley-Blackwell, Oxford.

Websites

Perioperative Management of the Female Patient. http://emedicine.medscape.com/article/285544-overview#a1 [accessed 19 September 2014]

Perioperative Management of the Geriatric Patient. http://emedicine.medscape.com/article/285433-overview [accessed 19 September 2014]

Perioperative Patient Care Flashcards. http://www.cram.com/flashcards/perioperative-patient-care-2708692 [accessed 19 September 2014]

Recommendations for the Perioperative Care of Patients Selected for Day Care Surgery (Australian). http://www.anzca.edu.au/resources/professional-documents/pdfs/ps15-2010-recommendations-for-the-perioperative-care-of-patients-selected-for-day-care-surgery.pdf [accessed 19 September 2014]

Videos

Clinical anaesthesia – preoperative patient assessment and management. http://www.youtube.com/watch?v=WuGiuGagkNk [accessed 19 September 2014]

Clinical pathway overview. http://www.youtube.com/watch?v=obmag6JTSu8 [accessed 19 September 2014]

Creating a caring environment in preoperative education. http://www.youtube.com/watch?v=z1Q0zqvXBUo [accessed 19 September 2014]

Medication safety in perioperative care. http://www.youtube.com/watch?v=enMSkLAmRwQ [accessed 19 September 2014]

NHS patient care pathways. http://www.youtube.com/watch?v=TK5jiYPub_Y [accessed 19 September 2014]

Patient care plans and pathways. http://www.youtube.com/watch?v=2lPZJQJvja4 [accessed 19 September 2014]

6–7 Surgical safety checklist

References

Carter (2009) RCN welcomes WHO Surgical Safety Checklist requirement Cardiff: RCN. (online). Available: http://www.rcn.org.uk/newsevents/press_releases/uk/rcn_welcomes_who_surgical_safety_checklist_requirement [accessed 20 July 2013]

Curley, M., Kalisch, B. & Stefanov, S. (2007) An intervention to enhance nursing staff teamwork and engagement. *Journal of Nursing Administration*, 37 (2), 77–84.

Cvetic, E. (2011) Communication in the perioperative setting. *AORN Journal*, 94 (3), 261–270.

Haynes, A. B., Weiser, T. G., Berry, W. R. & Lipsitz, S. R. (2009) A surgical safety checklist to reduce morbidity and mortality in a global population. *New England Journal of Medicine*, 360 (5), 491–499.

Hunter, D. N. & Finney, S J. (2011) Follow surgical checklists and take time out, especially in a crisis. *British Medical Journal*, 334, d8194.

Middleton, J. (2007) Communication skills (Essence of Care benchmark). *Nursing Times*, 13 December. http://www.nursingtimes.net/whats-new-in-nursing/communication-skills-essence-of-care-benchmark/361127.article [accessed 21 July 2013]

National Patient Safety Agency (2009) *WHO Surgical Safety Checklist*. NPSA, London. http://www.nrls.npsa.nhs.uk/resources/?EntryId45=59860 [accessed 21 July 2013]

World Health Organization (2009a) *Pilot Evaluation of the "WHO Surgical Safety Checklist"*. WHO, Geneva. http://www.who.int/patientsafety/safesurgery/pilot_sites/en/index.html [accessed 30 June 2013]

World Health Organization (2009b) *WHO Surgical Safety Checklist*. WHO, Geneva. http://whqlibdoc.who.int/publications/2009/9789241598590_eng_Checklist.pdf [accessed 29 September 2013]

World Health Organization (2013) *Implementation Manual*. WHO, Geneva. http://www.who.int/patientsafety/safesurgery/ss_checklist/en/ [accessed 21 July 2013]

Further reading

Haynes, A. B., Weiser, T. G., Berry, W. R. *et al.* (2009) Surgical safety checklist to reduce morbidity and mortality in a global population. *New England Journal of Medicine*, 360, 491–299. http://www.nejm.org/doi/full/10.1056/NEJMsa0810119 [accessed 19 September 2014]

Helmreich, R. L., Merritt, A. C. & Wilhelm, J. A. (1999) The evolution of crew resource management training in commercial aviation. *International Journal of Aviation Psychology*, 9 (1), 19–32.

Kao, L. S. & Thomas, E. J. (2008) Research review: Navigating towards improved surgical safety using aviation strategies. *Journal of Surgical Research*, 145, 327–335.

Websites

Safe Surgery Saves Lives. http://www.who.int/patientsafety/safesurgery/en/ [accessed 19 September 2014]

Surgical Safety Checklist is no magic bullet. http://www.wellcome.ac.uk/News/Media-office/Press-releases/2013/WTP053546.htm [accessed 19 September 2014]

Videos

5 steps to safer surgery. http://www.nrls.npsa.nhs.uk/patient-safety-videos/five-steps-to-safer-surgery/ [accessed 19 September 2014]

How to do the WHO Surgical Safety Checklist. http://www.youtube.com/watch?v=CsNpfMldtyk [accessed 19 September 2014]

How NOT to do the WHO Surgical Safety Checklist. http://www.youtube.com/watch?v=REyers2AAeI [accessed 19 September 2014]

How to implement the Surgical Safety Checklist. http://www.youtube.com/watch?v=pFG9ihbPT-A [accessed 19 September 2014]

8 Legal and professional accountability

References

Dimond, B. (2008) *Legal Aspects of Nursing*. Pearson Education, Harlow.

Highfield, M. (2013) *Professional Nurse Accountability*. California State University, Northridge, CA.

Linda, S. (2012) *Legal Issues in Nursing* (PowerPoint slides). http://www.slideshare.net/lindadevi1/legal-issues-in-nursing-ppt [accessed 29 September 2013]

Further reading

Hendrick, J. (2006) *Law and Ethics in Nursing and Healthcare* (2nd edn). Nelson Thornes, Cheltenham.

Herring, J. (2006) *Medical Law and Ethics*. Oxford University Press, Oxford.

Holland, J. & Burnett, S. (2006) *Employment Law*. Oxford University Press, Oxford.

Tingle, J. & Cribb, A. (2007) *Nursing Law and Ethics* (3rd edn). Blackwell, Oxford.

Websites

Health and Care Professions Council, www.hpc-uk.org
Human Rights. https://www.justice.gov.uk/human-rights [accessed 19 September 2014]

Videos

An example of hospital staff negligence. http://www.youtube.com/watch?v=yX5Y056Lfjw [accessed 19 September 2014]
Informed consent. http://www.youtube.com/watch?v=qp6PwBx5AJE [accessed 19 September 2014]
I signed a consent form before surgery. What does it mean? http://www.youtube.com/watch?v=NPFZSKjZ0Ng [accessed 19 September 2014]
Legal and ethical issues in nursing. http://www.youtube.com/watch?v=zjzfPARpI4Q [accessed 19 September 2014]
Nursing ethics movie. http://www.youtube.com/watch?v=5yYNOokQ2l8 [accessed 19 September 2014]

9 Interprofessional teamworking

References

College of Nurses of Ontario (2008) *Interprofessional Collaboration among Health Colleges and Professions.* College of Nurses of Ontario, Ontario. http://www.hprac.org/en/projects/resources/hprac-1433may28collegeofnurses.pdf [accessed 31 July 2013]
Coombs, M. A. (2004) *Power and Conflict between Doctors and Nurses.* Routledge, New York.
Hawley, G. (2007) Start at go. In: G. Hawley (ed.), *Ethics in Clinical Practice: An Inter-professional Approach.* Pearson Education, Harlow.
Health Education England (2013) *Better Training Better Care.* Health Education England, London. http://hee.nhs.uk/wp-content/blogs.dir/321/files/2012/09/US.pdf [accessed 31 July 2013]
Howkins, E. & Bray, J. (2008) *Preparing for Interprofessional Teaching: Theory and Practice.* Radcliffe, Oxford.
Kalisch, B. J. & Kalisch, P. A. (1977) An analysis of the sources of physician–nurse conflict. *Journal of Nursing Administration*, 1, 177–179.
MacDonald, B. M., Bally, J. M., Ferguson, L. M., Murray, L. B. & Fowler-Kerry, S. E. (2010) Knowledge of the professional role of others: A key interprofessional competency. *Nursing in Practice Education*, 10 (4), 238–242.
Osbiston, M. (2013) Interprofessional collaborative teamwork facilitates patient centred care: A student practitioner's perspective. *Journal of Perioperative Practice*, 23 (5), 110–113.
Reel, K. & Hutchings, S. (2007) Being part of a team: Interprofessional care. In: G. Hawley (ed.), *Ethics in Clinical Practice: An Interprofessional Approach.* Pearson Education, Harlow.
Stein, L. (1967) The doctor nurse game. *Archives of General Psychiatry.* 16, 699–703.
Tame, S. (2012) The relationship between continuing professional education and horizontal violence in perioperative practice. *Journal of Perioperative Practice*, 22 (7), 220–225.

Further reading

Hughes, S. & Mardell, A. (2012) *Oxford Handbook of Perioperative Practice.* Oxford University Press, Oxford.
Kenward, L. (2011) Promoting interprofessional care in the peri-operative environment. *Nursing Standard*, 25 (41), 35–39. http://nursingstandard.rcnpublishing.co.uk/archive/article-promoting-interprofessional-care-in-the-peri-operative-environment [accessed 19 September 2014]
Quick, J. (2011) Modern perioperative teamwork: An opportunity for interprofessional learning. *Journal of Perioperative Practice.* 21 (11), 387–390.

Websites

Collaborative Care Guidelines for Perioperative Nurses. http://novascotia.ca/dhw/mocins/docs/Collaborative_Care_Guidelines_for_Perioperative_Nurses_in_Nova_Scotia.pdf [accessed 19 September 2014]
Professional Communication and Team Collaboration. http://www.ncbi.nlm.nih.gov/books/NBK2637/ [accessed 19 September 2014]

Videos

Hybrid operating room simulation training. http://www.youtube.com/watch?v=OS5d2xwzM3Q [accessed 19 September 2014]
MX Webinar: Why interprofessional team training is important in reducing medical errors. http://www.youtube.com/watch?v=Dp6tXGv4qZw [accessed 19 September 2014]
UQ Interprofessional practice: Harness the power of healthcare teams. http://www.youtube.com/watch?v=iLwFrMYttz4 [accessed 19 September 2014]

10 Preparing anaesthetic equipment

References

Al-Shaikh, B. & Stacy, S. (2002) *Essentials of Anaesthetic Equipment.* Churchill Livingstone, London.
Association of Anaesthetists of Great Britain and Ireland (2009) *Recommendations for Standards of Monitoring during Anaesthesia and Recovery.* AAGBI, London.
Association of Anaesthetists of Great Britain and Ireland (2012) *Checking Anaesthetic Equipment.* AAGBI, London.
Diba, A. (2005) Infusion equipment and intravenous anaesthesia. In: A. Davey & A. Diba (eds), *Wards Anaesthetic Equipment.* Elsevier Saunders, London.
Hughes, S. J. & Mardell, A. (2012) *Oxford Handbook of Perioperative Practice.* Oxford University Press, Oxford.

Further reading

Association of Anaesthetists of Great Britain and Ireland (2009) *Safe Management of Anaesthetic Related Equipment.* AAGBI, London. http://www.aagbi.org/publications/guidelines/safe-management-anaesthetic-related-equipment-aagbi-safety-guideline [accessed 18 August 2013]
Association for Perioperative Practice (2011) *Perioperative Practice: In Your Pocket.* Association for Perioperative Practice, Harrogate.
Cassidy, C. J., Smith, A. & Arnot-Smith, J. (2011) Critical incident reports concerning anaesthetic equipment: Analysis of the UK National Reporting and Learning System (NRLS) data from 2006–2008. *Anaesthesia*, 66, 879–888.

Websites

Association of Anaesthetists of Great Britain and Ireland, http://www.aagbi.org/
British Anaesthetic and Recovery Nurses Association, http://www.barna.co.uk/
Royal College of Anaesthetists, http://www.rcoa.ac.uk/

Videos

Anaesthetic monitoring. http://www.youtube.com/watch?v=3Rvfjfj8ah4 [accessed 19 September 2014]
Blood pressure readings. http://www.youtube.com/watch?v=t0IngUYN2OA [accessed 19 September 2014]
How does a pulse oximeter work? http://www.youtube.com/watch?v=vtR65nHxQos [accessed 19 September 2014]
NIBP100D noninvasive blood pressure system. http://www.youtube.com/watch?v=c2H6UHB273Q [accessed 19 September 2014]
Tracheostomy care. http://www.youtube.com/watch?v=6lKHOtAim28 [accessed 19 September 2014]
Tracheostomy tube. http://www.youtube.com/watch?v=_dBg8s-Exx8 [accessed 19 September 2014]
Understanding ventilator settings. http://www.youtube.com/watch?v=6nERo9g5sBU [accessed 19 September 2014]
What is an endotracheal tube, Part 1 of 3. http://www.youtube.com/watch?v=wgyANXkG8IM [accessed 19 September 2014]

11 Checking the anaesthetic machine

References

Al-Shaikh, B. & Stacey, S. (2002) *Essentials of Anaesthetic Equipment* (2nd edn). Churchill Livingstone, London.

Association of Anaesthetists of Great Britain and Ireland (2012) *Checklist for Anaesthetic Equipment*. AAGBI, London. http://www.aagbi.org/sites/default/files/checklist_for_anaesthetic_equipment_2012.pdf [accessed 2 September 2013]

Cheng, C. J. C. & Bailey, A. R. (2002) Flow reversal through the anaesthetic machine back bar: An unusual assembly fault. *Anaesthesia*, 57 (1), 82–101.

Kumar, B. (1998) *Working in the Operating Department*. Churchill Livingstone, New York.

Membership of the Working Party: A. Hartle (Chair), Anderson, E., Bythell, V., Gemmell, L., Jones, H., McIvor, D., Pattinson, A., Sim, P. and Walker, I. (2012), Checking Anaesthetic Equipment 2012. *Anaesthesia*, 67: 660–668. doi:10.1111/j.1365-2044.2012.07163.x

Wicker, P. & Smith, B. (2008) Checking the anaesthetic machine. *Journal of Perioperative Practice*, 18 (8), 354–359.

Further reading

Euliano, T. Y. & Gravenstein, J. S. (2004) *Essential Anaesthesia: From Science to Practice*. Cambridge University Press, Cambridge.

Hughes, S. J. & Mardell, A. (2012) *Oxford Handbook of Perioperative Practice*. Oxford University Press, Oxford.

Websites

Checking Anaesthetic Machines. http://www.anaesthesia.med.usyd.edu.au/resources/lectures/gas_supplies_clt/checkingmachines.html [accessed 19 September 2014]

Videos

Anaesthesia machine check. http://www.youtube.com/watch?v=eRJZx158Q3I [accessed 19 September 2014]

Anaesthetic machine check Part 1. http://www.youtube.com/watch?v=07xAC81ACqk [accessed 19 September 2014]

Anaesthetic machine check Part 2. http://www.youtube.com/watch?v=qAid8c6-KNc [accessed 19 September 2014]

How to leak test an anaesthesia machine. http://www.youtube.com/watch?v=YALyurDifvc [accessed 19 September 2014]

Understanding ventilator settings. http://www.youtube.com/watch?v=6nERo9g5sBU [accessed 19 September 2014]

12 Anatomy and physiology of the respiratory and cardiovascular systems

References

Francis, C. (2009) *Respiratory Care*. Blackwell, Oxford.

Wicker, P. (2010) Chapter 1: Perioperative homeostasis. In: P. Wicker & J. O'Neill (2010) *Caring for the Perioperative Patient*. Wiley-Blackwell, Chichester.

Further reading

Clancy, J., McVicar, A. J. & Baird, N. (2002) *Perioperative Practice: Fundamentals of Homeostasis*. Routledge, London.

Jardins, T. (2007) *Cardiopulmonary Anatomy and Physiology* (4th edn). Delmar, New York.

Marieb, E. N. (2006) *Essentials of Human Anatomy and Physiology* (8th edn). Pearson, London.

Tortora, G. J. (2008) *Principles of Anatomy and Physiology* (12th edn). John Wiley & Sons Ltd, Oxford.

Websites

Cardiovascular System. http://www.innerbody.com/image/cardov.html [accessed 19 September 2014]

Circulatory System. http://www.bbc.co.uk/schools/gcsebitesize/pe/appliedanatomy/0_anatomy_circulatorysys_rev1.shtml [accessed 19 September 2014]

Electrocardiography. http://en.wikipedia.org/wiki/Electrocardiography [accessed 19 September 2014]

Respiratory System. http://www.innerbody.com/anatomy/respiratory [accessed 19 September 2014]

Respiratory System. http://en.wikipedia.org/wiki/Respiratory_system [accessed 19 September 2014]

Videos

Anatomy and physiology help: Chapter 20 Cardiovascular system. http://www.youtube.com/watch?v=MiVx8K8SIBw [accessed 19 September 2014]

Anatomy and physiology help: Chapter 23 Respiratory system. http://www.youtube.com/watch?v=Zsw6lZehmJM [accessed 19 September 2014]

Respiratory anatomy. http://www.youtube.com/watch?v=DCVIEMNPe1E [accessed 19 September 2014]

Respiratory system. http://www.youtube.com/watch?v=hc1YtXc_84A [accessed 19 September 2014]

13 Anaesthetic drugs

References

Andrews, J. J. & Johnston, R. V. (1993) The new Tec 6 desflurane vaporizer. *Journal of Anaesthesia and Analgesia*. 76, 1338.

British National Formulary (2012) http://www.bnf.org/bnf/index.htm [accessed 19 September 2014]

Cox, F. & Bhudia, N. (2009) Anaesthetic medicines: Back to basics. *Journal of Perioperative Practice*. 19 (11), 387–394.

Lupton, T. & Pratt, O. (2012) *Intravenous Drugs Used for Induction of Anaesthesia* Anaesthesia UK. http://www.frca.co.uk/Documents/107%20-%20IV%20induction%20agents.pdf [accessed 19 September 2014]

Simpson, P. & Popat, M. (2002) *Understanding Anaesthesia*. Butterworth-Heinemann, Oxford.

Further reading

Goodman, T. & Spry, C. (2013) *Essentials of Perioperative Nursing* (5th edn). Jones & Bartlett Learning, Burlington, MA.

NHS Choices (2011) *Anaesthesia – Definition*. NHS Choices. http://www.nhs.uk/Conditions/Anaesthesia/ [accessed 4 October 2013]

O'Neill, J. (2010) Chapter 8: Patient care during anaesthesia. In: P. Wicker & J. O'Neill (2010) *Caring for the Perioperative Patient*. Wiley-Blackwell, Chichester.

Websites

All about Opioids. http://www.medicalnewstoday.com/info/oic/ [accessed 19 September 2014]

Pharmokinetics of Inhalational Agents Relevant to the Anaesthetist. http://www.slideshare.net/drpothula/pharmacokinetics-of-inhalational-agents-relevant-to-anaestheist [accessed 19 September 2014]

Review of Currently Used Inhalation Anaesthetics. http://www.uam.es/departamentos/medicina/anesnet/journals/ija/vol3n2/inhal1.htm [accessed 19 September 2014]

Sedation or Induction Agents for Rapid Sequence Intubation in Adults. http://www.uptodate.com/contents/sedation-or-induction-agents-for-rapid-sequence-intubation-in-adults [accessed 19 September 2014]

Skeletal Muscle Relaxants. http://accesspharmacy.mhmedical.com/content.aspx?bookid=388&sectionid=45764249 [accessed 19 September 2014]

Videos

General anaesthetic drugs. http://www.youtube.com/watch?v=0FQNC_5wYh0 [accessed 19 September 2014]

General anaesthetics. http://www.youtube.com/watch?v=UR5YvTZopMA [accessed 19 September 2014]

Induction of anaesthesia. http://www.youtube.com/watch?v=Bbynl2IbmwM&list=PLF712157EF9F3FB01 [accessed 19 September 2014]

Rapid sequence induction. http://www.youtube.com/watch?v=DvFFL2Jctu4 [accessed 19 September 2014]

14 Perioperative fluid management

References

Bamboat & Bordeianou (2009) Perioperative Fluid Management. *Clinics in Colon and Rectal Surgery Journal.* Feb; *22*(1): 28–33.

Clancy, J., McVicar, A. J. & Baird, N. (2002) *Perioperative Practice: Fundamentals of Homeostasis.* Routledge, London.

English, W. A., English, R. E. & Wilson, I. H. (2013) *Perioperative Fluid Balance.* http://web.squ.edu.om/med-Lib/med/net/E-TALC9/html/clients/WAWFSA/html/acrobat/update20.pdf [accessed 19 September 2014]

Quilley, C. P., Lin, Y. S. & McGill, J. C. (1993) Chloride anion concentration as a determinant of renal vascular responsiveness to vasoconstrictor agents. *British Journal of Pharmacology, 108* (1), 106–110.

Wicker, P. (2010) Chapter 1: Perioperative homeostasis. In: P. Wicker & J. O'Neill (2010) *Caring for the Perioperative Patient.* Wiley-Blackwell, Chichester.

Further reading

Chappell, D., Jacob, M., Hofmann-Kiefer, K., Conzen, P. & Rehm, M. (2008) A rational approach to perioperative fluid management. *Anesthesiology. 109* (4), 723–740.

Grocott, M. P., Mythen, M. G. & Gan, T. J. (2005) Perioperative fluid management and clinical outcomes in adults. *Anesthesia and Analgesia, 100* (4), 1093–1106.

Websites

Approaches to Fluid Management. http://www.openanesthesia.org/w/index.php?title=Fluid_Management [accessed 19 September 2014]

Intraoperative Fluid Management and Blood Transfusion. http://www.ucdenver.edu/academics/colleges/medicalschool/education/degree_programs/MDProgram/clinicalcore/peri-operativecare/Documents/FluidMgmt.pdf [accessed 19 September 2014]

Videos

Fluid electrolyte balance. http://www.youtube.com/watch?v=pQe7Tb7NVYE [accessed 19 September 2014]

Isotonic, hypotonic, hypertonic IV fluids. http://www.youtube.com/watch?v=4r1G_oLH-Pw [accessed 19 September 2014]

Perioperative fluid therapy. http://www.youtube.com/watch?v=LFz43_fKkIM [accessed 19 September 2014]

15 Monitoring the patient

References

Association of Anaesthetists of Great Britain and Ireland (2007) *Recommendations for Standards of Monitoring during Anaesthesia and Recovery* (4th edn). AAGBI, London.

Australian and New Zealand College of Anaesthetists (2013) *Recommendations on Monitoring during Anaesthesia.* ANZCA, Melbourne. http://www.anzca.edu.au/resources/professional-documents/pdfs/ps18-2013-recommendations-on-monitoring-during-anaesthesia.pdf [accessed 14 November 2013]

O'Neill (2010) Chapter 8: Patient care during anaesthesia. In: P. Wicker & J. O'Neill (2010) *Caring for the Perioperative Patient* (2nd edn, pp. 271–338). Wiley-Blackwell, Chichester.

Strachan, A. N. & Richmond, M. N. (1997) Ether in an isoflurane vaporizer and the use of vapour analysers in safe anaesthesia. *British Journal of Anaesthesia.* 78, 107–108.

Further reading

Euliano, T. Y. & Gravenstein, J. S. (2004) *Essential Anesthesia: From Science to Practice.* Cambridge University Press, Cambridge.

Merry, A. F., Cooper, J. B., Soyannwo, O., Wilson, I. H. & Eichhorn, J. H. (2010) International standards for a safe practice of anaesthesia. *Canadian Journal of Anesthesia. 57* (11), 1027–1034. http://link.springer.com/article/10.1007%2Fs12630-010-9381-6?LI=true#page-1 [accessed 19 September 2014]

Smith, B., Rawling, P., Wicker, P. & Jones, C. (2006) *Operating Department Practice: Anaesthesia and Critical Care.* Cambridge University Press, Cambridge.

Yentis, S. M., Hirsch, N. P. & Smith, G. B. (1995) *Anaesthesia A to Z.* Butterworth-Heinemann, Oxford.

Websites

Pulse Oximetry. http://en.wikipedia.org/wiki/Pulse_oximetry [accessed 19 September 2014]

Pulse Oximetry – World Health Organization. http://www.who.int/patientsafety/safesurgery/pulse_oximetry/en/ [accessed 19 September 2014]

Videos

Anaesthesia induction monitor. http://www.youtube.com/watch?v=QRwRZJhifCE [accessed 19 September 2014]

Cardiac monitor. http://www.youtube.com/watch?v=PRHclb8PPzo [accessed 19 September 2014]

How to use a pulse oximeter. http://www.youtube.com/watch?v=irVEYvEIb6o [accessed 19 September 2014]

How to use digital blood pressure monitor. http://www.youtube.com/watch?v=YM3iXS146Yc [accessed 19 September 2014]

Monitoring general anaesthesia. http://www.youtube.com/watch?v=YBbI3oYa3sU [accessed 19 September 2014]

16 General anaesthesia

References

EBME (2013) *Total Intravenous Anaesthesia.* http://www.ebme.co.uk/articles/clinical-engineering/95-total-intravenous-anaesthesia-tiva [accessed 17 November 2013]

Goodman, T. & Spry, C. (2014) *Essentials of Perioperative Nursing* (5th edn). Jones and Bartlett Learning, Burlington, MA.

Hughes, J. H. & Mardell, A. (2012) *Oxford Handbook of Perioperative Practice.* Oxford University Press, Oxford.

Larson, M. D. (2008) *Guedel's Anaesthetic Depth Chart.* http://www.csahq.org/pdf/bulletin/guedel_57_4.pdf [accessed 18 November 2013]

Further reading

Francis, C. (2006) *Respiratory Care.* Blackwell, Oxford.

Websites

General Anaesthesia. http://www.docstoc.com/docs/6149109/GENERAL-ANAESTHESIA [accessed 19 September 2014]

Geriatric Anaesthesia. http://www.authorstream.com/Presentation/drmizan076250-1571727-geriatric-anaesthesia/ [accessed 19 September 2014]

History of Anaesthesia. http://www.rcoa.ac.uk/about-the-college/history-of-anaesthesia [accessed 19 September 2014]

History of General Anesthesia. http://en.wikipedia.org/wiki/History_of_general_anesthesia [accessed 19 September 2014]

Videos

Airway management. http://www.youtube.com/
watch?v=v8AX0u4N22A [accessed 19 September 2014]
General anaesthetic. http://www.youtube.com/watch?v=_
hof4z9MYTI [accessed 19 September 2014]
Intubation procedure. http://www.youtube.com/
watch?v=mKrl3I3Z28s [accessed 19 September 2014]
Stages of general anaesthesia. http://www.youtube.com/watch?v=
Bbynl2IbmwM&list=PLF712157EF9F3FB01 [accessed 19
September 2014]
Understanding ventilator settings. http://www.youtube.com/
watch?v=6nERo9g5sBU [accessed 19 September 2014]

17 Local anaesthesia

References

Coventry, D. M. (2007) Local anaesthetic techniques. In: A. R.
Aitkenhead, D. J. Rowbotham & G. Smith (eds) *Textbook of
Anaesthesia* (5th edn, pp. 315–344). Churchill Livingstone,
Edinburgh.
Gavin, R. (2008) *Local Anaesthesia for Minor Procedures*. Auckland
District Health Board, Auckland. http://www.adhb.govt.nz/
starshipclinicalguidelines/Local%20Anaesthesia%20for%
20minor%20procedures.htm [accessed 20 November 2013]
Hopley, L. & Van Schalkwyk, J. (2006) *Local Anaesthetic Agents*.
http://www.anaesthetist.com/anaes/drugs/Findex.htm#locals.htm
[accessed 10 November 2013]
O'Neill, J. (2010) Chapter 8: Patient care during anaesthesia. In:
P. Wicker & J. O'Neill *Caring for the Perioperative Patient*
(2nd edn, pp. 271–338). Wiley-Blackwell, Chichester.

Further reading

Davey, A. & Ince, C. (2005) *Fundamentals of Operating Department
Practice*. Greenwich Medical, London.

Websites

Local Anaesthetic. http://www.nhs.uk/conditions/Anaesthetic-local/
Pages/Introduction.aspx [accessed 19 September 2014]
Local and Regional Anesthesia. http://emedicine.medscape.com/
article/1831870-overview [accessed 19 September 2014]
Local Anesthetics (Ester and Amide-Type). http://www.globalrph.com/
local-anesthetics.htm [accessed 19 September 2014]

Videos

Injection of local anesthetic. http://www.youtube.com/
watch?v=Uxav0kAWU14 [accessed 19 September 2014]
Local anaesthesia for venous cannulation. http://www.youtube.com/
watch?v=NDWWvkKX8n4 [accessed 19 September 2014]
Local anesthetics. http://www.youtube.com/watch?v=6oiIxzda5sk
[accessed 19 September 2014]
Pharmacology – local anaesthetic. http://www.youtube.com/
watch?v=K_qjguv2Wtg [accessed 19 September 2014]

18 Regional anaesthesia

References

Burkard, J., Lee Olson, R. & Vacchiano, C. A. (2005) Regional
anesthesia. In: J. J. Nagelhout & K. L. Zaglaniczny (eds), *Nurse
Anesthesia* (3rd edn, pp. 977–1030). Elsevier Saunders, St Louis, MO.
Hadzic, A. (2007) *Textbook of Regional Anaesthesia and Acute Pain
Management*. McGraw-Hill, New York.
Morgan, G. E. & Mikhail, M. (2006). Peripheral nerve blocks. In:
G. E. Morgan, M. S. Mikhail & M. J. Murray (eds), *Clinical
Anesthesiology* (4th edn, pp. 283–308). Lange Medical Books, New
York.
O'Neill, J. (2010) Patient care during anaesthesia. In: P. Wicker &
J. O'Neill (eds), *Caring for the Perioperative Patient* (2nd edn).
Wiley-Blackwell, Chichester. doi: 10.1002/9781444323290.ch8

Rosenberg, P. H. & Heavner, J. E. (1985). Multiple and
complementary mechanisms produce analgesia during
intravenous regional anesthesia. *Anesthesiology*, 62, 840–842.
Wedel, D. J. & Horlocker, T. T. (2005) Nerve blocks. In: R. D. Miller
(ed.), *Miller's Anesthesia* (6th edn, pp. 1685–1715). Elsevier,
Philadelphia, PA.

Further reading

Euliano, T. Y. & Gravenstein, J. S. (2004) *Essential Anesthesia: From
Science to Practice*. Cambridge University Press, Cambridge.

Websites

Bier Block. http://www.ifna-int.org/ifna/e107_files/downloads/
lectures/H16BierBlock.pdf [accessed 19 September 2014]
Epidural Techniques. http://www.ifna-int.org/ifna/e107_files/
downloads/lectures/H12Epidural.pdf [accessed 19 September 2014]
Local Anaesthetics Used in Spinal Anaesthesia. http://www.
pharmacell.com/cms/wp-content/uploads/2012/02/8-local-
anesthetics-used-for-spinal-anesthesia.pdf [accessed 19
September 2014]

Videos

Ankle block. http://www.youtube.com/watch?v=7PYreMxoKPo
[accessed 19 September 2014]
Bier block. http://www.youtube.com/watch?v=BhdVZOoS83o
[accessed 19 September 2014]
Caudal anaesthesia. http://www.youtube.com/
watch?v=I0hwZGcmuic [accessed 19 September 2014]
Epidural spinal anaesthesia. http://www.youtube.com/
watch?v=rM1aQC-HAX0 [accessed 19 September 2014]
Spinal anesthesia technique before surgery. http://www.youtube.com/
watch?v=LpLlK2XmbVc [accessed 19 September 2014]
What is an epidural? http://www.youtube.com/
watch?v=uNDcf3Vw1vo [accessed 19 September 2014]

19 Roles of the circulating and scrub team

References

Gruendemann, B. J. & Fernsebner, B. (1995) *Comprehensive
Perioperative Nursing. Vol. 1: Principles*. Jones and Bartlett
Learning, London.
Phillips, N. (2007) *Berry and Kohn's Operating Room Technique*
(11th edn). Mosby Elsevier, St Louis, MO.
Smith, C. (2005) Chapter 12: Care of the patient undergoing surgery.
In: K. Woodhead & P. Wicker (eds), *A Textbook of Perioperative
Care* (pp. 161–180). Elsevier, Edinburgh.
Wicker, P. & Nightingale, A. (2010) Patient care during surgery. In.
P. Wicker & J. O'Neill (eds), *Caring for the Perioperative Patient*
(2nd edn, pp. 339–378). Wiley-Blackwell, Chichester.

Further reading

Conway, N., Ong, P., Bowers, M. & Grimmett, N. (2014) *Clinical
Pocket Reference: Operating Department Practice* (2nd edn).
Clinical Pocket Reference, Oxford. www.clinicalpocketreference.
com
Goodman, T. & Spry, C. (2014) *Essentials of Perioperative Nursing*.
Jones and Bartlett Learning, Burlington, MA.

Websites

Circulating Nurse Role. http://www.rch.org.au/uploadedFiles/Main/
Content/mcpc/Circulating_Nurse_Role.pdf [accessed 19
September 2014]
Operating Department Practice. http://www.edgehill.ac.uk/health/
odp/ [accessed 19 September 2014]
Perioperative Nursing. http://www.nsna.org/Portals/0/Skins/NSNA/
pdf/Career_Berter4.pdf [accessed 19 September 2014]
Role of the Circulating Nurse. http://nursingcrib.com/nursing-notes-
reviewer/role-of-circulating-nurse/ [accessed 19 September 2014]

Videos

Perioperative nursing – how to set a table. http://www.youtube.com/watch?v=-NsZPuqxr9U [accessed 19 September 2014]

Preparing the operating room for the patient. http://www.youtube.com/watch?v=OxJMRUHJrJU [accessed 19 September 2014]

Responsibilities of the circulating nurse. http://www.youtube.com/watch?v=pRCyeayKdqg [accessed 19 September 2014]

Surgical sponges left inside patients pose big risk. http://www.youtube.com/watch?v=oSzy3-wl9qU [accessed 19 September 2014]

The surgical count. http://www.youtube.com/watch?v=s4RCzhdQlVA [accessed 19 September 2014]

What is an operating department practitioner (ODP)? http://www.youtube.com/watch?v=lPbP7rToi7c [accessed 19 September 2014]

20 Basic surgical instruments

References

Gruendemann, B. J. & Fernsebner, B. (1995) *Comprehensive Perioperative Nursing*. Jones and Bartlett Learning, London.

Phillips, N. (2007) *Berry and Kohns Operating Room Technique* (11th edn). Mosby Elsevier, St Louis, MO.

Whalan, C. (2006) *Assisting at Surgical Operations*. Cambridge University Press, Cambridge.

Further reading

Cuschieri, A., Grace, P. A., Darzi, A., Borley, N. & Rowley, D. I. (2005) *Clinical Surgery*. Blackwell, Oxford.

Rothrock, J. C. (1999) *The RN First Assistant* (3rd edn). Lipincott, New York.

Woodhead, K. (2005) Managing risk of swab and instrument retention. *Clinical Services Journal*. 4 (1), 49–51.

Websites

Laparotomy Instruments. https://www.google.co.uk/patents/WO1999015084A1?cl=en&dq=laparotomy+instrument+sets&hl=en&sa=X&ei=g0qWUpCwHae7ygO3gYGwCA&ved=0CGgQ6AEwBg [accessed 19 September 2014]

Surgical Instrument. http://en.wikipedia.org/wiki/Surgical_instrument [accessed 19 September 2014]

Surgical Instruments. http://cal.vet.upenn.edu/projects/surgery/1000.htm [accessed 19 September 2014]

Surgical Instruments. http://www.slideshare.net/amir9935/surgical-instruments [accessed 19 September 2014]

Surgical Instruments (Flashcards). http://www.cram.com/flashcards/surgical-instruments-389257 [accessed 19 September 2014]

Videos

Common surgical instruments. http://www.youtube.com/watch?v=qm4IGZac6cs [accessed 19 September 2014]

Surgical instruments. http://www.youtube.com/watch?v=u3G71-lb-HQ [accessed 19 September 2014]

The surgical count. http://www.youtube.com/watch?v=s4RCzhdQlVA [accessed 19 September 2014]

21 Surgical scrubbing

References

Ayliffe, GA., Babb, JR., Quoraishi, AH. (1978) A test for 'hygienic' hand disinfection. *Journal of Clinical Pathology*. 31: 923–928.

Chow, A., Arah, O. A., Chan, S. P., Poh, B. F., Krishnan, P., Ng, W. K., Choudhury, S., Chan, J. and Ang, B. (2012) Alcohol handrubbing and chlorhexidine handwashing protocols for routine hospital practice: A randomized clinical trial of protocol efficacy and time effectiveness. *American Journal of Infection Control*, 40 (9), 800–805.

Horton, R. (1995) Handwashing: The fundamental infection control principle. *British Journal of Nursing*. 4 (16), 926–933.

World Health Organization (2006) *WHO Guidelines on Hand Hygiene in Health Care*. WHO, Geneva. http://www.who.int/patientsafety/information_centre/Last_April_versionHH_Guidelines%5B3%5D.pdf [accessed 28 November 2013]

Further reading

Gruendemann, BJ. (1990) *Illustrated guide to surgical scrubbing, gowning, and gloving*. Texas. Johnson & Johnson Medical Inc.

Rothrock, J. (2011) *Alexander's Care of the Patient in Surgery (4th Ed)*. Elsevier Mosby. St Louis, Missouri.

Wicker, P. & Nightingale, A. (2010) Patient care during surgery (Chapter 9). In: *Wicker P & O'Neill J (2010) Caring for the Perioperative Patient (2nd Ed) Chichester*. Wiley-Blackwell

World Health Organisation (2009) *HO Guidelines on Hand Hygiene in Health Care: First Global Patient Safety Challenge Clean Care Is Safer Care*. [Accessed September 2014] Available: http://www.ncbi.nlm.nih.gov/books/NBK144036/

Websites

A Guide to "Scrubbing In": http://www.medscape.com/viewarticle/725336_7

How To Perform Surgical Hand Scrubs: http://www.infectioncontroltoday.com/articles/2001/05/how-to-perform-surgical-hand-scrubs.aspx

Operating Department Practitioners: http://en.wikipedia.org/wiki/Operating_Department_Practitioners#Surgical_stage

Surgical nursing: http://en.wikipedia.org/wiki/Surgical_nursing

Videos

How to – Surgical Hand Scrubbing – Step by Step | Ansell Medical: http://www.youtube.com/watch?v=x6E92fGgdH4

Scrubbing 101: http://www.youtube.com/watch?v=QvRk5ZE7iRg

Scrubbing, Gloving, Gowning – Pre OP: http://www.youtube.com/watch?v=FGcLXOIxFfI

22 Surgical positioning

References

Phillips, N. (2007) *Berry and Kohn's Operating Room Technique* (11th edn). Mosby Elsevier, St Louis, MO.

Pirie, S. (2010) Patient care in the perioperative environment. *Journal of Perioperative Practice*, 20 (7), 245–248.

Wicker, P. & Nightingale, A. (2010) Patient care during surgery. In: P. Wicker & J. O'Neill (eds), *Caring for the Perioperative Patient* (pp. 339–378). Wiley-Blackwell, Chichester.

Further reading

Aschemann, D. (2005) *Positioning Techniques in Surgical Applications*. Springer, Berlin.

Beckwett, A. E. (2010) Are we doing enough to prevent patient injury caused by positioning for surgery? *Journal of Perioperative Practice*. 20 (1), 26–29.

Ellenbogen, R. G. & Abdulrauf, S. I. (2012) *Principles of Neurological Surgery. Chapter 4: Principles of surgical positioning*. Elsevier, St Louis, MO. http://www.expertconsultbook.com/expertconsult/ob/book.do?method=display&type=bookPage&decorator=none&eid=4-u1.0-B978-1-4377-0701-4..00004-X&isbn=978-1-4377-0701-4 [accessed 30 November 2013]

Knight, D. J. W. & Mahajan, R. P. (2004) Patient positioning in anaesthesia. *Continuing Education in Anaesthesia, Critical Care & Pain*, 4 (5), 160–163. http://ceaccp.oxfordjournals.org/content/4/5/160.full [accessed 19 September 2014]

Websites

Patient Positioning. https://www.ecri.org/Documents/PSA/February_2011/SurgAn6.pdf [accessed 19 September 2014]

Recommended Standards of Practice for Surgical Positioning. http://www.ast.org/uploadedFiles/Main_Site/Content/About_Us/Standard%20Surgical%20Positioning.pdf [accessed 19 September 2014]

Videos

Basic principles of patient positioning. http://www.youtube.com/watch?v=5_97uVDeO7Q [accessed 19 September 2014]

Lithotomy positioning in surgery. http://www.youtube.com/watch?v=oFPqkuOzJWg [accessed 19 September 2014]

Patient positioning. http://www.youtube.com/watch?v=LskwFQ19-5k [accessed 19 September 2014]

Positioning the prone surgical patient. http://www.youtube.com/watch?v=Vu5htEF5IXQ [accessed 19 September 2014]

23 Maintaining the sterile field

References

Manley, K. & Bellman, L. (2013) *Surgical Nursing: Advancing Practice*. Churchill Livingstone, Edinburgh.

Meara, G. & Reive, R. (2013) *Surgical Aseptic Technique and Sterile Field*. Alberta Health Services, Alberta. http://www.albertahealthservices.ca/EnvironmentalHealth/wf-eh-surgical-aseptic-technique-sterile-field.pdf [accessed 2 December 2013]

Rothrock, J. (2011) *Alexander's Care of the Patient in Surgery* (14th edn). Mosby, Toronto.

Further reading

Kumar, B. (1998) *Working in the Operating Department*. Churchill Livingstone, Edinburgh.

Monahan, F., Sands, J., Neighbors, M., Marek, J. & Green-Nigro, C. (2006) *Phipp's Medical Surgical Nursing*. Mosby, St Louis, MO.

Websites

Asepsis and Aseptic Practices in the Operating Room. http://www.infectioncontroltoday.com/articles/2000/07/asepsis-and-aseptic-practices-in-the-operating-ro.aspx [accessed 19 September 2014]

Aseptic Technique in Theatre. http://www.gosh.nhs.uk/health-professionals/clinical-guidelines/aseptic-technique-in-theatre/ [accessed 19 September 2014]

OR Basics: The Sterile Field. http://www.massdevice.com/blogs/lisa-mccallister/or-basics-sterile-field [accessed 19 September 2014]

Videos

Draping. http://www.youtube.com/watch?v=lLUHycgF09c [accessed 19 September 2014]

Draping instruction for BARRIER® universal surgical drapes. http://www.youtube.com/watch?v=QgO7ur25hXM [accessed 19 September 2014]

Preparation of the sterile field. http://www.youtube.com/watch?v=nulUT_5tMMI [accessed 19 September 2014]

Sterile field set-up. http://www.youtube.com/watch?v=CgP1fXxOAj8 [accessed 19 September 2014]

Sterile gowning and gloving technique. http://www.youtube.com/watch?v=jACKu5qGVRM [accessed 19 September 2014]

24 Sterilisation and disinfection

References

California Department of Public Health (2013) Cleaning, Disinfection, and Sterilization. CDPH, Richmond, CA. http://www.cdph.ca.gov/programs/hai/Documents/Slide-Set-13-Cleaning-Disinfection-Sterilization.pdf [accessed 2 December 2013]

Centre for Healthcare Related Infection Surveillance and Prevention (2008) *Disinfection and Sterilization Infection Control Guidelines (Version 2)*. CHRISP, Queensland. http://www.health.qld.gov.au/chrisp/sterilising/section_1.pdf [accessed 2 December 2013]

Healthcare Infection Control Practices Advisory Committee (2008) *Guideline for Disinfection and Sterilization in Healthcare Facilities*. HICPAC, Atlanta, GA. http://www.cdc.gov/hicpac/pdf/guidelines/disinfection_nov_2008.pdf [accessed 3 December 2013]

Lines, S. (2003) Decontamination and control of infection in theatre. *British Journal of Perioperative Nursing*. 13 (2), 70–75.

Meredith, S. J. & Sjorgen, G. (2008) Decontamination: Back to basics. *Journal of Perioperative Practice*, 18 (7), 285–288.

Further reading

Mehar, Z. K. (2011) *Surgical Instrument and Sterilization Guidebook: A Manual of Surgical Instruments Which Are Primarily Used in Operation Theaters and Standard Protocol for Sterilization*. Lambert Academic Publishing, Saarbrucken.

Russell, H. (1982) *Principles and Practice of Disinfection, Preservation and Sterilisation*. Wiley-Blackwell, Chichester.

Rutala, W. A. & Weber, D. J. (2004) Disinfection and sterilization in health care facilities: What clinicians need to know. *Clinical Infectious Diseases*. 39 (5), 702–709.

Websites

Guidelines for Cleaning, Disinfection and Sterilisation. http://www.nhsdg.scot.nhs.uk/Departments_and_Services/Infection_Control/Infection_Control_Files/Local_Policies/Misc/Guidelines_for_Cleaning__Disinfection_and_Sterilisation_of_Patient_Care_Equipment_Staff_Responsibilities.pdf [accessed 19 September 2014]

Infection Control Today. http://www.infectioncontroltoday.com/topics/disinfection-and-sterilization.aspx [accessed 19 September 2014]

Sterilisation and Disinfection. http://www.surgical-tutor.org.uk/default-home.htm?principles/microbiology/sterilisation.htm~right [accessed 19 September 2014]

Videos

CDC principles of cleaning and disinfecting environment surfaces. http://www.youtube.com/watch?v=DYG5lGdxpmU [accessed 19 September 2014]

Cleaning of minimally invasive surgical instruments (MIS). http://www.youtube.com/watch?v=M55lZBZi_08 [accessed 19 September 2014]

Equipment disinfection in operating theatres and hospital clinic. http://www.youtube.com/watch?v=KrPZ12M5BX4 [accessed 19 September 2014]

Of critical importance: Sterilization protocols. http://www.youtube.com/watch?v=4gPPD-rygOM [accessed 19 September 2014]

25 Swab and instrument counts

References

Bell, R. (2012) Hide and seek, the search for a missing swab: A critical analysis. *Journal of Perioperative Practice*, 22 (5), 151–156.

Coates, T. (2012) Retained swabs? A never event or a 'clever' event that has the potential to act as a fundamental driver to improve practice and systems. *Journal of Perioperative Practice*, 22 (4), 112–113.

Gilmour, D. (2005) Perioperative care. In R. Pudner (ed.), *Nursing the Surgical Patient* (pp. 17–33). Balliere Tindall, Oxford. http://www.elsevierhealth.com/media/us/samplechapters/9780702027574/9780702027574.pdf [accessed 5 December 2013]

Gilmour, D. (2012) Swab and instrument count. In: K. Woodhead & L. Fudge (eds), *Manual of Perioperative Care*. Wiley Blackwell, Chichester. doi:10.1002/9781118702734.ch18

Smith, C. (2005) Chapter 12: Care of the patient undergoing surgery. In: K. Woodhead & P. Wicker (eds), *A Textbook of Perioperative Care* (pp. 161–180). Elsevier, Edinburgh.

Further reading

East Cheshire NHS Trust (2013) *Swab, Instrument and Needle Counts*. East Cheshire NHS Trust, Macclesfield. http://www.eastcheshire.nhs.uk/About-The-Trust/policies/P/Perioperative%20count%20policy%201559.pdf [accessed 5 December 2013]

Lamont, T., Dougall, A., Johnson, S., Mathew, D., Scarpello, J. & Mossis, E. (2010) Reducing the risk of retained swabs after vaginal birth: Summary of a safety report from the National Patient Safety Agency. *British Medical Journal.* 341, c3679. http://www.bmj.com/content/341/bmj.c3679 [accessed 5 December 2013]

Saunders, S. (2004) Practical measures to ensure health and safety in theatres. *Nursing Times.* 100 (11), 32. http://www.nursingtimes.net/nursing-practice/clinical-zones/management/practical-measures-to-ensure-health-and-safety-in-theatres/204462.article [accessed 5 December 2013]

Websites

Instruments Left Inside Patients. http://www.bbc.co.uk/news/10194990 [accessed 19 September 2014]

WHO Guidelines for Safe Surgery 2009. http://whqlibdoc.who.int/publications/2009/9789241598552_eng.pdf [accessed 19 September 2014]

Videos

Counting integrity. http://www.youtube.com/watch?v=GLjFFauuuao [accessed 19 September 2014]

Preventing retained surgical items. http://www.youtube.com/watch?v=JBsk9Xw_pJI [accessed 19 September 2014]

Surgical counts. http://www.youtube.com/watch?v=uhsS9AwAwcM [accessed 19 September 2014]

Surgical sponges left inside patients pose big risk. http://www.youtube.com/watch?v=oSzy3-wl9qU [accessed 19 September 2014]

Surgical tool left in body. http://www.youtube.com/watch?v=HmsBFDFOqT0 [accessed 19 September 2014]

The surgical count. http://www.youtube.com/watch?v=s4RCzhdQlVA [accessed 19 September 2014]

26 Working with electrosurgery

References

Association for Perioperative Practice (2011) *Standards and Recommendation for Safe Perioperative Practice.* AFPP, Harrogate.

Hainer, B. L. (1991) Fundamentals of electrosurgery. *Journal of the American Board of Family Practice.* 4 (6), 419–426.

Lee, J. (2002) Update on electrosurgery. *Outpatient Surgery Magazine,* III (2). http://www.outpatientsurgery.net/issues/2002/02/update-on-electrosurgery [accessed 28 May 2013]

McCormick, P. W. (2008) Bovie smoke: A perilous plume. *Neurosurgeon.* 17 (1), 10–12.

O'Riley, M. (2010) Electrosurgery in perioperative practice. *Journal of Perioperative Practice.* 20 (9), 329–333.

Prasad, R., Quezado, Z., St Andre, A. & O'Grady, N. P. (2006) Fires in the operating room and intensive care unit: Awareness is the key to prevention. *Anesthesia and Analgesia.* 102, 172–174.

Sanderson, C. (2012) Surgical smoke. *Journal of Perioperative Practice.* 22 (4), 122–128.

Soon, S. L. & Washington, C. V., Jr (2010) Electrosurgery, electrocoagulation, electrofulguration, electrodessication, electrosection, electrocautery. In: J. K. Robinson, C. W. Hanke, D. M. Siegel & A. Fratila (eds), *Surgery of the Skin: Procedural Dermatology* (pp. 137–152). Mosby Elsevier, St Louis, MO.

Tucker, R. D. (2000). Principles of electrosurgery. In: M. V. Sivak (ed.), *Gastroenterologic Endoscopy* (2nd edn, pp. 125–135). WB Saunders, Philadelphia, PA.

Valleylab (2013) Principles of electrosurgery. http://www.asit.org/assets/documents/Prinicpals_in_electrosurgery.pdf [accessed 19 September 2014]

Watson, D. (2010) Surgical smoke evacuation during laparoscopic surgery. *AORN Journal.* 92 (3), 347–350.

Wicker, P. (2000) Back to basics – electrosurgery in perioperative practice. *British Journal of Perioperative Nursing.* 10 (4), 221–226.

Wicker, P. & O'Neill, J. (2010) *Caring for the Perioperative Patient.* Wiley-Blackwell, Oxford.

Further reading

Boulay, B. & Carr-Locke, D. (2010) Current affairs: Electrosurgery in the endoscopy suite. *Gastrointestinal Endoscopy,* 72 (5), 1044–1046.

Bovie, W. T. & Cushing, H. (1928) Electrosurgery as an aid to the removal of intracranial tumors with a preliminary note on a new surgical-current generator. *Surgery, Gynecology & Obstetrics.* 47, 751–784.

Morris, M. L., Tucker, R. D., Baron, T. H., Song, L. M. W. K. (2009) Electrosurgery in gastrointestinal endoscopy: Principles to practice. *American Journal of Gastroenterology.* 104 (6), 1563–1574.

Pollack, S. V., Carruthers, A. & Grekin, R. C. (2000) The history of electrosurgery. *Dermatologic Surgery.* 26 (10), 904–098.

Wicker, P. (1991) *Working with Electrosurgery.* National Association of Theatre Nurses, Harrogate.

Websites

Complications and Recommended Practices for Electrosurgery in Laparoscopy. http://www.chimei.org.tw/main/cmh_department/57726/07/data/19.%20Complications%20and%20recommended%20practices%20for%20electrosurgery%20in%20laparoscopy.pdf [accessed 19 September 2014]

Electrosurgery e-Learning Module. http://www.mhra.gov.uk/ConferencesLearningCentre/LearningCentre/Deviceslearningmodules/Electrosurgery/ [accessed 19 September 2014]

Safe Use of Monopolar Electrosurgical Devices during Minimally Invasive Surgery. http://laparoscopy.blogs.com/prevention_management/chapter_03_safe_use_of_electrosurgical_devices/ [accessed 19 September 2014]

Videos

Electrosurgery in laparoscopic surgery. http://www.youtube.com/watch?v=mqmvaKxfq3A [accessed 19 September 2014]

Electrosurgery in minimal access surgery. http://www.youtube.com/watch?v=EVIEnNP4qdA [accessed 19 September 2014]

Electrosurgical principles. http://www.youtube.com/watch?v=7LW78yoaEe0 [accessed 19 September 2014]

Fundamentals of electrosurgery. http://www.youtube.com/watch?v=hYxta20bpW0 [accessed 19 September 2014]

Gloves in electrosurgery – accidental burns. http://www.youtube.com/watch?v=56kO-iJxh5g [accessed 19 September 2014]

27 Tourniquet management

References

Klenerman, L. (2003) *The Tourniquet Manual: Principles and Practice.* Springer Verlag, London.

Rhys-Davies, N. C. & Stotter, A. T. (1985) The Rhys-Davies exsanguinator. *Annals of the Royal College of Surgeons of England.* 67 (3), 193–195.

Richey, S. L. (2007) Tourniquets for the control of traumatic hemorrhage: A review of the literature. *World Journal of Emergency Surgery,* 2 (28). doi:10.1186/1749-7922-2-28

Sharma, J. P. & Salhotra, R. (2012) Tourniquets in orthopedic surgery. *Indian Journal of Orthopaedics.* 46 (4), 377–383. http://www.ncbi.nlm.nih.gov/pmc/articles/PMC3421924/ [accessed 6 December 2013]

Wakai, A., Winter, D. C., Street, J. T. & Redmond, P. H. (2001) Pneumatic tourniquets in extremity surgery. *Journal of the American Academy of Orthopaedic Surgeons.* 9 (5), 345–351.

Wikipedia (2013) *Tourniquet.* http://en.wikipedia.org/wiki/Tourniquet [accessed 6 December 2013]

Further reading

Kam, P. C. A., Kavanagh, R. & Yoong, F. F. Y. (2001) The arterial tourniquet: Pathophysiological consequences and anaesthetic implications. *Anaesthesia,* 56, 534–545.

Noordin, S., McEwan, J., Kragh, J. F., Eisen, A. & Masri, B. A. (2009) Surgical tourniquets in orthopaedics. *Journal of Bone and Joint Surgery*, 91 (12), 2958–2967. http://jbjs.org/article. aspx?articleid=29047 [accessed 6 December 2013]

Odensson, A. & Finsen, V. (2002) The position of the tourniquet on the upper limb. *Journal of Bone and Joint Surgery*, 84B, 202–204.

Yousif, N. J., Grunert, B. K., Forte, R. A., Marloub, H. S. & Sanger, J. R. (1993) A comparison of upper and forearm tourniquet tolerance. *Journal of Hand Surgery*, 18B, 639–641.

Websites

Arterial Tourniquets. http://www.aagbi.org/sites/default/files/200-Arterial-Tourniquets.pdf [accessed 19 September 2014]

Recommended Standards of Practice for Safe Use of Pneumatic Tourniquets. http://www.ast.org/uploadedFiles/Main_Site/Content/About_Us/Standards%20Pneumatic%20Tourniquets.pdf [accessed 19 September 2014]

Tourniquet Safety in Lower Leg Applications. http://www.tourniquets.org/pdf/Lower%20Leg%20Applications.pdf [accessed 19 September 2014]

Videos

Pneumatic tourniquet. http://www.youtube.com/watch?v=vCK8Lrpat8I [accessed 19 September 2014]

Pneumatic tourniquet along with handpump and 3 cuffs. http://www.youtube.com/watch?v=2WsaiozYFTc [accessed 19 September 2014]

Safe use of pneumatic tourniquet cuffs. http://www.youtube.com/watch?v=1IUPmZGq5LE [accessed 19 September 2014]

Why to consider managing tourniquet time. http://www.youtube.com/watch?v=1XkPVbBwU7A [accessed 19 September 2014]

28 Wounds and dressings

References

Ignatavicius, D. & Workman, M. L. (2013) *Medical-Surgical Nursing* (7th edn). Elsevier, Oxford.

Pulman, K. (2004) Dressings in the management of open surgical wounds. *British Journal of Perioperative Nursing*. 14 (8), 354–360.

Rothrock, J. C. (2010) *Alexander's Care of the Patient in Surgery* (14th edn). Mosby- Elsevier, St Louis, MO.

Siddique, K., Mirza, S. & Housden, P. (2011) Effectiveness of hydrocolloid dressing in postoperative hip and knee surgery: Literature review and our experience. *British Journal of Perioperative Nursing*, 21 (8), 275–278.

Further reading

Clarke, P. & Jones, J. (1998) *Brigden's Operating Department Practice*. Churchill Livingstone, Edinburgh.

Websites

Clinical Practice Guidelines. http://www.rch.org.au/clinicalguide/guideline_index/Wound_dressings_acute_traumatic_wounds/ [accessed 19 September 2014]

Treatment Options for Surgical Wounds. http://www.smith-nephew.com/australia/healthcare/treatment-options/treatment-options-for-surgical-wounds/ [accessed 19 September 2014]

Wound Dressing Selection Guide. http://www.mhcwoundcare.com/education_resources/Wound_Dressing_Selection_Guide_for_Surgical_Procedures.pdf [accessed 19 September 2014]

Videos

Complex surgical wound care. http://www.youtube.com/watch?v=8rLlVFdJAiY [accessed 19 September 2014]

Foam wound dressings. http://www.youtube.com/watch?v=7-PzOzXj6GE [accessed 19 September 2014]

Gauze wound dressings. http://www.youtube.com/watch?v=mon9-LXlh0A [accessed 19 September 2014]

Hydrocolloid wound dressings. http://www.youtube.com/watch?v=8-cRBU6Zgt0 [accessed 19 September 2014]

Post surgery dressing. http://www.youtube.com/watch?v=paxeVCy7-0A [accessed 19 September 2014]

Transparent film wound dressings. http://www.youtube.com/watch?v=4xDvFgvvgog [accessed 19 September 2014]

29 Introducing the recovery room

References

Hatfield, A. & Tronson, M. (2009) *The Complete Recovery Book* (4th edn). Oxford University Press, Oxford.

Smedley & Quine (2012)

Wicker, P. & Cox, F. (2010) Chapter 10: Patient care during recovery. In: P. Wicker & J. O'Neill (eds), *Caring for the Perioperative Patient* (pp. 379–412). Wiley-Blackwell, Chichester.

Woodhead, K. & Fudge, L. (2012) *Manual of Perioperative Care: An Essential Guide*. Wiley-Blackwell, Chichester.

Further reading

Gilmour, D. (2005) Perioperative care. In R. Pudner (ed.), *Nursing the Surgical Patient* (pp. 17–33). Balliere Tindall, Oxford. http://www.elsevierhealth.com/media/us/samplechapters/9780702027574/9780702027574.pdf [accessed 5 December 2013]

Pirie, S. (2005) New procedures in the recovery unit. *British Journal of Perioperative Nursing*, 15 (10), 414–419.

Radford, M., County, B. & Oakley, M. (2004) *Advancing Perioperative Practice*. Nelson Thornes, Cheltenham.

Scott, B. (2012) Airway management in post anaesthetic care. *Journal of Perioperative Practice*. 22 (4), 135–138.

Websites

Recovery Room Care of the Surgical Patient. http://www.brooksidepress.org/Products/Nursing_Care_of_the_Surgical_Patient/lesson_3_Section_1.htm [accessed 19 September 2014]

Videos

Post anesthesia care unit. http://www.youtube.com/watch?v=ZrdaVEsz9MY&list=TLQs9I4bNGCC5KBGfH1cQn4STtQX-8bDlt [accessed 19 September 2014]

Postoperative recovery. http://www.youtube.com/watch?v=BLKEUHYr9Is [accessed 19 September 2014]

Pre and post-operative care. http://www.youtube.com/watch?v=XZq1gExGh8k [accessed 19 September 2014]

Pre/postoperative anxiety, pain, and behavioral recovery in child surgery. http://www.youtube.com/watch?v=4qmYTHWTmhk [accessed 19 September 2014]

Risk factors for PONV. http://www.youtube.com/watch?v=ft58EsCi1bg [accessed 19 September 2014]

30 Patient handover

References

Hatfield, A. & Tronson, M. (2009) *The Complete Recovery Book* (4th edn). Oxford University Press, Oxford.

Hughes, S. J. & Mardell, A. (2009) *Oxford Handbook of Perioperative Practice*. Oxford University Press, Oxford.

Smith, B. & Hardy, D. (2007) Discharge criteria in recovery – 'just in case'. *Journal of Perioperative Practice*. 17 (3), 102–107.

Wicker, P. & Cox, F. (2010) Chapter 10: Patient care during recovery. In: P. Wicker & J. O'Neill (eds), *Caring for the Perioperative Patient* (pp. 379–412). Wiley Blackwell, Chichester.

Younker, J. (2008) Care of the intubated patient in the PACU: The ABCDE approach. *Journal of Perioperative Practice*. 14 (2), 74–80.

Further reading

Anwari, J. S. (2002) Quality of handover to the postanaesthesia care unit nurse. *Anaesthesia*. 57, 488–493.

Horn, J., Bell, M. D. D. & Moss, E. (2004) Handover of responsibility for the anaesthetised patient –opinion and practice. *Anaesthesia*, 59, 658–663.

Royal College of Anaesthetists (2012) *Raising the Standard: A Compendium of Audit Recipes.* Section 3 Postoperative Care (pp. 111–133). RCOA, London.

Segall, N., Bonifacio, A. S., Schroeder, R. A. et al. (2012) Can we make postoperative patient handovers safer? A systematic review of the literature. *Anesthesia and Analgesia*, 115 (1), 102–115. http://www.hadassah-med.com/media/2021648/perativePatientHandoversSafer.pdf [accessed 19 September 2014]

Smith, A. F., Pope, C., Goodwin, D. & Mort, M. (2008) Interprofessional handover and patient safety in anaesthesia: Observational study of handovers in the recovery room. *British Journal of Anaesthesia.* 101 (3), 332–337.

Websites

The Effect of a Checklist on the Quality of Post-anaesthesia Patient Handover. http://www.medscape.com/viewarticle/810540_1 [accessed 19 September 2014]

Videos

Communication handoff: ED to inpatient. http://www.youtube.com/watch?v=YBvtCs7xdJ0 [accessed 19 September 2014]

Communication handoff: PACU to inpatient. http://www.youtube.com/watch?v=Q2ZtB4HSiYU [accessed 19 September 2014]

Know the plan, share the plan, review the risk. http://www.youtube.com/watch?v=H6BSace51Zg [accessed 19 September 2014]

31 Postoperative patient care – Part 1

References

Anderson, I. (2003) *Care of the Critically Ill Surgical Patient* (2nd edn). Arnold, London.

Hatfield, A. & Tronson, M. (2009) *The Complete Recovery Book* (4th edn). Oxford University Press, Oxford.

Jevon, P. & Ewens, B. (2002) *Monitoring the Critically Ill Patient.* Blackwell Science, Oxford.

National Confidential Enquiry into Patient Outcome and Death (2001) *Changing the Way We Operate.* NCEPOD, London.

National Patient Safety Agency (2007) *Safer Care for the Acutely Ill Patient: Learning from Serious Incident.* 5th Report from the Patient Safety Observatory. NPSA, London. http://www.nrls.npsa.nhs.uk/resources/?EntryId45=59828 [accessed 13 December 2013]

Further reading

NetCE (2013) *Postoperative Complications.* CME Resource, Sacramento, CA. http://www.netce.com/coursecontent.php?courseid=797 [accessed 17 December 2013]

Rose, D. K., Cohen, M. M. & DeBoer, D. P. (1996) Cardiovascular events in the postanesthesia care unit: Contribution of risk factors. *Anesthesiology.* 84 (4), 772–781.

Websites

Medication Safety Alert. http://www.ismp.org/Newsletters/acutecare/showarticle.asp?id=44 [accessed 19 September 2014]

Postoperative Care. http://www.surgeryencyclopedia.com/Pa-St/Postoperative-Care.html [accessed 19 September 2014]

Recovery Care. http://www.networks.nhs.uk/nhs-networks/staffordshire-shropshire-and-black-country/documents/Recovery%202013.pdf [accessed 19 September 2014]

Statement on the Handover Responsibilities of the Anaesthetist. http://www.anzca.edu.au/resources/professional-documents/pdfs/ps53-2013-statement-on-the-handover-responsibilities-of-the-anaesthetist.pdf [accessed 19 September 2014]

Videos

Enhanced recovery after surgery. http://www.youtube.com/watch?v=9Ec_CsdjbP4 [accessed 19 September 2014]

Mechanical ventilation nursing management. http://www.youtube.com/watch?v=5l6kBs2nvRs [accessed 19 September 2014]

32 Postoperative patient care – Part 2

References

Alfaro, N. I. (2013) *Roles of the Postanesthesia Care Unit Nurse.* Slideshare. http://www.slideshare.net/najr2006/roles-of-the-postanesthesia-care-unit-nurse [accessed 16 December 2013]

American Society of PeriAnesthesia Nurses (2001) Clinical guidelines for the prevention of unplanned perioperative hypothermia. *Journal of PeriAnesthesia Nursing.* 16, 305–314.

Hatfield, A. & Tronson, M. (2009) *The Complete Recovery Book* (4th edn). Oxford University Press, Oxford.

Kiekkas, P., Poulopoulou, M., Papahatzi, A. & Souleles, P. (2005) Effects of hypothermia and shivering on standard PACU monitoring of patients. *Journal of the American Association of Nurse Anaesthetists.* 73, 47–53.

National Institute of Health and Clinical Excellence (2008) *Inadvertent Perioperative Hypothermia.* NICE, London.

Stanhope, N. (2006) Temperature measurement in the Phase 1 PACU. *Journal of PeriAnesthesia Nursing.* 21 (1), 27–36.

Further reading

Sohn, V. Y. & Steele, S. R. (2009) Temperature control and the role of supplemental oxygen. *Journal of Clinical Colon Rectal Surgery*, 22 (1), 21–27.

Websites

Inadvertent perioperative hypothermia. http://www.nice.org.uk/guidance/cg65 [accessed 16 December 2013]

Post-operative Care. https://www.rcoa.ac.uk/system/files/CSQ-ARB2012-SEC3.pdf [accessed 16 December 2013]

Recovery Room Care of the Surgical Patient. http://www.brooksidepress.org/Products/Nursing_Care_of_the_Surgical_Patient/lesson_3_Section_1.htm [accessed 16 December 2013]

Videos

Postoperative care assessment. http://www.youtube.com/watch?v=jd3HkGIj-hY [accessed 19 September 2014]

Postoperative care content map. http://www.youtube.com/watch?v=ayYRWiyRlFU [accessed 19 September 2014]

Post op initial assessment. http://www.youtube.com/watch?v=sdnM5ZuPfl0 [accessed 19 September 2014]

Pre and post-operative care. http://www.youtube.com/watch?v=XZq1gExGh8k [accessed 19 September 2014]

33 Monitoring in recovery

References

Hatfield, A. & Tronson, M. (2009) *The Complete Recovery Book* (4th edn). Oxford University Press, Oxford.

Joanna Briggs Institute (JBI) (2011) Post-anesthetic discharge scoring criteria. *Best Practice.* 15 (17), 1–4.

Jones, K. A., Lennon, R. L. & Hosking, M. P. (1992) Method of intraoperative monitoring of neuromuscular function and residual blockade in the recovery room. *Journal of Minnesota Medicine.* 75 (7), 23–26.

Rawlinson, A., Kitchingham, N., Hart, C., McMahon, G., Ong, S. L. & Khanna, A. (2012) Mechanisms of reducing postoperative pain, nausea and vomiting: A systematic review of current techniques. *Journal of Evidence Based Medicine.* 17, 75–80.

Royal College of Physicians and Royal College of Psychiatrists (2003) *The Psychological Care of Medical Patients: A Practical Guide.* RCP/RCP, London. http://www.rcpsych.ac.uk/files/pdfversion/cr108.pdf [accessed 17 December 2013]

Shepherd, A. (2011) Measuring and managing fluid balance. *Nursing Times.* 107 (28), 12–16.

Smith, H. S., Smith, E. J. & Smith, B. R. (2012) Postoperative nausea and vomiting. *Annals of Palliative Medicine, 1* (2), 94–102.

Further reading
McGrath, C. D. & Huner, J. M. (2006) Monitoring of neuromuscular block. *Continuing Education in Anaesthesia, Critical Care & Pain.* 6 (1), 7–12. http://ceaccp.oxfordjournals.org/content/6/1/7.full [accessed 19 September 2014]

Reid, J., Robb, E., Stone, D., Bowen, P., Baker, R., Irving, S. & Waller, M. (2004) Improving the monitoring and assessment of fluid balance. *Nursing Times.* 100 (20), 36–39.

Scales, K. & Pilsworth, J. (2008) The importance of fluid balance in clinical practice. *Nursing Standard, 22* (47), 50–57.

Smith, J. & Roberts, R. (2011) *Vital Signs for Nurses: An Introduction to Clinical Observations.* Wiley-Blackwell, Oxford.

Task Force on Postanesthetic Care (2002) Care practice guidelines for postanesthetic care. *Anesthesiology. 96,* 742–752.

Websites
Respiratory Monitoring. http://anaesthesia.co.in/wp-content/uploads/2012/05/Respiratory-Monitoring.ppt [accessed 19 September 2014]

Standards of Monitoring during Anaesthesia and Recovery. http://www.aagbi.org/sites/default/files/standardsofmonitoring07.pdf [accessed 19 September 2014]

Videos
C-section surgery pain management & recovery. http://www.youtube.com/watch?v=3dutQ5hgkdE [accessed 19 September 2014]

Recovery – pain management. http://www.youtube.com/watch?v=O2xNscJME74 [accessed 19 September 2014]

Risk factors for PONV. http://www.youtube.com/watch?v=ft58EsCi1bg [accessed 19 September 2014]

34 Maintaining the airway

References
Aitkenhead, A. R., Smith, G. & Rowbotham, D. J. (2007) *Textbook of Anaesthesia.* Churchill Livingstone Elsevier, Oxford.

Association of Anaesthetists of Great Britain and Ireland (2013a) *Guidance on the Provision of Anaesthesia Services for Post-operative Care.* AAGBI, London. http://www.rcoa.ac.uk/document-store/guidance-the-provision-of-anaesthesia-services-post-operative-care-2013 [accessed 18 December 2013]

Association of Anaesthetists of Great Britain and Ireland (2013b) *Immediate Post-anaesthesia Recovery.* AAGBI, London. www.aagbi.org/sites/default/files/immediate_post-anaesthesia_recovery_2013.pdf [accessed 18 December 2013]

Dolenska, S., Dalal, P. & Taylor, A. (2004) *Essentials of Airway Management.* Greenwich Medical Media, London.

Scott, B. (2012) Airway management in post anaesthetic care. *Journal of Perioperative Practice, 22* (4), 135–138.

West, J. B. (2008) *Respiratory Physiology: The Essentials.* Lippincott Williams & Wilkins, Baltimore, MD.

Further reading
Cook, T. M., Woodall, N. & Frerk, C. (2011) Results of the Fourth National Audit Project of the Royal College of Anaesthetists and the Difficult Airway Society. Part 1: Anaesthesia. *British Journal of Anaesthesia, 106* (5), 617–631.

Mimoz, O., Benard, T., Gaucher, A., Frasca, D. & Debaene, B. (2012) Accuracy of respiratory rate monitoring using a non-invasive acoustic method after general anaesthesia. *British Journal of Anaesthesia.* Advance access online. http://bja.oxfordjournals.org/content/early/2012/02/08/bja.aer510.full.pdf [accessed 17 December 2013]

Pinnock, C., Lin, T. & Smith, T. (2009) *Fundamentals of Anaesthesia.* Greenwich Medical Media, London.

Roberts, K., Whalley, H. & Bleetman, A. (2005) The nasopharyngeal airway: Dispelling myths and establishing the facts. *Emergency Medicine Journal. 22* (6), 394–396.

Websites
Airway Management. http://en.wikipedia.org/wiki/Airway_management [accessed 19 September 2014]

Airway Management. http://www.sgna.org/issues/sedationfactsorg/patientcare_safety/airwaymanagement.aspx [accessed 19 September 2014]

Airway Management in the Recovery Room. http://prezi.com/n6baqorap_or/airway-management-in-the-recovery-room/ [accessed 19 September 2014]

Major Complications of Airway Management in the United Kingdom. http://www.rcoa.ac.uk/system/files/CSQ-NAP4-Section1.pdf [accessed 19 September 2014]

Recovery Positioning. http://en.wikipedia.org/wiki/Recovery_position [accessed 19 September 2014]

Videos
Airway management with simple adjuncts – respiratory medicine. http://www.youtube.com/watch?v=U4FrtssdyEQ [accessed 19 September 2014]

35 Common postoperative problems

References
American College of Chest Physicians/Society of Critical Care Medicine Consensus Conference (1992) Definitions for sepsis and organ failure and guidelines for the use of innovative therapies in sepsis. *Critical Care Medicine, 20* (6), 864–874.

Garner, J. S., Jarvis, W. R., Emori, T. G., Horan, T. C., Hughes, J. M. (1988) CDC definitions for nosocomial infections, 1988. *American Journal of Infection Control. 16* (3), 128–140. Erratum in: *American Journal of Infection Control, 16* (4), 177.

Hatfield, A. & Tronson, M. (2009) *The Complete Recovery Book* (4th edn). Oxford University Press, Oxford.

Henry, M. M. & Thomson, J. N. (2012) *Clinical Surgery.* Elsevier, Edinburgh.

Hood, P., Tarling, M. & Turner, S. (2011) *AFPP in Your Pocket: Perioperative Practice.* Association for Perioperative Practice, Harrogate.

Lobo, S. M., Rezende, E., Knibel, M. F. *et al.* (2008) Epidemiology and outcomes of non-cardiac surgical patients in Brazilian intensive care units. *Revista Brasileira de Terapia Intensiva. 20* (4), 376–384. http://www.scielo.br/scielo.php?script=sci_arttext&pid=S0103-507X2008000400010&lng=en [accessed 19 September 2014]

Wicker, P. & Cox, F. (2010) Chapter 10: Patient care during recovery. In: P. Wicker & J. O'Neill (eds), *Caring for the Perioperative Patient* (pp. 379–412). Wiley-Blackwell, Chichester.

Further reading
Gruendemann, B. J. & Fernsebner, B. (1995) *Comprehensive Perioperative Nursing.* Jones and Bartlett Learning, London.

Manley, K. & Bellman, L. (2000) *Surgical Nursing: Advancing Practice.* Churchill Livingstone, Edinburgh.

Web sites
8 Common Surgery Complications. http://www.webmd.com/healthy-aging/features/common-surgery-complications [accessed 19 September 2014]

Common Postoperative Complications. http://www.patient.co.uk/doctor/common-postoperative-complications [accessed 19 September 2014]

Postoperative Complications. https://www.inkling.com/read/clinical-surgery-henry-thompson-3rd/chapter-7/postoperative-complications [accessed 19 September 2014]

Post-operative Complications. http://www.surgwiki.com/wiki/Post-operative_complications [accessed 19 September 2014]

Special Problems of Pre- and Post-operative Care. http://www.ncbi.nlm.nih.gov/pmc/articles/PMC2377617/pdf/annrcse00274-0041.pdf [accessed 19 September 2014]

Videos

Postoperative complications. http://www.youtube.com/watch?v=JqoVZCNIeXY [accessed 19 September 2014]

Surgical sponges left inside patients pose big risk. http://www.youtube.com/watch?v=oSzy3-wl9qU [accessed 19 September 2014]

The incidence and management of postoperative haemorrhage. http://www.youtube.com/watch?v=DSU2tX7LArM [accessed 19 September 2014]

When surgery tools are left behind. http://www.youtube.com/watch?v=RxFy9Zd8I9U [accessed 19 September 2014]

36 Managing postoperative pain

References

Etches, R. C. (1994) Respiratory depression associated with patient-controlled analgesia: A review of eight cases. *Canadian Journal of Anaesthesia*. 41, 125–132.

Hatfield, A. & Tronson, M. (2009) *The Complete Recovery Book* (4th edn). Oxford University Press, Oxford.

Kehlet, H. (1998) Modification of response to surgery and anesthesia by neural blockade: Clinical implications. In: M. T. Cousins & P. O. Bridebaugh (eds), *Neural Blockade in Clinical Anesthesia and Management of Pain* (3rd edn). Lippincott, Philadelphia, PA.

Ramsay, M. A. E. (2000) Acute postoperative pain management. *BUMC Proceedings Journal*. 13 (3), 244–247. http://www.ncbi.nlm.nih.gov/pmc/articles/PMC1317048/ [accessed 23 December 2013]

Wicker, P. & Cox, F. (2010) Chapter 10: Patient care during recovery. In: P. Wicker & J. O'Neill (2010) *Caring for the Perioperative Patient*. Wiley-Blackwell, Oxford.

Further reading

Layzell, M. (2005) Improving the management of postop pain. *Nursing Times*. 101 (26), 34. http://www.nursingtimes.net/nursing-practice/clinical-zones/pain-management/improving-the-management-of-postoperative-pain/203791.article [accessed 23 December 2013]

Mackintosh, C. (2007) Assessment and management of patients with post-operative pain. *Nursing Standard*. 22, 5, 49–55. http://www.nurseone.ca/docs/NurseOne/Private%20Documents/rural_and_remote/PostOperative.pdf [accessed 19 September 2014]

Management of Postoperative Pain Working Group (2002) *Clinical Practice Guidelines for the Management of Postoperative Pain*. Veterans Health Association, Washington, DC. http://www.healthquality.va.gov/guidelines/Pain/pop/pop_fulltext.pdf [accessed 23 December 2013]

Ramsay, M. A. E. (2000) Acute postoperative pain management. *Proceedings of the Baylor University Medical Centre*. 13 (3), 244–247. http://www.ncbi.nlm.nih.gov/pmc/articles/PMC1317048/ [accessed 19 September 2014]

Websites

Acute Postoperative Pain Management. http://www.nps.org.au/__data/assets/pdf_file/0014/70052/OKA5301_NPS_APOP_EVC_FINAL.pdf [accessed 19 September 2014]

Postoperative Pain Management. http://www.guideline.gov/content.aspx?id=23897 [accessed 19 September 2014]

Videos

New treatments for postoperative pain. http://www.youtube.com/watch?v=x0EJQ1txcjQ [accessed 19 September 2014]

Perioperative pain management: Improved strategies. http://www.youtube.com/watch?v=u83gQTlrS0k [accessed 19 September 2014]

Post operative pain management. http://www.youtube.com/watch?v=EIyXAaw2Ers [accessed 19 September 2014]

37 Managing postoperative nausea and vomiting

References

Chetterjee, S., Rudra, A. & Sengupta, S. (2011) Current concepts in the management of postoperative nausea and vomiting. *Anesthesiology Research and Practice, 2011*. http://www.hindawi.com/journals/arp/2011/748031/ [accessed 27 December 2013]

Mathias, J. M. (2008) Protect your patients from nausea, vomiting. *OR Manager*, 24 (4), 27–28.

Miaskowski, C. (2009) A review of the incidence, causes, consequences, and management of gastrointestinal effects associated with postoperative opioid administration. *Journal of Perianesthia Nursing*, 4 (4), 222–228.

Smith, H. S., Smith, E. J. & Smith, B. R. (2012) Postoperative nausea and vomiting. *Annals of Palliative Medicine*. 1 (2). http://www.amepc.org/apm/article/view/1035/1261 [accessed 27 December 2013]

Tinsley, M. H. & Barone, C. P. (2012) Preventing postoperative nausea and vomiting. *OR Nurse*. 6 (3), 18–25.

Wilhelm, S. M., Dehoorne-Smith, M. & Kale-Pradhan, P. B. (2007) Prevention of postoperative nausea and vomiting. *Annals of Pharmacotherapy*. 41 (1), 68–78.

Further reading

Chandrakantan, A. & Glass, P. S. A. (2011) Multimodal therapies for postoperative nausea and vomiting, and pain, *British Journal of Anaesthesia*. 107 (suppl. 1), 127–140. http://bja.oxfordjournals.org/content/107/suppl_1/i27.full [accessed 19 September 2014]

Drug Therapy Committee. *Postoperative Nausea and Vomiting: Treatment Strategies*. Massachusetts General Hospital, Boston, MA. http://www2.massgeneral.org/pharmacy/Newsletters/2002/March%202002/Postoperative%20Nausea%20and%20Vomiting.htm [accessed 27 December 2013]

Gan, T. J. (2006) Risk factors for postoperative nausea and vomiting. *Anesthesia and Analgesia*, 102 (6), 1884–1898.

Jokinen, J., Smith, A. F., Roewer, N., Eberhart, L. H. & Kranke, P. (2012) Management of postoperative nausea and vomiting: How to deal with refractory PONV. *Anesthesiology Clinics*, 30 (3), 481–493.

Kovac, A. L. (2000) Prevention and treatment of postoperative nausea and vomiting. *Drugs*, 59 (2), 213–243.

Steinbrook, R. A., Garfield, F., Batista, S. H. & Urman, R. D. (2013) Caffeine for the prevention of postoperative nausea and vomiting. *Journal of Anaesthesiology Clinical Pharmacology*. 29 (4), 526–529. http://www.joacp.org/article.asp?issn=0970-9185;year=2013;volume=29;issue=4;spage=526;epage=529;aulast=Steinbrook [accessed 19 September 2014]

Websites

Guidelines on the Prevention of Post-operative Vomiting in Children. http://www.apagbi.org.uk/sites/default/files/APA_Guidelines_on_the_Prevention_of_Postoperative_Vomiting_in_Children.pdf [accessed 19 September 2014]

PONV/PDNV Clinical Guideline. http://www.aspan.org/Clinical-Practice/Clinical-Guidelines/PONV-PDNV [accessed 19 September 2014]

Postoperative Nausea and Vomiting. http://www.slideshare.net/WahidAltaf/ponv-anaesthesia-managment [accessed 19 September 2014]

Videos

Nausea vomiting antiemetics. http://www.youtube.com/watch?v=ztc4JQqk8TY [accessed 19 September 2014]

Physiology of vomiting. http://www.youtube.com/watch?v=L92VzBWfSEw [accessed 19 September 2014]

PONV Dr. Joseph Pergolizzi. http://vimeo.com/54224867 [accessed 19 September 2014]

Risk factors for PONV. http://www.youtube.com/
watch?v=ft58EsCi1bg [accessed 19 September 2014]
Understanding surgery/PONV. http://www.youtube.com/
watch?v=5rzDTdRUDzU [accessed 19 September 2014]

38 Caring for the critically Ill

References

Bhattacharyya, T., Iorio, R. & Healy, W. L. (2002) Rate of and risk factors for acute inpatient mortality after orthopaedic surgery. *Journal of Bone and Joint Surgery.* 84, 562–572.

Findlay, G. P., Goodwin, A. P. L., Protopapa, K., Smith, N. C. E. & Mason, M. (2011) *Knowing the Risk: A Review of the Perioperative Care of Surgical Patients.* National Confidential Enquiry into Patient Outcome and Death, London.

Greene, K. A., Wilde, A. H. & Stulberg, B. N. (1991) Preoperative nutritional status of total joint patients. Relationship to postoperative wound complications. *Journal of Arthroplasty.* 6, 321–325.

Pearse, R. M., Harrison, D. A., James, P., Watson, D., Hinds, C., Rhodes, A., Grounds, R. M. & Bennett, E. D. (2006) Identification and characterisation of the high-risk surgical population in the United Kingdom. *Journal of Critical Care.* 10 (3), R81.

Schwarzkopf, R., Takemoto, R. C., Immerman, I., Slover, J. D. & Bosco, J. A. (2010) Prevalence of Staphylococcus aureus colonization in orthopaedic surgeons and their patients: A prospective cohort controlled study. *Journal of Bone and Joint Surgery.* 92, 1815–1819.

Simpson, J. C. & Moonesinghe, S. R. (2013) Introduction to the postanaesthetic care unit. *Perioperative Medicine.* 2, 5. http://www.perioperativemedicinejournal.com/content/2/1/5 [accessed 2 January 2014]

Vizcaychipi, M. P. (2013) A descriptive review of magnesium in homeostasis. *Journal of Operating Department Practice.* 1 (1), 40–45.

Wu, W. C., Schifftner, T. L., Henderson, W. G. *et al.* (2007) Preoperative hematocrit levels and postoperative outcomes in older patients undergoing noncardiac surgery. *Journal of the American Medical Association.* 297, 2481–2488.

Further reading

Hatfield, A. & Tronson, M. (2009) *The Complete Recovery Book* (4th edn). Oxford University Press, Oxford.

Websites

Common Illnesses of Critically Ill Patients. http://www.thoracic.org/clinical/critical-care/patient-information/common-illnesses-of-critically-ill-patients.php [accessed 19 September 2014]

Initial Assessment of the Critically Ill Patient. http://www.chest.mohealth.gov.eg/mawared/day42.pdf [accessed 19 September 2014]

Videos

Crashing patient: The critically ill obese patient. http://www.youtube.com/watch?v=EAGzHjyfh04 [accessed 19 September 2014]

Critically ill patient. http://www.youtube.com/watch?v=sXeTppCcuuo [accessed 19 September 2014]

Recognising the critically ill patient. http://www.youtube.com/watch?v=uqQVGHihjpI [accessed 19 September 2014]

39 Airway problems

References

Ball, D. R. (2011) *Surgical Critical Care and Trauma Part 2: Airway Management in Trauma and Critical Care.* http://ptolemy.library.utoronto.ca/sites/default/files/reviews/2012/February%20-%20Airway%20Management.pdf [accessed 3 January 2013]

Jevon, P. & Ewens, J. S. (2002) *Monitoring the Critically Ill Patient.* Blackwell Science, Oxford.

Loftus, I. (2010) *Care of the Critically Ill Surgical Patient* (3rd edn). CRC Press, Boca Raton, FL.

Further reading

Hagberg, C., Georgi, R. & Krier, C. (2005) Complications of managing the airway. *Best Practice & Research Clinical Anaesthesiology.* 19 (4), 641–659. http://clinicaldepartments.musc.edu/anesthesia/education/medicalstudent/Outline/airway%20complications.pdf [accessed 19 September 2014]

Henderson, J. J., Popat, M. T., Latto, I. P. & Pearce, A. C. (2004). Difficult Airway Society guidelines for the management of the unanticipated difficult intubation. *Anaesthesia.* 59, 675–694.

Hillman, D. R., Platt, P. R. & Eastwood, P. R. (2004) The upper airway during anaesthesia, *British Journal of Anaesthesia.* 91 (1), 31–39. http://bja.oxfordjournals.org/content/91/1/31.long [accessed 19 September 2014]

Mort, T. (2004) Emergency tracheal intubation: Complications associated with repeated laryngoscopic attempts. *Journal of Anesthesiology and Analgesia.* 99, 607–613.

Ross, A. K. & Ball, D. R. (2009). Equipment for airway management. *Anaesthesia and Intensive Care Medicine.* 10, 471–475.

Websites

Airway Management in the Critically Ill. http://www.docstoc.com/docs/115935016/Airway-Management-in-the-Critically-Ill-%28PowerPoint%29 [accessed 19 September 2014]

Obese Patients and Airways. http://www.sciencedaily.com/releases/2011/03/110329192328.htm [accessed 19 September 2014]

Videos

Anesthesia: Airway management in sleep apnea. http://www.youtube.com/watch?v=GGKL6Qe1_8E [accessed 19 September 2014]

Anesthesia issues in children for upper airway surgery. http://www.youtube.com/watch?v=mt7HuoTeOqY [accessed 19 September 2014]

Problems in extubation after anesthesia. http://www.youtube.com/watch?v=lE5b_roHbEY [accessed 19 September 2014]

40 Rapid sequence induction

References

Association of Anaesthetists of Great Britain and Ireland (2009) *Pre-hospital Anaesthesia.* AAGBI, London.

Difficult Airway Society (2014) *Rapid Sequence Induction.* DAS, London. http://www.das.uk.com/guidelines/rsi.html [accessed 5 January 2014]

Hein, C. & Owen, H. (2005) The effective application of cricoid pressure. *Journal of Emergency Primary Health Care,* 3 (1), 1–7. http://ro.ecu.edu.au/jephc/vol3/iss1/7/ [accessed 5 January 2014]

Hernandez, A., Wolf, S. W., Vijayakumar, V., Solanki, D. R. & Mathru, M. (2004) Sellick's maneuver for the prevention of aspiration – is it effective. *Anesthesiology.* 101, A1542.

Perry, J. J., Lee, J. S., Sillberg, V. A. & Wells, G. A. (2008) Rocuronium vs Succinylchlorine for rapid sequence induction intubation. *Cochrane Database of Systematic Reviews 2008.* 2, CD002788. DOI:10.1002/14651858.CD002788.pub2

Further reading

Bair, A. E. (2014) Rapid sequence intubation in adults. http://www.uptodate.com/contents/rapid-sequence-intubation-in-adults [accessed 5 January 2014]

Moos, D. (2007) Ineffective cricoid pressure – the critical role of formalised training. *British Journal of Anaesthetic and Recovery Nursing,* 8 (3), 43–50.

University of Missouri (2014) *Rapid Sequence Intubation: Medications, Dosages, and Recommendations.* University of

Missouri, Columbus, MO. http://med.umkc.edu/docs/em/ Intubation_Chart.pdf [accessed 5 January 2014]

Websites

Rapid sequence intubation. http://www.scdhec.gov/health/docs/rsi. pdf [accessed 19 September 2014]

Rapid sequence intubation. http://www.scottishintensivecare.org.uk/ uploads/2014-07-08-00-14-41-RSIbrochurepdf-76814.pdf [accessed 19 September 2014]

Videos

Anaesthesia CME – RSI – Rapid sequence induction. http://www. youtube.com/watch?v=DvFFL2Jctu4 [accessed 19 September 2014]

Endotracheal intubation: RSI with rocuronium/ketamine. http://www.youtube.com/watch?v=kTd7km_jnKw [accessed 19 September 2014]

Rapid sequence intubation – Parts 1–6: (1) http://www.youtube.com/ watch?v=5c8S2VaG4ZA; (2) http://www.youtube.com/watch?v= -T5kL2F-b30; (3) http://www.youtube.com/watch?v =QRPivxf90Zw; (4) http://www.youtube.com/ watch?v=IjLCJAKjjkU; (5) http://www.youtube.com/ watch?v=2PUL-2aleCE; (6) http://www.youtube.com/ watch?v=VePNGHSMRQc [accessed 19 September 2014]

RSI Drugs 101: EM in 5. http://www.youtube.com/watch? v=wbUDS_OrDiY [accessed 19 September 2014]

41 Bleeding problems

References

Chee, Y. L., Crawford, J. C., Watson, H. G. & Greaves, M. (2008) Guidelines on the assessment of bleeding risk prior to surgery or invasive procedures. *British Journal of Haematology*, 140 (5), 496–504.

Gallop, D. G. (2005) Catastrophic intraoperative hemorrhage: 5-step action plan. *OBG Management*, June. http://www. obgmanagement.com/fileadmin/obg_archive/ pdf/1706/1706OBGM_Article1.pdf [accessed 7 January 2014]

Hatfield, A. & Tronson, M. (2009) *The Complete Recovery Room Book* (4th edn). Oxford University Press, Oxford.

Kozek-Langenecker, S. A., Afshari, A., Albaladejo, P. *et al.* (2013) Management of severe perioperative bleeding. *European Journal of Anaesthesiology*, 30, 270–38. http://anest-rean.lt/wp-content/ uploads/2013/05/Management_of_severe_perioperative_ bleeding_.2.pdf [accessed 7 January 2014]

Mansour, J., Graf, K. & Lafferty, P. (2012) Bleeding disorders in orthopedic surgery. *Orthopedics*. 35 (12), 1053–1062. http://www. healio.com/orthopedics/journals/ortho/%7B9b321b20-5acf-4781- a026-1fa3b93547b5%7D/bleeding-disorders-in-orthopedic- surgery# [accessed 7 January 2014]

Martinowitz, U., Kenet, G., Segal, E., Luboshitz, J., Lubetsky, A., Ingerslev, J. & Lynn, M. (2001) Recombinant activated factor VII for adjunctive hemorrhage control in trauma. *Journal of Trauma*. 51 (3), 431–439.

Rossaint, R., Bouillon, B., Cerny, V. *et al.* (2010) Management of bleeding following major trauma: An updated European guideline. *Critical Care*. 14, R52. http://ccforum.com/content/pdf/ cc8943.pdf [accessed 7 January 2014]

Further reading

Assessment of perioperative bleeding risk. http://gmurrell.com.au/ ACES/Assessment%20of%20perioperative%20bleeding% 20risk.ppt [accessed 19 September 2014]

Koh, M. B. & Hunt, B. J. (2003) The management of perioperative bleeding. *Blood Reviews*. 17 (3), 179–185. http://www.ncbi.nlm. nih.gov/pubmed/12818228 [accessed 19 September 2014]

Surgical bleeding and haemostasis. http://www.authorstream.com/ Presentation/drkansals-510688-surgical-bleeding-haemostasis/ [accessed 19 September 2014]

Websites

Perioperative Bleeding. http://www.cslbehring.com/products/ bleeding-disorders-perioperative-bleeding-causes.htm [accessed 19 September 2014]

Perioperative Management of Patients on Chronic Antithrombotic Therapy. http://asheducationbook.hematologylibrary.org/ content/2012/1/529.full.pdf [accessed 19 September 2014]

Strategies for Preventing and Treating Uncontrolled Perioperative Bleeding. http://www.medscape.org/viewarticle/571999 [accessed 19 September 2014]

Videos

Surgical bleeding. http://www.youtube.com/watch?v=APJK7okrKuw [accessed 19 September 2014]

The Incidence and Management of Post-Operative Hemorrhage after Laparoscopic Gastric Bypass. http://www.youtube.com/ watch?v=DSU2tX7LArM [accessed 19 September 2014]

42 Malignant hyperthermia

References

Genetics Home Reference (2007) *Central Core Disease*. GHR, Bethesda, MD. http://ghr.nlm.nih.gov/condition/central-core- disease [accessed 12 January 2014]

Glahn, K. P. E., Ellis, F. R., Halsall, P. J., Müller, C. R., Snoeck, M. M. J., Urwyler, A. & Wappler, F. (2010) Recognizing and managing a malignant hyperthermia crisis: Guidelines from the European Malignant Hyperthermia Group. *British Journal of Anaesthesia*. 105 (4), 417–420. http://bja.oxfordjournals.org/content/105/4/417. long [accessed 12 January 2014]

Heller, J. L. (2011) Malignant hyperthermia. *Medline Plus*. http:// www.nlm.nih.gov/medlineplus/ency/article/001315.htm [accessed 12 January 2014]

Jungbluth, H. (2007) Multi-minicore disease. *Orphanet Journal of Rare Diseases, 2*, 31. http://www.ojrd.com/content/2/1/31 [accessed 12 January 2014]

Malignant Hyperthermia Association of the United States (2013) *Guide to Malignant Hyperthermia in an Anesthesia Setting: Postoperative Procedure*. MHAUS, Sherbourne, New York. http:// www.mhaus.org/healthcare-professionals/be-prepared/post- operative-procedure [accessed 12 January 2014]

University of California San Francisco Medical Centre (2013) *Chem-20*. UCSF Medical Centre, San Francisco, CA. http:// www.ucsfhealth.org/tests/003468.html [accessed 12 January 2014]

Further reading

Association of Anaesthetists of Great Britain and Ireland (2013) *UK National Core Competencies for Post-anaesthesia Care 2013: Immediate Post-anaesthesia Recovery 2013 Supplement*. AAGBI, London. http://www.aagbi.org/sites/default/files/Immediate% 20Post-anaesthesia%20recovery%202013% 20supplement.pdf [accessed 12 January 2014]

Pollock, N., Langton, E., Stowell, K., Simpson, C. & McDonnell, N. (2004) Safe duration of postoperative monitoring for malignant hyperthermia susceptible patients. *Journal of Anaesthesia and Intensive Care*. 32, 502–509.

Pollock, N., Langton, E., McDonnell, N., Tiemessen, J. & Stowell, K. (2006) Malignant hyperthermia and day stay surgery. *Anaesthesia and Intensive Care*, Feb 1. http://www.thefreelibrary.com/ Malignant+hyperthermia+and+day+stay+surgery.-a0188739645 [accessed 12 January 2014]

Websites

AAGBI Malignant Hyperthermia Publication Guidelines. http:// www.aagbi.org/publications/publications-guidelines/M/R [accessed 19 September 2014]

Malignant Hyperthermia. http://www.drugs.com/health-guide/ malignant-hyperthermia.html [accessed 19 September 2014]

Malignant Hyperthermia. http://www.medicinenet.com/malignant_hyperthermia/article.htm [accessed 19 September 2014]

Videos

Malignant hyperthermia. http://www.youtube.com/watch?v=F_fo9lbcMNs [accessed 19 September 2014]

Malignant hyperthermia: Intraoperative video – case report. http://www.youtube.com/watch?v=Q0FighAIizQ [accessed 19 September 2014]

Malignant hyperthermia presentation. http://www.youtube.com/watch?v=nppeo1ugEI8 [accessed 19 September 2014]

The preparation of dantrolene. http://www.youtube.com/watch?v=kSOvl1IzSNY [accessed 19 September 2014]

43 Cardiovascular problems

References

Aresti, N. A., Malik, A. A., Ihsan, K. M., Aftab, S. M. E. & Khan, W. S. (2014) Perioperative management of cardiac disease. *Journal of Perioperative Practice*, 24 (1&2), 9–14.

European Society of Cardiology (ESC) (2009) Guidelines for pre-operative cardiac risk assessment and perioperative cardiac management in non-cardiac surgery. *European Heart Journal*. 30, 2769–2812. http://eurheartj.oxfordjournals.org/content/30/22/2769.full.pdf [accessed 13 January 2014]

Fleisher, L. A., Beckman, J. A., Brown, K. A. *et al.* (2007) Guidelines on perioperative cardiovascular evaluation and care for noncardiac curgery. *Journal of the American College of Cardiology*, 50 (17), 159–231.

Goldman, L., Caldera, D. L., Nussbaum, S. R. *et al.* (1977) Multifactorial index of cardiac risk in noncardiac surgical procedures. *New England Journal of Medicine*, 297 (16), 845–850.

Qazizada, A. A. & Higgins, J. C. (2013) Preoperative evaluation and care: The cardiac patient undergoes noncardiac surgery. *Consultant 360*, 53 (*12*), 878–882. http://www.consultant360.com/articles/preoperative-evaluation-and-care-cardiac-patient-undergoes-noncardiac-surgery [accessed 17 January 2014]

Sear, J. W. & Higham, H. (2002) Issues in the perioperative management of the elderly patient with cardiovascular disease. *Journal of Drugs and Aging*. 19 (6), 429–51. http://www.ncbi.nlm.nih.gov/pubmed/12149050# [accessed 19 September 2014]

Further reading

Hatfield, A. & Tronson, M. (2009) *The Complete Recovery Book* (4th edn). Oxford University Press, Oxford.

Scott, I. A., Shohag, H. A., Kam, P. C. A., Jelinek, M. V. & Khadem, G. M. (2013) Preoperative cardiac evaluation and management of patients undergoing elective non-cardiac surgery. *Medical Journal of Australia*. 199 (10), 667–673. https://www.mja.com.au/journal/2013/199/10/preoperative-cardiac-evaluation-and-management-patients-undergoing-elective-non [accessed 19 September 2014]

SIGN (2004) *Postoperative Management in Adults: A Practical Guide to Postoperative Care for Clinical Staff*. Scottish Intercollegiate Guidelines Network, Edinburgh.

Website

Perioperative Cardiac Management. http://emedicine.medscape.com/article/285328-overview [accessed 19 September 2014]

Videos

Heart disease and heart attacks. http://www.youtube.com/watch?v=vYnreB1duro [accessed 19 September 2014]

Preoperative cardiovascular assessment of patients for non-cardiac surgery. http://www.youtube.com/watch?v=AaGCreSuVgQ [accessed 19 September 2014]

Prevention of perioperative cardiac morbidity. http://www.youtube.com/watch?v=rLriDDVTloU [accessed 19 September 2014]

44 Electrosurgical burns

References

Association for Perioperative Practice (2011). *Standards and Recommendation for Safe Perioperative Practice*. AFPP, Harrogate.

Demircin et al. (2013). Medicolegal aspects of surgical diathermy burns: A case report and review. *Romanian Journal of Legal Medicine 21*(3): 173–176.

Dhebri, A. R. & Afify, S. E. (2002) Free gas in the peritoneal cavity: The final hazard of diathermy. *Postgraduate Medical Journal*, 78, 496-497. http://pmj.bmj.com/content/78/922/496.full [accessed 7 June 2014]

Jiang, J., Zhu, F. Q., Luo, J., Wang, L. F. & Jiang, Q. (2004) Severe burn of penis caused by excessive short-wave diathermy. *Asian Journal of Andrology*. 6, 377–378.

National Reporting and Learning System (2012) *Risk of Skin Prep Related Fire in Operating Theatres*. NRLS. http://www.nrls.npsa.nhs.uk/resources/?entryid45=132981 [accessed 8 January 2014]

O'Riley, M. (2010) Electrosurgery in perioperative practice. *Journal of Perioperative Practice*. 20 (9), 329–333.

Prasad, R., Quezado, Z., St Andre, A. & O'Grady, N. P. (2006). Fires in the operating room and intensive care unit: Awareness is the key to prevention. *Anesthesia and Analgesia*. 102, 172–174.

Valleylab (2013) *Principles of Electrosurgery*. Covidien, Dublin. http://www.asit.org/assets/documents/Prinicpals_in_electrosurgery.pdf [accessed 19 September 2014]

Wicker, C. P. (1991) *Working with Electrosurgery*. National Association of Theatre Nurses, Harrogate.

Further reading

Association of Surgical Technologists (2012) *Recommended Standards of Practice for Use of Electrosurgery Association of Surgical Technologists*. AST, Littleton, CO. http://www.ast.org/uploadedFiles/Main_Site/Content/About_Us/Standard%20Electrosurgery.pdf [accessed 19 September 2014]

Dennis, V. (2004) Protecting patients from laparoscopic burns. *Encision*, August. http://encision.com/news/electrosurgery-in-the-news/protecting-patients-from-laparoscopic-burns/ [accessed 19 September 2014]

Endonurse (2007) Cautery and electrosurgery. *Endonurse*, Feb. 1. http://www.endonurse.com/articles/2007/02/cautery-and-electrosurgery.aspx [accessed 19 September 2014]

Websites

Burns caused by fire. http://www.rcsed.ac.uk/journal/svol1_2/10200010.html [accessed 19 September 2014]

Intraoperative Fires. http://www.ncbi.nlm.nih.gov/pubmed/18504243 [accessed 19 September 2014]

Risk of Skin-Prep Related Fire in Operating Theatres. http://www.nrls.npsa.nhs.uk/resources/?EntryId45=132981 [accessed 19 September 2014]

Videos

Fires in the operating room. http://www.youtube.com/watch?v=Pt6rqc7wyTA [accessed 19 September 2014]

Gloves in electro surgery – reducing risk. http://www.youtube.com/watch?v=56kO-iJxh5g [accessed 19 September 2014]

Oxygen alcohol prep surgical fire simulation. http://www.youtube.com/watch?v=BjvgKPqsfSY [accessed 19 September 2014]

Surgery gas explosion and evil eye phobia. http://www.youtube.com/watch?v=hrq_vnzsAHE [accessed 19 September 2014]

45 Venous thromboembolism

References

Agnelli, G. (2004) Prevention of venous thromboembolism in surgical patients. *Circulation*. 110, IV-4–IV12. http://circ.ahajournals.org/content/110/24_suppl_1/IV-4.full [accessed 19 September 2014]

Augistinos, P. & Ouriel, K. (2004) Treatment of venous thromboembolism. *Circulation, 110*, 1–27. http://circ.ahajournals.org/content/110/9_suppl_1/I-27.full [accessed 22 January 2014]

Department of Health (2010) *Venous Thromboembolism (VTE) Risk Assessment Gateway Reference no. 10278.* DH, London. http://webarchive.nationalarchives.gov.uk/20130107105354/http://www.dh.gov.uk/en/Publicationsandstatistics/Publications/PublicationsPolicyAndGuidance/DH_088215 [accessed 22 January 2014]

Desciak, M. C. & Martin, D. E. (2011) Perioperative pulmonary embolism: Diagnosis and anesthetic Management. *Journal of Clinical Anesthesia, 23*, 153–165. http://www.cinj.org/sites/cinj/files/documents/PerioperativePulmonaryEmbolism.pdf [accessed 22 January 2014]

Narani, K. K. (2010) Deep vein thrombosis and pulmonary embolism – prevention, management, and anaesthetic considerations. *Indian Journal of Anaesthesia. 54* (1), 8–17. http://www.ncbi.nlm.nih.gov/pmc/articles/PMC2876903/ [accessed 22 January 2014]

National Institute for Health and Care Excellence (2011) *Venous Thromboembolism: Reducing the Risk of Venous Thromboembolism (Deep Vein Thrombosis and Pulmonary Embolism) in Patients Undergoing Surgery.* NICE, London. http://guidance.nice.org.uk/CG92 [accessed 22 January 2014]

Wienert, P., Gallenkemper, G., Junger, M. & Rabe, E. (2005). Guideline: Intermittent pneumatic compression. *Phlebologie. 34* (3), 176–180.

Further reading

American Operating Room Nurses (2007) AORN guidelines for prevention of venous stasis. *AORN. 85* (3), 607–624.

Eisele, R., Kinzl, L. & Koelsch, T. (2007) Rapid-inflation intermittent pneumatic compression for prevention of deep venous thrombosis. *Journal of Bone and Joint Surgery, 89* (5), 1050–1056.

Van Wicklin, S. A., Ward, K. S. & Cantrell, S. W. (2006) Implementing a research utilization plan for prevention of deep vein thrombosis. *AORN. 83* (6), 1351–1362.

Websites

Deep Venous Thrombosis. www.oocities.org/shcraz1978us/dvt.ppt [accessed 19 September 2014]

Videos

A look at deep vein thrombosis and pulmonary embolism. http://www.youtube.com/watch?v=2K0WskqBWdw [accessed 19 September 2014]

Anti DVT deep vein thrombosis leg inflatable compressors. http://www.youtube.com/watch?v=4xsuKcVc-mI [accessed 19 September 2014]

Deep vein thrombosis (DVT) and pulmonary embolism (PE). http://www.youtube.com/watch?v=0PEhvACEROI [accessed 19 September 2014]

Prevention of DVT in orthopaedic trauma. http://www.youtube.com/watch?v=KaGlLtBIMi0 [accessed 19 September 2014]

46 Latex allergy

References

Brown, K. (1999) Care of the latex sensitive patient in theatre. *British Journal of Theatre Nursing. 9* (4), 170–173.

Katz, J. D. (2005) *Natural Rubber Latex Allergy.* American Society of Anesthesiologists, Schaumburg, IL. http://ecommerce.asahq.org/publicationsAndServices/latexallergy.pdf [accessed 22 January 2014]

Mercurio, J. (2011) Creating a latex perioperative environment. *OR Nurse November, 5* (6), 18–25. http://www.nursingcenter.com/lnc/pdf?AID=1253787&an=01271211-201111000-00006&Journal_ID=682710&Issue_ID=1253733 [accessed 23 January 2014]

Sussman, G. & Gold, M. (2014) *Guidelines for the Management of Latex Allergies and Safe Latex Use in Health Care Facilities.* American College of Allergy, Asthma & Immunology, Arlington

Heights, IL. http://www.acaai.org/allergist/allergies/Types/latex-allergy/Pages/latex-allergies-safe-use.aspx [accessed 23 January 2014]

Further reading

Duger, C., Kol, I. O., Kaygusuz, K., Gursoy, S., Ersan, I. & Mimaroglu, C. (2012) A perioperative anaphylactic reaction caused by latex in a patient with no history of allergy. *Anaesthesia Pain & Intensive Care. 16* (1), 71–73. http://www.apicareonline.com/?p=1118 [accessed 20 January 2014]

Royal Children's Hospital Melbourne (2012) *Latex – Management of a Patient at Risk of or with a Known Latex Allergy.* Royal Children's Hospital, Melbourne. http://www.rch.org.au/rchcpg/hospital_clinical_guideline_index/Latex_management_of_a_patient_at_risk_of_or_with_a_known_latex_allergy/ [accessed 21 January 2014]

Websites

Guidelines for the Anaesthetic Management of Patients with Latex Allergy. http://www.rcht.nhs.uk/DocumentsLibrary/RoyalCornwallHospitalsTrust/Clinical/Anaesthetics/GuidelinesForTheAnaestheticManagementOfPatientsWithLatexAller.pdf [accessed 19 September 2014]

Operating Suite Guidelines for Latex Allergic Patients. http://www.allergy.org.au/health-professionals/papers/management-of-latex-allergic-patients/operating-suite [accessed 19 September 2014]

Videos

Latex allergies: What you need to know. http://www.youtube.com/watch?v=R9GJ-FixkuM [accessed 19 September 2014]

Latex allergy. http://www.youtube.com/watch?v=4RQE4mMgqgI [accessed 19 September 2014]

Latex allergy association. http://www.youtube.com/watch?v=a4WlElqQnM4 [accessed 19 September 2014]

Nursing assessment – latex allergy. http://www.youtube.com/watch?v=-4iyle5PgRM [accessed 19 September 2014]

47 Assisting the surgeon

References

College of Operating Department Practitioners (2011) *Curriculum Document, Bachelor of Science (Hons) in Operating Department Practice – England, Northern Ireland and Wales; Bachelor of Science in Operating Department Practice – Scotland.* CODP, London.

Department of Health (2006) *The Curriculum Framework for the Surgical Care Practitioner.* DH (National Practitioner Programme), London.

Holmes, S. (1994) Development of the cardiac surgeon assistant. *British Journal of Nursing. 3* (5), 204–210.

Jones, A., Arshad, H. & Nolan, J. (2011) Surgical care practitioner practice: One team's journey explored. *Journal of Perioperative Practice, 22* (1), 19–23.

Perioperative Care Collaborative (2012) *Surgical First Assistant.* PCC, Harrogate.

Royal College of Surgeons of England (2011) *Position Statement – Surgical Assistants.* RCS, London. www.rcseng.ac.uk/publications/docs/rcs-position-statement-surgical-assistants [accessed 26 January 2014]

Whalan, C. (2006) *Assisting at Surgical Operations: A Practical Guide.* Cambridge University Press, Cambridge.

Further reading

Beesley, J. (2005) Much care needed over advanced practitioner roles. *Health Estate*, July. http://www.healthestatejournal.com/story/473/much-care-needed-over-advanced-practitioner-roles [accessed 19 September 2014]

Brame, K. (2011) The advanced scrub practitioner role: A student's reflection. *Journal of Perioperative Practice. 21* (4), 118–122.

Bruce, C. A., Bruce, I. A. & Williams, L. (2006) The impact of surgical care practitioners on surgical training. *Journal of the Royal Society of Medicine*, 99 (9), 432–433. http://www.ncbi.nlm.nih.gov/pmc/articles/PMC1557893/ [accessed 19 September 2014]

Halliwell, G. L. (2012) Becoming an advanced scrub practitioner: My personal journey. *Journal of Perioperative Practice*. 22 (12), 393–397.

Quick, J. (2013) The role of the surgical care practitioner within the surgical team. *British Journal of Nursing*. 22 (13), 759–765.

Rothrock, J. C. (1999) *The RN First Assistant: An Expanded Perioperative Nursing Role*. Lippincott Williams & Wilkins, Philadelphia, PA.

Rothrock, J. C. & Seifert, P. C. (2009) *Assisting in Surgery: Patient Centred Care*. Competency & Credentialing Institute, Denver, CO.

Websites

Advanced Practice. http://www.afpp.org.uk/news/resources/Advanced-Practice [accessed 19 September 2014]

Surgical Care Practitioner Curriculum. http://www.rcseng.ac.uk/surgeons/training/accreditation/surgical-careers-practitioners-scps [accessed 19 September 2014.

The surgeons who are not doctors. http://www.bbc.co.uk/news/health-20629396 [accessed 19 September 2014]

Videos

Draping. http://www.youtube.com/watch?v=lLUHycgF09c [accessed 19 September 2014]

Medical assistant training prepare for minor surgical procedures. http://www.youtube.com/watch?v=-ggM1sTpYaM [accessed 19 September 2014]

Perspective of a surgical assistant. http://www.youtube.com/watch?v=afjvWWS3r84 [accessed 19 September 2014]

Surgical assistant. http://www.youtube.com/watch?v=-_S5ZHoyJpE [accessed 19 September 2014]

What is a surgical assistant? http://www.youtube.com/watch?v=gscvcBfmJVw [accessed 19 September 2014]

48 Shaving, marking, prepping and draping

References

Association of Surgical Technologists (2008) *Recommended Standards of Practice for Skin Prep of the Surgical Patient*. AST, Littleton, CO. http://www.ast.org/uploadedFiles/Main_Site/Content/About_Us/Standard_Skin_Prep.pdf [accessed 30 January 2014]

Davidson, K., Dobb, M. & Tanner, J. (2003) UK surgical draping practices. *British Journal of Perioperative Practice*. 13 (3), 109–114.

Hemani, M. L. & Lepor, H. (2009) Skin preparation for the prevention of surgical site infection: Which agent is best? *Reviews in Urology*. 11 (4), 190–195.

PPSA (2008) Surgical site markers: Putting your mark on patient safety. *Pennsylvania Patient Safety Advisory Journal*. 5 (4), 130–135. http://patientsafetyauthority.org/ADVISORIES/AdvisoryLibrary/2008/Dec5%284%29/Pages/130.aspx [accessed 30 January 2014]

Whalan, C. (2006) *Assisting at Surgical Operations*. Cambridge University Press, Cambridge.

Further reading

Cullan, D. & Wongworawat, M. (2007) Sterility of the surgical site marking between the ink and the epidermis. *Journal of the American College of Surgery*. 205 (2), 319–321.

Digison, M. B. (2007) A review of antiseptic agents for pre-operative skin preparation. *Plastic Surgical Nursing*. 27, 185–189.

Moore, D. T. (2004) Clinical issues: Nurses administering propofol; OR temperature and humidity; OR internet use; OR cleaning; approved skin markers. *AORN Journal*, 80 (5), 929–934.

Websites

Positioning, Skin Preparation and Draping. http://www.slideshare.net/BeaGalang/positioning-skin-prep-incision-draping [accessed 19 September 2014]

Surgical Site Marking Protocols and Policy. http://www.ruh.nhs.uk/about/policies/documents/clinical_policies/blue_clinical/Blue_7021.pdf [accessed 19 September 2014]

Wash but Don't Shave before Surgery, Patients Told. http://www.telegraph.co.uk/health/10415993/Wash-but-dont-shave-before-surgery-patients-told.html [accessed 19 September 2014]

Videos

Betadine scrub and paint. http://www.youtube.com/watch?v=2GAoHDDScC8 [accessed 19 September 2014]

Patient prep. http://www.youtube.com/watch?v=iM_V0FUSjeA [accessed 19 September 2014]

Surgical drapes – cardiothoracic drape. http://www.youtube.com/watch?v=f-mSYn0EfsM [accessed 19 September 2014]

Surgical marking and anaesthesia. http://www.youtube.com/watch?v=orDpgREl-V4 [accessed 19 September 2014]

Surgical positioning, prepping and draping. http://www.youtube.com/watch?v=VB1ufcUCr6c [accessed 19 September 2014]

49 Retraction of tissues

References

Goodman, T. & Spry, C. (2014) *Essentials of Perioperative Nursing*. Jones & Bartlett Learning, Burlington, MA.

Kirkup, J. (1996) The history and evolution of surgical instruments. VII. Spring forceps (tweezers), hooks and simple retractors. *Annals of the Royal College of Surgeons of England*. 78 (6), 544–552. http://www.ncbi.nlm.nih.gov/pmc/articles/PMC2502851/pdf/annrcse01604-0070.pdf [accessed 1 February 2014]

Spera, P., Lloyd, J. D., Hernandez, E., Hughes, N., Peterson, C., Nelson, A. & Spratt, D. G. (2011) Tissue retraction in the perioperative setting. *AORN Journal*. 94, 54–58.

Whalan, C. (2006) *Assisting at Surgical Operations*. Cambridge University Press, Cambridge.

Further reading

Berquer, R., Smith, W. D. & Davis, D. (2002) An ergonomic study of the optimum operating table height for laparoscopic surgery. *Surgical Endoscopy*, 16 (3), 416–421.

Rothrock, J. C. (1999) *The RN First Assistant: An Expanded Perioperative Nursing Role* (3rd edn). Lippincott, Philadelphia, PA.

Websites

Retractor (Medical). http://en.wikipedia.org/wiki/Retractor_%28medical%29 [accessed 19 September 2014]

Surgical Retractors. http://www.orsupply.com/medical/category/Surgical-Instruments/872/category/Surgical-Retractors/910 [accessed 19 September 2014]

Videos

Maintenance of the Greenberg retractor and handrest. http://www.youtube.com/watch?v=UWQxmKXByjM&list=PLvMr0jivPc4aDT4FL-jDF-3txVKz4ezbC [accessed 19 September 2014]

Mini self retaining retractor for metacarpals. http://www.youtube.com/watch?v=_z6F3OrnyT4 [accessed 19 September 2014]

The Doxpal – self retaining surgical retractors. https://www.youtube.com/watch?v=eQnt9zk0zdE [accessed 19 September 2014]

Thompson Kurulum (table mounted retractor). http://www.youtube.com/watch?v=ueVa2TxBZec [accessed 19 September 2014]

Wound retractor. http://www.youtube.com/watch?v=0klbEKKKP-M&list=PLvMr0jivPc4aDT4FL-jDF-3txVKz4ezbC [accessed 19 September 2014]

50 Suture techniques and materials

References

Asali, E. A. (2014) *Sutures and Suturing*. International University for Science & Technology, Damascus. http://iust.edu.sy/

courses/Sutures%20and%20Suturing.pdf [accessed 1 February 2014]

McDermott, C. (2014) *Suture Materials*. CIS Self Study Plan, Purdue University, West Lafayette, IN. https://www.distance.purdue.edu/training/cssp/cis/pdf/CIS230.pdf [accessed 4 February 2014]

Semer, N. B. (2001) Suturing: The basics. In: N. B. Semer, *Practical Plastic Surgery for Nonsurgeons*, Hanley & Belfus, Philadelphia, PA. http://practicalplasticsurgery.org/docs/Practical_01.pdf [accessed 2 February 2014]

STO (2014) *Suture Materials*. Surgical tutor.org.uk. http://www.surgical-tutor.org.uk/default-home.htm?principles/technique/sutures.htm~right [accessed 2 February 2014]

Whalan, C. (2006) *Assisting at Surgical Operations*. Cambridge University Press, Cambridge.

Further reading

Suture materials comparison chart. http://en.wikipedia.org/wiki/Suture_materials_comparison_chart [accessed 19 September 2014]

Suture types. http://www.upstate.edu/surgery/pdf/education/clerkship/suture_types.pdf [accessed 19 September 2014]

Websites

Pocket Guide to Suture Materials, Techniques and Knots. http://www.fmdental.pl/uploads/20110107131642.pdf [accessed 19 September 2014]

Surgical Knot Tying Manual. http://www.covidien.com/imageServer.aspx?contentID=11850&contenttype=application/pdf [accessed 19 September 2014]

Suturing Techniques. http://dermnetnz.org/procedures/suturing.html [accessed 19 September 2014]

Videos

3 interrupted sutures: Simple, vertical mattress, & horizontal mattress. http://www.youtube.com/watch?v=qGU4Pn4UnME [accessed 19 September 2014]

8 common suture techniques for skin closure. http://www.youtube.com/watch?v=-ZWUgKiBxfk [accessed 19 September 2014]

How to tie a surgeon's knot. http://www.youtube.com/watch?v=TIhPxjMFlTI [accessed 19 September 2014]

Suture types part 1. http://www.youtube.com/watch?v=BW91H41w8ts [accessed 19 September 2014]

Two handed surgical square knot with explanations! http://www.youtube.com/watch?v=o-dkb-YX3-E [accessed 19 September 2014]

Types of sutures. http://www.youtube.com/watch?v=yJLkoORmeYI [accessed 19 September 2014]

51 Haemostatic techniques

References

Hakim, N. S. & Canelo, R. (2007) *Haemostasis in Surgery*. Imperial College Press, London.

Moss, R. (2013) *Management of Surgical Hemostasis: An Independent Study Guide*. Association of Peri-Operative Registered Nurses, Denver, CO.

Niles, J. (1999) Surgical haemostasis. *In Practice*, 21, 196–204.

Samudralla, S. (2008) Topical hemostatic agents in surgery: A surgeon's perspective. *AORN Journal*, 88 (3), S2–S11.

Further reading

Boonstra, E. A., Molenaar, I. Q., Porte, R. J. & T de Boer, M. (2009) Topical haemostatic agents in liver surgery: Do we need them? *International Hepato-Pancreato-Biliary Association Journal*. 11 (4), 306–310. http://www.ncbi.nlm.nih.gov/pmc/articles/PMC2727083/ [accessed 3 February 2014]

Henley, J. & Brewer, J. D. (2013) Newer hemostatic agents used in the practice of dermatologic surgery. *Dermatology Research and Practice Journal*. 2013, 279289. http://www.hindawi.com/journals/drp/2013/279289/ [accessed 3 February 2014]

Moumoulidis, I., Martinez Del Pero, M., Brennan, L. & Jani, P. (2010) Haemostasis in head and neck surgical procedures. *Annals of the Royal College of Surgeons of England*. 92 (4), 292–294. http://www.ncbi.nlm.nih.gov/pubmed/20501015 [accessed 19 September 2014]

Websites

Haemostasis in Breast Surgery. http://www.rydygier.cm-uj.krakow.pl/essurg/docs/turin_2010/2611/Presentazioni/26112010Sella/Hemostasisinsurgery/Iovino.pdf [accessed 19 September 2014]

Surgical Bleeding and Homeostasis. http://www.authorstream.com/Presentation/drkansals-510688-surgical-bleeding-haemostasis/ [accessed 19 September 2014]

Videos

Blood coagulation techniques and hemostasis in oral surgery. http://www.youtube.com/watch?v=7OTNbDyCLCc [accessed 19 September 2014]

Controlling hemostasis during open liver resection. http://www.youtube.com/watch?v=bYPQ-1ORjrA [accessed 19 September 2014]

Hemostasis. http://www.youtube.com/watch?v=GAcAPDVD3C0 [accessed 19 September 2014]

Hemostasis lecture in HD. http://www.youtube.com/watch?v=dGdK45-4tIg [accessed 19 September 2014]

Surgical hemostasis, litigation in continuity. http://www.youtube.com/watch?v=-vIAYuglIcM [accessed 19 September 2014]

Total laparoscopic hysterectomy. http://www.youtube.com/watch?v=S7bk-k5NuOw [accessed 19 September 2014]

52 Laparoscopic surgery

References

Bradley, J. P. (2014) *Camera Holding Skills and the Role of the ASP*. http://www.slideshare.net/Telepresence/camera-holding-skills-and-the-role-of-the-asp [accessed 6 February 2014]

Chiu, A., Bowne, W. B., Sookraj, K. A., Zenilman, M. E., Fingerhut, A. & Ferzli, G. S. (2008) The role of the assistant in laparoscopic surgery: Important considerations for the apprentice-in-training. *Surgical Innovation*. 15 (3), 229–236. http://www.ncbi.nlm.nih.gov/pubmed/18757384 [accessed 1 February 2014]

Ferzli, G. S. (2011) Role of the Assistant in Lap Surgery: Important Considerations for the Apprentice in Training. http://www.slideshare.net/drferzli/assistant-role-laparoscopicsurgery [accessed 6 February 2014]

Kaar, J. (1999) The RN first assistant's role in a laparoscopic cholecystectomy. *AORN Journal*, 70 (3), 455–460.

Rothrock, J. C. (1999) *The RN First Assistant* (3rd edn). Lippincott, Williams & Wilkins, Philadelphia, PA.

Further reading

Aesculap (2010) *Laparoscopic Instruments*. Aesculap, Center Valley, PA. http://www.aesculapusa.com/assets/base/doc/DOC465_REV_F_Laparoscopic_Catalog.pdf [accessed 4 February 2014]

Aggarwal, M. (2014) *Anaesthesia for Laparoscopic Surgery* (PowerPoint). http://www.google.com/url?sa=t&rct=j&q=surgical%20assistant%20in%20laparoscopic%20surgery%20ppt&source=web&cd=1&ved=0CCMQFjAA&url=http%3A%2F%2Fanaesthesia.co.in%2Fwp-content%2Fuploads%2F2012%2F05%2F9.-Laparoscopic-Surgery.ppt&ei=PgTxUoSqIKSs7QbgwIGQCg&usg=AFQjCNHd3NB74TtTSLe6g6TPuNi9jWO3MA&cad=rja [accessed 4 February 2014]

Rahman, M. N. & Mishra, R. K. (2011) The camera-holding robotic device in laparoscopy surgery. *World Journal of Laparoscopic Surgery*. 4 (3), 132–135. http://www.jaypeejournals.com/eJournals/ShowText.aspx?ID=2345&Type=FREE&TYP=TOP&IN=_eJournals/images/JPLOGO.gif&IID=194&isPDF=YES [accessed 4 February 2014]

Websites

Helping at Lap Surgery. http://mpatkin.org/surg_lap/lap_helping1. htm [accessed 19 September 2014]

Laparoscopic Cholecystectomy. http://emedicine.medscape.com/ article/1582292-overview [accessed 19 September 2014]

Tips for When One Is Struggling with Laparoscopic Surgery. http://academicobgyn.com/2013/01/29/tips-for-when-one-is-struggling-with-laparoscopic-surgery/ [accessed 19 September 2014]

Videos

Complication during laparoscopic surgery. http://www.youtube.com/ watch?v=2ea0AbjQYHM [accessed 19 September 2014]

Laparoscopic camera holder. http://www.youtube.com/ watch?v=VY812VHl5Xk [accessed 19 September 2014]

Laparoscopic cholecystectomy. http://www.youtube.com/ watch?v=ecQCvZb9qUA [accessed 19 September 2014]

Laparoscopic (keyhole surgery) removal of an ovarian cyst. http:// www.youtube.com/watch?v=WySe52jOj40 [accessed 19 September 2014]

53 Orthopaedic surgery

References

American Academy of Orthopaedic Surgeons (2011) *Total Hip Replacement*. AAOS, Rosemont, IL. http://orthoinfo.aaos.org/ topic.cfm?topic=a00377 [accessed 8 February 2014]

American Academy of Orthopaedic Surgeons (2012) *Total Knee Replacement*. AAOS, Rosemont, IL. http://orthoinfo.aaos.org/ topic.cfm?topic=a00389 [accessed 8 February 2014]

Jones, A., Arshad, H. & Nolan, J. (2012) Surgical care practitioner practice: One team's journey explored. *Journal of Perioperative Practice*. 22 (1), 19–23.

Palan, J., Gulati, A., Andrew, J. G., Murray, D. W. & Beard, D. J. (2009) The trainer, the trainee and the surgeons' assistant. *Journal of Bone and Joint Surgery*. 91 (7), 928–934. http://www. bjj.boneandjoint.org.uk/content/91-B/7/928.full [accessed 19 September 2014]

Rothrock, J. C. (1999) *The RN First Assistant* (3rd edn). Lipincott Williams & Wilkins, Philadelphia, PA.

Whalan, C. (2006) *Assisting at Surgical Operations*. Cambridge University Press, Cambridge.

Further reading

British Orthopaedic Association (2006) *Primary Total Hip Replacement: A Guide to Good Practice*. BOA, London.

Hayler, D. (1999) A step in the right direction – orthopaedic trauma. *British Journal of Theatre Nursing*. 9 (5), 222–224.

Lindsay, W., Bigsby, E. & Bannister, G. (2011) Prevention of infection in orthopaedic joint replacement. *Journal of Perioperative Practice*, 21 (6), 206–209.

Waller, C. S. (2010) *Knee Arthroscopy*. http://www. hipandkneesurgery.com.au/wp-content/themes/craig-waller/pdf/ knee-arthroscopy-brochure.pdf [accessed 8 February 2014]

Wand, R. J., Dear, K. E. A., Bigsby, E. & Wand, J. S. (2012) A review of shoulder replacement surgery. *Journal of Perioperative Practice*, 22 (11), 354–359.

Websites

Hip Replacement. http://www.nhs.uk/conditions/hip-replacement/ Pages/Introduction.aspx [accessed 19 September 2014]

Knee Arthroscopic Surgery for Meniscal Tears. http://www. dukehealth.org/health_library/advice_from_doctors/bodies-in-motion/meniscal-tears [accessed 19 September 2014]

Knee Arthroscopy. http://orthoinfo.aaos.org/topic.cfm?topic=a00299 [accessed 19 September 2014]

Knee Replacement. http://www.nhs.uk/conditions/Knee-replacement/Pages/Kneereplacementexplained.aspx [accessed 19 September 2014]

Videos

Arthroscopic knee surgery. http://www.youtube.com/ watch?v=kpW2MOOI5yw [accessed 19 September 2014]

Hip replacement surgery. http://www.youtube.com/ watch?v=BYwVaKkRdF4 [accessed 19 September 2014]

Horrific crash aftermath in hospital. http://www.youtube.com/ watch?v=kOaezU-TAQs [accessed 19 September 2014]

Knee arthroscopy. http://www.youtube.com/watch?v=pguNCtOwzEc [accessed 19 September 2014]

Total hip replacement. http://www.youtube.com/ watch?v=Mv5O2J1jf2o [accessed 19 September 2014]

Total hip replacement surgery. http://www.youtube.com/watch?v=0-O8IFzV8Nc [accessed 19 September 2014]

Trauma surgery. http://www.youtube.com/watch?v=MxrQQ6NVok4 [accessed 19 September 2014]

54 Cardiac surgery

References

Goldman, M. A. (2008) *Pocket Guide to the Operating Room* (3rd edn). F.A. Davis, Philadelphia, PA.

Phillips, N. (2007) *Berry and Kohn's Operating Room Technique* (11th edn). Mosby Elsevier, St Louis, MO.

Rothrock, J. C. (1999) *The RN First Assistant* (3rd edn). Lipincott Williams & Wilkins, Philadelphia, PA.

Whalan, C. (2006) *Assisting at Surgical Operations*. Cambridge University Press, Cambridge.

Further reading

Alex, J., Rao, V. P., Cale, A. R., Griffin, S. C., Cowen, M. E. & Guvendik, L. (2004) Surgical nurse assistants in cardiac surgery: A UK trainee's perspective. *European Journal of Cardiothoracic Surgery*, 25, 111–115.

Cuschieri, A., Grace, P. A., Darzi, A., Borley, N. & Rowley, D. I. (2003) *Clinical Surgery* (2nd edn). Blackwell, Oxford.

Websites

Association of Physician Assistants in Cardiovascular Surgery, http:// www.apacvs.org/

Cardiac Surgeries. http://www.slideshare.net/AmrutaPai/cardiac-surgeries-22838733?from_search=2 [accessed 19 September 2014]

What Is Heart Surgery? http://www.nhlbi.nih.gov/health/health-topics/topics/hs/ [accessed 19 September 2014]

Videos

Aortic valve replacement. http://www.youtube.com/ watch?v=5jLfPlQBYuw [accessed 19 September 2014]

Coronary bypass surgery. http://www.youtube.com/ watch?v=7PpidBmoA4c [accessed 19 September 2014]

Heart surgery: Minimally invasive aortic valve replacement. http:// www.youtube.com/watch?v=B9b_VCjI3n0 [accessed 19 September 2014]

Open heart surgery. http://www.youtube.com/ watch?v=tRFMEeQCkpA [accessed 19 September 2014]

Right thoracotomy approach for minimally invasive mitral valve surgery. http://www.youtube.com/watch?v=EnJQh_W3r3A [accessed 19 September 2014]

55 Things to do after surgery

References

Perioperative Care Collaborative (2012) *Surgical First Assistant*. PCC, Harrogate.

Rothrock, J. C. (1999) *The RN First Assistant* (3rd edn). Lipincott Williams & Wilkins, Philadelphia, PA.

Rothrock, J. C. & Seifert, P. C. (2009) *Assisting in Surgery: Patient Centred Care*. Competency and Credentialing Institute, Denver, CO.

Whalan, C. (2006) *Assisting at Surgical Operations*. Cambridge University Press, Cambridge.

Further reading

Deighton, C. (2007) A reflection on the development of the advanced scrub practitioner. *Journal of Perioperative Practice. 17* (10), 485–492.

Fleming, E. & Carberry, M. (2011) Steering a course towards advanced nurse practitioner: A critical care perspective. *Nursing in Critical Care. 16* (2), 67–76.

Livesley, J., Waters, K. & Tarbuck, P. (2009) The management of advanced practitioner preparation: A work-based challenge. *Journal of Nursing Management. 17* (5), 584–593.

Websites

How to become a Surgical Care Practitioner: http://www.plymouth.ac.uk/files/extranet/docs/FoH/SCP%20Flowchart.pdf

Surgical Care Practitioner (SCP): https://www.rcseng.ac.uk/surgeons/training/accreditation/surgical-care-practitioners-scps

Surgical First Assistant Modules: http://www.edgehill.ac.uk/health/cpd-modules/surgical-first-assistance-operative-procedures-hea3055/

The Curriculum Framework for the Surgical Care Practitioner: http://www.rcseng.ac.uk/surgeons/training/docs/surgical-care-practitioner-curriculum

The Surgical Care Practitioner: A Feasible Alternative: http://www.ncbi.nlm.nih.gov/pmc/articles/PMC1963525/

Videos

Surgical assistants training: http://www.youtube.com/watch?v=yn9NE9-YsTw

Welcome to theatre part 1: http://www.youtube.com/watch?v=IE0c-kvOeaU

Welcome to theatre part 2: http://www.youtube.com/watch?v=56QdTyhXczw

What is an Operating Department Practitioner: http://www.youtube.com/watch?v=lPbP7rToi7c

What is a Surgical Assistant?: http://www.youtube.com/watch?v=gscvcBfmJVw

Index

ABCDE approach 67, 69
accountability 16–17
acupuncture 79
airway maintenance
    anaesthesia 22
    emergency
        procedures 86–87
    recovery 65, 67, 69, 73, 74–75
allergic reactions
    anaesthesia 37
    latex allergy 100–101
    recovery 77
    Safe Surgery Checklist 15
anaesthesia 21–39
    adverse effects 37
    care plans 10–11
    checking the anaesthetic
        machine 24–25
    complications 35
    consumable items 22–23
    drugs 28–29, 34–35
    fluid warmers 23
    general anaesthesia 34–35,
        65, 93
    latex allergy 101
    local anaesthesia 36–37
    malignant hyperthermia 93
    medical gas cylinders 23
    monitoring devices 22–23,
        32–33
    patient positioning 49
    perioperative fluid
        management 30–31
    preparing and managing
        equipment 9, 22–23
    recovery 65
    regional anaesthesia 38–39,
        65
    respiratory and
        cardiovascular
        systems 26–27
    Safe Surgery Checklist 14–15
    topical anaesthesia 37
    two-bag test 24–25
analgesics 28–29, 34–35, 73, 79
anti-emetics 81
aortic stenosis 95
aortic valve replacement 118
arm boards 49
arrhythmias 95
arthroscopy 118–119
aspirators 45
assault 17

bandages 58–61
Better Training Better Care
    (BTBC) 18–19
Bier's block 39
bipolar electrosurgery 56–57, 96
bleeding
    coagulation 112
    emergency
        procedures 90–91
    haemostatic
        techniques 112–113
    monitoring in recovery 73
blood and blood byproducts 31
blood-borne viruses 7
blood chemistry 2
blood gases 2

capnography 33
cardiac surgery 118–119
cardiogenic shock 69
cardiopulmonary bypass
    (CBP) 119
cardiovascular system
    anatomy and
        physiology 26–27
    emergency
        procedures 94–95
    recovery 68–69, 73
care pathways 11
care plans 2–3, 10–11, 70–71
CARESCAPE Monitor B850 32
caudal epidural block 38–39
central venous pressure (CVP)
    line 23
chemical sterilisation 53
circulating practitioners 42–43,
    50–51
cleaning and hygiene
    circulating and scrub
        team 42–43, 50–51
    preventing infection
        transmission 6–7
    scrub procedures 46–47
    standard precautions 6
    sterile field 50–51
    sterilisation and
        disinfection 52–53
clinical governance 19
coagulation of blood 112
colloids 30–31, 91
conflicts 19
congestive heart failure 95
consent 17

contractual
    accountability 16–17
core surgical trainees
    (CST) 18–19
coronary circulation 27
cough etiquette 6
critical bleeding 90–91
critically ill patients 84–85
crystalloids 30–31
cuffed tracheostomy tube 22

deep vein thrombosis (DVT) 99
delayed hypersensitivity 101
dextrose 31
diagnostic screening 3
diathermy burns 96–97
discharge 65, 67, 75
disinfection 52–53
documentation 67
drainage 73
draping 51, 106–107
dressings 60–61

elective joint replacement 119
electrical stimulation of
    peripheral nerves 79
electrocardiogram
    (ECG) 26–27, 33
electrosurgery 56–57
electrosurgical burns 96–97
emergency procedures 83–101
    airway problems 86–87
    bleeding problems 90–91
    cardiovascular
        problems 94–95
    caring for the critically
        ill 84–85
    electrosurgical burns 96–97
    latex allergy 100–101
    malignant
        hyperthermia 92–93
    rapid sequence
        induction 88–89
    venous
        thromboembolism 98–99
endotracheal tubes 74, 88–89
environmental cleaning 6
epidural anaesthesia 38–39, 65
equipment
    anaesthesia 9, 22–23
    cleaning 7
    emergency procedures 86,
        88–89

patient care equipment 6
personal protective
    equipment 4–5, 6–7
preparing and
    managing 8–9, 22–23
recovery 74
surgical equipment 9,
    108–111
Esmarch bandages 58–59
eutectic mixture of local
    anaesthetics (EMLA) 36
explosion 97
eye protection 4

face masks 74, 86
filtration 53
fire 97
fluid management 30–31, 73
fluid warmers 23
footwear 5
forceps 45
Fowler position 48–49

gas exchange 26–27
general anaesthesia 34–35, 65, 93
gloves 4, 6, 46
glycaemic control 15
gowns 6
graduated compression
    stockings (GCS) 99
Guedel airway 22, 87
Guedel's signs 35

haematology 2
haemodynamics 69, 91, 119
haemorrhage 77, 91
haemostasis 112–113
hair removal 15
hand-held retractors 108–109
hand hygiene 6, 46–47
handover 66–67
Hartmann's solution 31
headwear 5
high-dependency units
    (HDU) 85
hip replacement 118
hospital requirements 17
hot-air ovens 53
human error 19
hygiene see cleaning and
    hygiene
hypertension 95
hyperthermia 71, 72–73

hypertonic saline 31
hypothermia 71, 72–73, 119
hypovoloemic shock 69, 91

immediate hypersensitivity 101
induction agents 29, 34–35
infection 6–7
  orthopaedic surgery 119
  postoperative
    complications 3
  standard precautions 6
  surgical site infection 15
  theatre scrubs and personal
    protective equipment 5, 6
  wounds and dressings 61
infiltration anaesthesia 37
inhalation agents 28–29
instrument counts 54–55
instrument trays 51
intensive care units (ICU) 85
intermittent compression
    devices (ICD) 99
intermittent pneumatic
    compression (IPC) 98–99
interprofessional
    teamworking 18–19
intraoperative care plans 10–11
intravascular catheters 77
intravenous cannulae 30, 36
irritation 101
ischaemic heart attack 94

jackknife position 49

knee replacement 118

laparoscopic surgery 114–115
laryngeal mask airways
    (LMA) 22–23
laryngospasm 75
lateral position 48–49
latex allergy 100–101
legal accountability 16–17
linens 6
lithotomy position 48–49
local anaesthesia 36–37

major bleeding 113
malignant hyperthermia
    (MH) 92–93
marking the patient 106–107
massage 79
massive blood loss 91
mechanical sterilisation 53
medical gas cylinders 23
methicillin-resistant
    Staphylococcus aureus
    (MRSA) 7, 61
microinstrumentation 45
minimally invasive
    techniques 119
minor bleeding 113
moist-heat sterilisation 53
monitoring devices 22–23,
    32–33, 72–73
monopolar
    electrosurgery 56–57, 96
muscle relaxants 28–29, 34–35

nasopharyngeal airway 74
National Confidential Enquiry
    into Patient Outcome and
    Death (NCEPOD) 69, 85

National Patient Safety Agency
    (NPSA) 13–15
nausea and vomiting
    (N&V) 73, 80–81
necrosis 96
needle stick injuries 6–7
negligence 17
nerve blockade 37
neuromuscular blockers
    (NMB) 88–89
neuromuscular junction 28
neuromuscular system 73
non-invasive blood pressure
    (NIBP) 33
non-ionising radiation 53
nonsteroidal anti-inflammatory
    drugs (NSAIDs) 79
normal saline (NS) 31
normothermia 15

opioids 28–29, 79
oral airways 22, 74, 86
orthopaedic surgery 118–119
osmosis 30

pain management 73, 78–79
paralysis with induction 89
patient dress 5
patient handover 66–67
patient notes 2, 68
patient outcomes 11
patient positioning 48–49
patient preparation 2–3
personal protective equipment
    (PPE) 4–5, 6–7
physical sterilisation 53
physiological lab values 2
platelet count 2
pneumatic tourniquets 58–59
post-anaesthetic care unit
    (PACU) 64–65
postoperative care 11, 68–71, 101
postoperative complications 3
postoperative duties 120–121
postoperative nausea and
    vomiting (PONV) 73, 80–81
powered surgical
    instruments 45
preoperative assessment 2–3, 95
preoperative investigations 3
preoperative patient
    checklist 10
prepping the patient 106–107
professional
    accountability 16–17
prone position 48–49
Pseudomonas aeruginosa 47
psychological status 73
pulse oximeters 33

rapid sequence induction
    (RSI) 88–89
recovery 63–81
  admission to recovery unit 67
  airway maintenance 65, 67,
    69, 73, 74–75
  allergic reactions 77
  cardiovascular status 68–69, 73
  care plans 70–71
  caring for the critically
    ill 84–85
  complications 75, 76–77
  critical bleeding 91

discharge 65, 67, 75
documentation 67
drainage and bleeding 73
fluid balance 73
general patient care 71
haemorrhage 77
initial assessment 67
intravascular catheters 77
monitoring 72–73
nausea and vomiting 73, 80–81
neuromuscular status 73
pain status 73, 78–79
patient handover 66–67
postoperative care 68–71
psychological status 73
recovery room 64–65
respiratory status 68–69, 73, 75
septic shock 77
temperature status 71, 72–73
urinary complications 77
urine output and voiding 73
wound dehiscence 77
regional anaesthesia 38–39, 65
regional analgesia 79
respiratory hygiene 6
respiratory system 26–27,
    68–69, 73, 75
retractors 45, 108–109
Rhys Davies exsanguinator 58–59

Safe Surgery Checklist
    (SSCL) 12–15
scalpels 45
scrub practitioners 42–43,
    50–51, 117
scrub procedures 46–47
scrubs 4–5
sedation 88–89
self and others
    accountability 16–17
self-retaining retractors 108–109
septic shock 77
sharps 6–7
shaving the patient 106–107
sign in/out 15
skin marking 106–107
skin prepping 106–107
spinal anaesthesia 38–39, 65
splash injuries 7
standard precautions 6
staplers 45
sterile field 50–51
sterilisation 52–53
sternotomy 119
stirrups 49
suction devices 45
supine position 48–49
surface anaesthesia 37
surgery 41–61
  advanced surgical
    practice 103–121
  assisting the
    surgeon 104–121
  basic surgical
    instruments 44–45
  cardiac surgery 118–119
  circulating and scrub
    team 42–43, 50–51
  complications 61
  critical bleeding 91
  electrosurgery 56–57
  haemostatic
    techniques 112–113

laparoscopic surgery 114–115
  orthopaedic
    surgery 118–119
  patient positioning 48–49
  postoperative duties 120–121
  retraction of tissues 108–109
  safety and hazards 57
  scrub procedures 46–47
  shaving, marking, prepping
    and draping 106–107
  sterile field 50–51
  sterilisation and
    disinfection 52–53
  suture techniques and
    materials 110–111
  swab and instrument
    counts 54–55
  tourniquet
    management 58–59
  wounds and dressings 60–61
surgical care practitioner
    (SCP) 104–121
surgical first assistant
    (SFA) 105–121
surgical masks 5, 6
Surgical Safety Checklist
    (SSCL) 12–15
surgical site infection (SSI) 15
sutures 45, 110–111
swab counts 54–55

table-mounted
    retractors 108–109
teamworking 18–19
temperature probes 33
temperature status 71, 72–73
theatre scrubs 4–5
thermal burns 97
time out 15
tissue retraction 108–109
topical anaesthesia 37
total intravenous anaesthesia
    (TIVA) 29, 35, 93
tourniquets 58–59
tracheostomy 74, 87
training and development 115
trauma 119
Trendelenburg position 48–49
two-bag test 24–25

urinalysis 2
urinary complications 77
urine output 73

vapour analysers 33
Velband bandages 58–59
venous thromboembolism
    (VTE) 15, 98–99
vertebral column 38–39
voiding 73
vomiting *see* nausea and
    vomiting

waste disposal 6
white blood cell count
    (WBC) 2
World Health Organization
    (WHO) 13–15
wounds
  closure 104
  dehiscence 77
  dressings 60–61
wrist bands 2